ODERN
VVOMAN'S
BODY

THE MODERN WOMAN'S BODY

Editor	Susan Pinkus
Art director	Micky Pledge
Typographer	Philip Patenall
Contributors	Caroline Bugler, Damian Grint, Jessica Johnson, Sue Johnson, Ann Kramer, Ruth Swan, Richard Walker
Indexer	David Harding
Consultants	Dr Katherine Anderson MB, BS, DRCOG, MRCP, Dr Frances Williams MA, MB, BChir, MRCP
Artists	Darren Bennett, Michael Bentley, James Dallas, Brian Hewson, Elly King, Anna Kostal, Pavel Kostal, Lee Lawrence, Kathleen McDougall, Paul McCauley, Graham Rosewarne
Administration	Carole Dease, Penelope Saavedra

Cover illustration by Pavel Kostal

ISBN 0–283–99982–9

Copyright © 1990 The Diagram Group

Part of this book was previously published by Paddington Press as *Woman's Body – An Owner's Manual* (© 1977 The Diagram Group).

Published by
Sidgwick & Jackson, 1 Tavistock Chambers, Bloomsbury Way, London WC1A 2SG

Printed in England by Butler & Tanner Ltd, Frome, Somerset

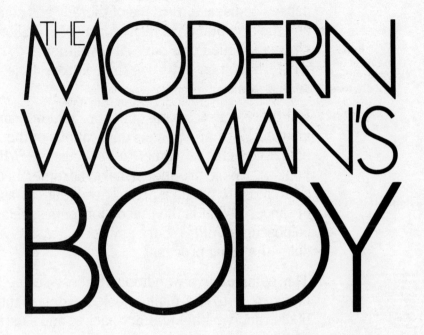

THE MODERN WOMAN'S BODY

THE DIAGRAM GROUP

Foreword

New understanding about the female physique, causes of disease, the role of therapy and counseling, and the acceptance of many forms of so-called alternative medicine have all revolutionized the western woman's attitude to health and fitness over recent years.

But there are still many questions that demand an answer. What are the real implications of the AIDS epidemic as far as women are concerned? What can you do to avoid pre-menstrual syndrome? Is the Pill a carcinogen, or can it actually prevent certain forms of cancer? What is the reason for tests such as colposcopy? And is there any perfectly safe way to delay the aging process?

This completely new edition of a best-selling guide takes an up-to-the-minute look at women, their bodies and well-being. Fact-packed and illustrated with hundreds of explanatory charts and diagrams, it takes us right from the very moment of conception through to retirement years and beyond, providing instant access to information about every aspect of female health, both physical and emotional.

Armed with this book, the woman of today will not only have a clearer understanding of how her body works, but will also discover how she can prevent many things that commonly go wrong. There are, she will find, many important decisions that the informed woman can make toward ensuring a longer, healthier and generally far more fulfilling life.

Contents

BEING A WOMAN

Is it true that men and women differ in the way they think as well as physiologically? What is a woman's current life expectancy? And, on a global level, what does being female in today's world – with its many cultural, social and economic differences – really imply for each and every one of us? The pages that follow trace the fascinating story of female physical and emotional development from the womb to mature womanhood.

Chapter one

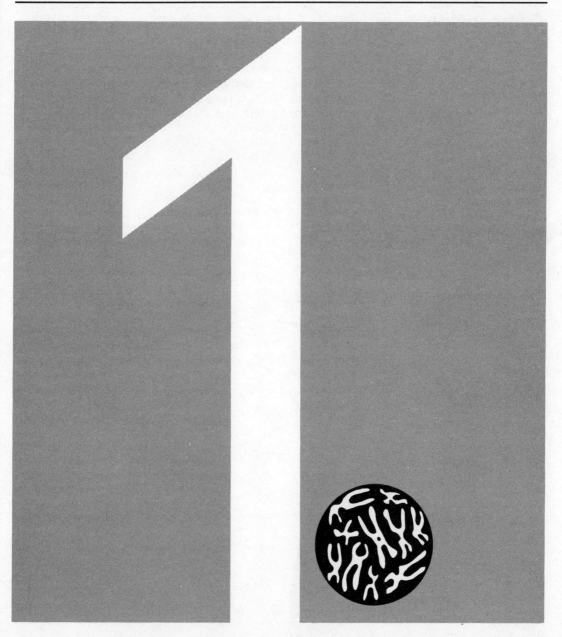

1.01 Physical development from ovum to adulthood

Conception

Below is shown the edge of a female ovum, magnified about 50,000 times. The ovum is by far the largest cell that the body produces (despite its minuteness, and great variations in its actual size).

Three spermatozoa are also shown here magnified in the same way. The ovum has just been fertilized by the topmost sperm. Immediately after fertilization, the ovum's outer wall hardens, to prevent any further sperm from entering. (For a description of the process of conception, see section 6.01.)

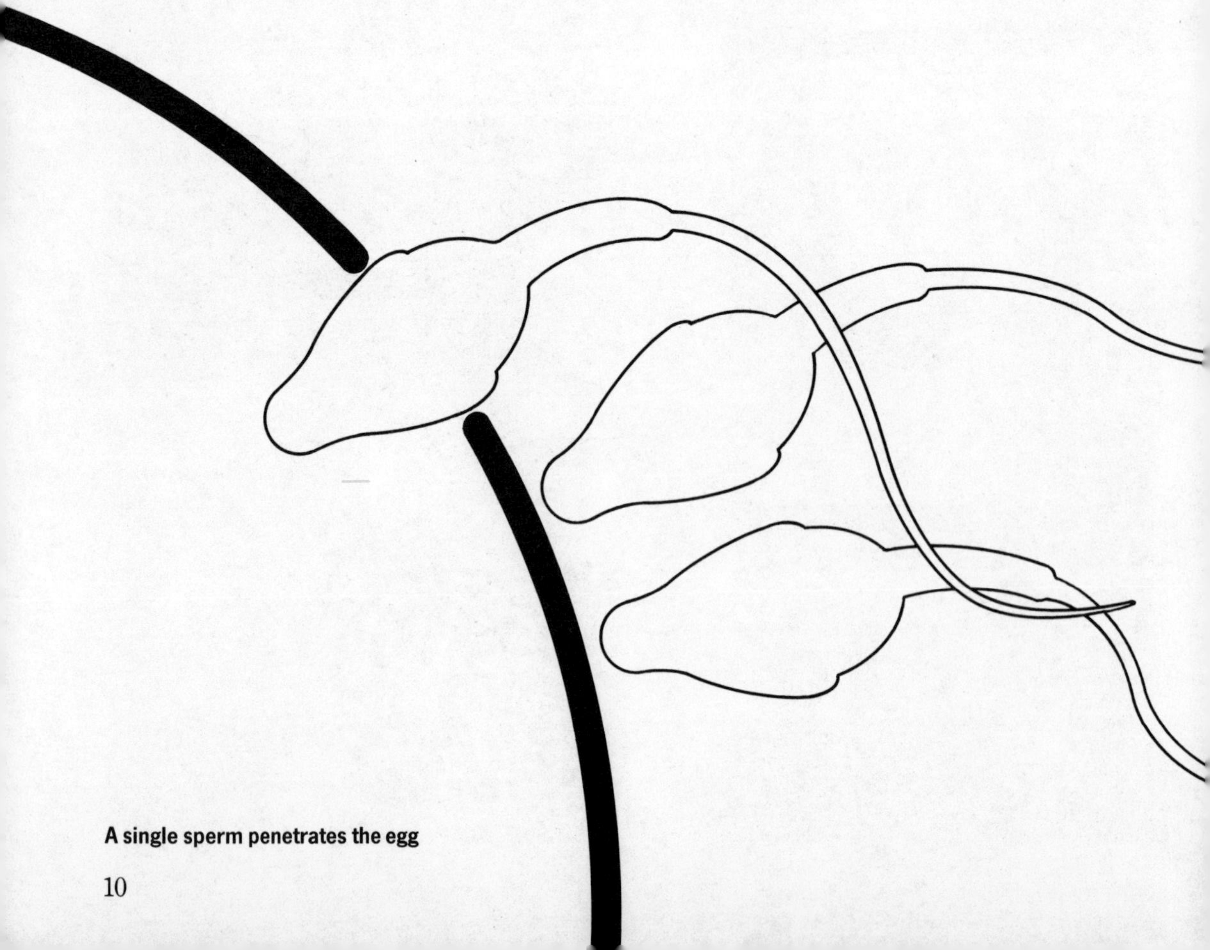

A single sperm penetrates the egg

Every body cell contains a "blueprint" of information, which decides how it functions. The information is carried on 23 pairs of chromosomes, which lie in the nucleus of the cell.

But because of special cell division, an ovum or a sperm contains only 23 single chromosomes. So when they unite, the new fertilized cell, from which the offspring grows, again contains 23 pairs of chromosomes – each parent having contributed half.

One pair of chromosomes decides the offspring's sex. The ovum always carries an X chromosome. But a sperm can carry either an X or a Y chromosome. So if the ovum is fertilized by an X sperm, the resulting XX combination produces a girl. (If it is fertilized by a Y sperm, the XY combination produces a boy.)

The chromosomes carried by the sperm will determine your baby's sex. But the alkalinity or acidity of your natural secretions is also thought to have some bearing on which sperm will fertilize the ovum. It is sometimes suggested, therefore, that douching with an alkaline solution may increase the chances of having a girl; with an acid solution, a boy. Certain foods have also been said to be influential in a similar way. However, there is little definite proof of this.

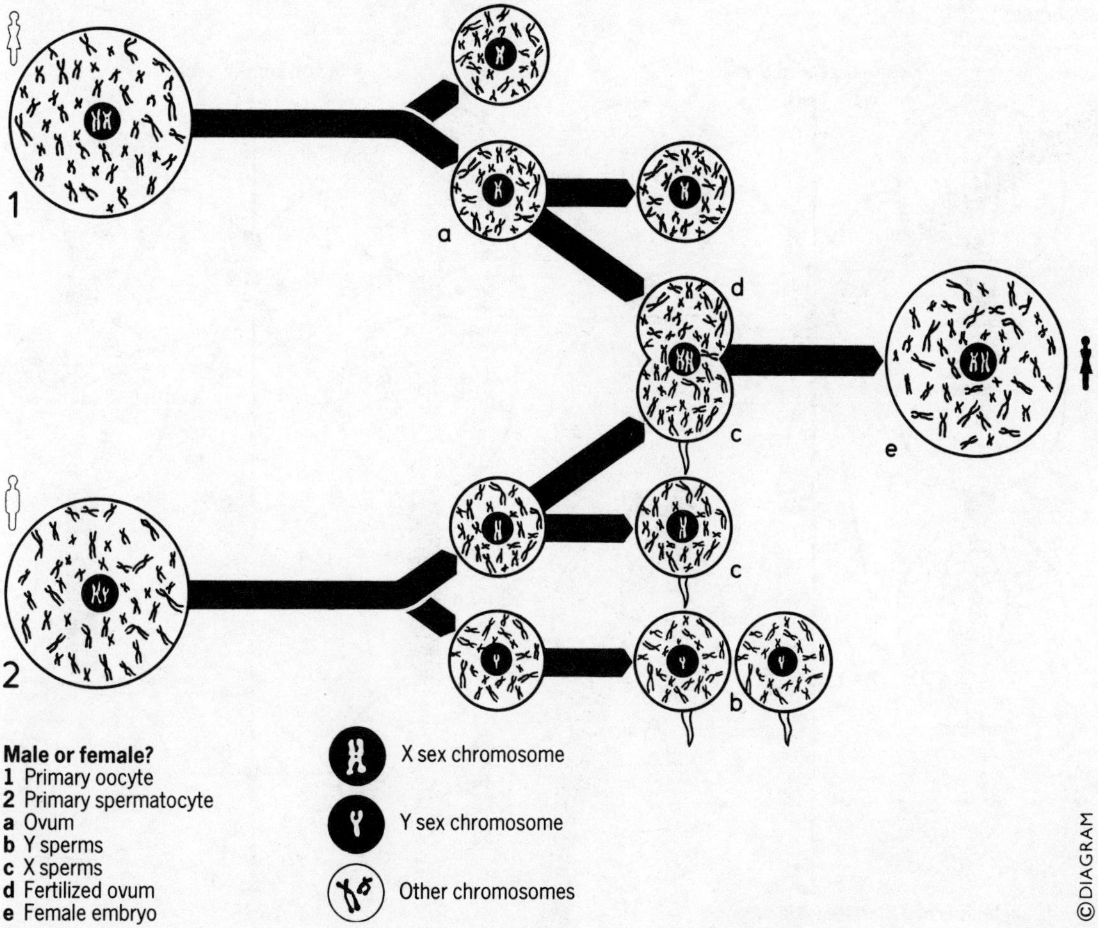

Male or female?
1 Primary oocyte
2 Primary spermatocyte
a Ovum
b Y sperms
c X sperms
d Fertilized ovum
e Female embryo

X sex chromosome

Y sex chromosome

Other chromosomes

© DIAGRAM

11

Fetal development

Until the 8th week after conception, a male and female fetus still appear exactly the same. One week later – when the fetus is still only 1¼in (3cm) long and weighs 0.07oz (2gm) – the external membrane has vanished from the genitals of the female fetus, giving entrance to a primitive vagina. Meanwhile, in the male, one end of the genital folds has begun to lengthen into a rudimentary penis. By the 11th week, the contrasting shapes of the external genitals are established.

Inside the fetus, the process is more complex and drawn out. In the undifferentiated fetus, there are two tube systems: the Müllerian and the Wolffian ducts. But in the female, between the 7th and 9th weeks, the Wolffian tubes almost disappear, while the lower Müllerian tubes combine to form the vagina. Then, more slowly, through to the 34th week, the undifferentiated sex glands (gonads) turn into primitive ovaries, and the upper Müllerian tubes become the Fallopian tubes. In the male, in contrast, it is the Müllerian tubes that disappear, the gonads migrate to the scrotum to become testes, and the Wolffian tubes each develop into a vas deferens.

Comparative development of male and female genital organs

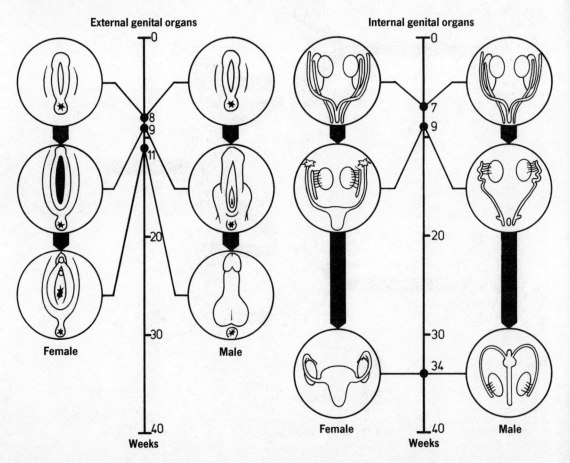

External genital organs

Female   Male

Weeks

Internal genital organs

Female   Male

Weeks

Human development in the nine months before birth is faster than at any time afterward. The drawings *below* show the development of an average fetus in stages, beginning with the 8th week. As the fetus grows, it also shifts its position within the womb.

An eight-week-old fetus begins to show a distinctly human form (**1**). Just over one inch long and weighing about one-thirtieth of an ounce, it depends entirely on food and oxygen conveyed from the mother, via the placenta and umbilical cord, to its rapidly growing tissues. The fetus is capable of moving about, since some of the major muscles have developed, but the movements are too slight to be detected.

By five months (**2**), the embryo is about eight inches (20cm) long and weighs about half a pound (226g). The lungs and digestive organs are not yet fully developed. The mother can now feel the baby as it turns and kicks.

At seven months (**3**), the fetus is about twelve inches (30.5cm) long and weighs two to three pounds (0.9–1.36kg). Calcium and iron from the mother are being used in the final formation of the skeleton and the blood.

At nine months (**4**), the fetus, now capable of an independent existence, moves into a vertical head-down position facing the mother's back. At birth, the baby usually weighs between six and eight pounds (2.7–3.6kg).

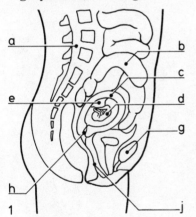

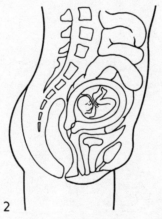

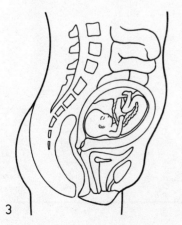

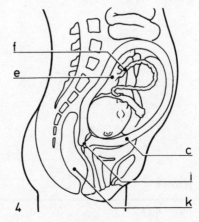

The growing fetus
a Spine
b Large intestine
c Uterus
d Fetus
e Placenta
f Umbilical cord
g Pubic bone
h Cervical plug
i Cervix
j Vagina
k Rectum

©DIAGRAM

Infant growth patterns

The 6ft (1.8m) kangeroo gives birth to a baby weighing less than 0.05oz (1gm): the blue whale produces offspring weighing nearly 10 tons. Human babies that have survived have ranged from under 1.1lb (0.5kg) to over 29lb (13.15kg) – but it is far healthier for the baby to be just an average 7lb 4oz (3.3kg).

In fact, the average for a girl is slightly lower (just over 7lb or 3.17kg), and for a boys correspondingly higher (7½lb or 3.4kg). Girls' hearts and lungs are marginally smaller at birth, too (though their livers are heavier). All this is not because girls are born after shorter pregnancies than boys. In fact, there is a slight tendency for there to be more girls among those babies born after unusually long pregnancies, and more boys among those born after unusually short ones.

However, "premature babies" were once often defined by birthweight, rather than length of pregnancy. On this criterion, slightly more female babies were termed "premature" as slightly more were under 5½lb (2.5kg) in weight. But really they were often "full-term, low birthweight." Whether underweight or overweight, babies that are far from the average have less likelihood of survival. Average-weight babies have under a 2% death rate; 6 or 9lb (2.72 or 4.08kg) babies, a 3% one; 4½ or 10½ pounders (2.04 or 4.76kg,) a 10% rate.

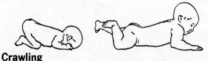
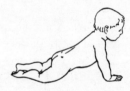

Crawling

Sitting

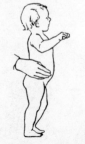

Walking

Age in months   3   6

DEVELOPMENT
Perfectly normal babies vary greatly in their rate of development. Sitting up for a few moments without support can start at any time between 5 months and a year; and walking without help, any time between 8 months and 4 years. Parents should not think that delay is always very serious, or that it is likely to have a lasting effect.

A newborn baby lies head down, hips high, knees tucked under her abdomen. If she is held in a sitting position, her back is rounded and her head droops. Between 1 and 3 months, she begins to lift her chin off the ground for a moment, and will lift her head for a moment if held sitting. But if held standing, she sags at the knees and hips. At about 6 months, she can support herself on her arms, lying or sitting, and can bear her own weight if held standing. Between 8 and 10 months, she begins to be able to crawl on hands and knees, to sit and lean forward without support, and to hold herself upright. At a year, she can creep like a bear, on hands and feet, turn around as she sits, and walk with one hand held. At 13 months, she can often walk alone but a push-along baby-walker may be very helpful.

Remember, though, that babies differ enormously in their development, and some perfectly normal babies may not yet be crawling on the first birthday.

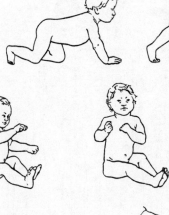

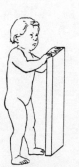

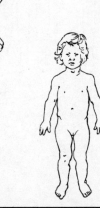

9   12   15

©DIAGRAM

Childhood development

HEIGHT AND WEIGHT

The first set of figures (**a**) gives typical heights and weights for western males and females. The second set of figures (**b**) indicates how much of her eventual height a girl is likely to have achieved at each age; for example, 83% at age 10. The third set of figures (**c**) indicates how much of her eventual weight a girl is likely to have achieved at each age; for example, 53% at age 10. (Boys' figures are always in brackets.) Of course, such predictions are only averages.

There are two reasons why a girl may be taller (or shorter) than average for her age. She may be going to be a tall (or short) adult. Or she may be advancing more quickly or more slowly than usual to an eventual average height: that is, she may be advanced (or behind) in her general development for her age.

The development of a child's permanent teeth gives a rough guide to this general rate of development. Compare the ages at which the teeth appear with the ages given on p.88 If they appear at the earlier age, the development is advanced; if at the later age, slow; if between, average.

It is interesting to note how much more slowly a child moves toward his or her eventual weight than height. At the age of 2, for instance, a child is already about one-half her adult height, but only about one-fifth her adult weight.

Comparative height and weight for females and males aged 2–22. (Figures for males are in brackets.)

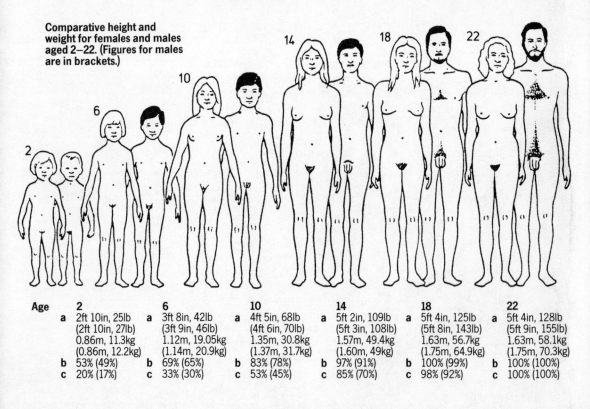

Age	2	6	10	14	18	22
a	2ft 10in, 25lb (2ft 10in, 27lb) 0.86m, 11.3kg (0.86m, 12.2kg)	3ft 8in, 42lb (3ft 9in, 46lb) 1.12m, 19.05kg (1.14m, 20.9kg)	4ft 5in, 68lb (4ft 6in, 70lb) 1.35m, 30.8kg (1.37m, 31.7kg)	5ft 2in, 109lb (5ft 3in, 108lb) 1.57m, 49.4kg (1.60m, 49kg)	5ft 4in, 125lb (5ft 8in, 143lb) 1.63m, 56.7kg (1.75m, 64.9kg)	5ft 4in, 128lb (5ft 9in, 155lb) 1.63m, 58.1kg (1.75m, 70.3kg)
b	53% (49%)	69% (65%)	83% (78%)	97% (91%)	100% (99%)	100% (100%)
c	20% (17%)	33% (30%)	53% (45%)	85% (70%)	98% (92%)	100% (100%)

Puberty

Puberty is the time when a young person starts to be able to have children. In a girl, eggs in the ovaries begin to mature, and menstruation – probably the most important physical development of puberty – begins. (In a boy, the testes start producing sperm.) But these are only two of the physical changes taking place. Other changes affect almost every part of the body; and there are important emotional and psychological developments, too, which gradually transform a child into an adult.

In the western world throughout this century, puberty has been starting younger and younger. But there is still a very wide variety of age of onset, which is difficult to explain. Several factors seem to contribute: traits inherited from parents; nutrition level; general living conditions; and the physical and psychological state. (Mental disturbance or long childhood illness can delay puberty.)

All these seem to be more important than any effect – if there is one – of race or climate. But the rate of puberty does vary with the season of the year: growth in height is fastest in spring; growth in weight, fastest in the fall.

MENSTRUATION

The changes that take place in a girl's body at puberty are controlled by the hypothalamus, a specific part of the brain. About two years before the onset of menstruation, the hypothalamus starts to secrete substances known as "releasing factors." These releasing factors travel to the pituitary gland at the base of the brain, and cause chemical substances, or "hormones," to be released. The first hormone produced is called **follicle-stimulating hormone (FSH)**, so called because it stimulates the growth of the follicles containing eggs in the ovaries. Stimulated by FSH, the follicles produce estrogen which helps the growth of breasts and genitals.

The rising level of estrogen in the bloodstream has an effect on the hypothalamus called "negative feedback." It causes a reduction in FSH releasing factor, but also makes the hypothalamus release a second substance – luteinizing hormone releasing factor. This in turn causes the pituitary to release **luteinizing hormone (LH)**.

Luteinizing hormone causes one of the follicles to burst and release its egg for possible fertilization. The remaining collapsed follicle, known as the "corpus luteum," continues to secrete estrogen, and also starts to secrete a new substance, progesterone, which prepares the lining of the uterus to receive and nourish a fertilized egg. If the egg is not fertilized, the levels of both estrogen and progesterone in the bloodstream fall, and cause the lining of the uterus to break down. The resulting bleeding constitutes the menstrual period. This cycle repeats itself about once every 28 days, from puberty to menopause.

On average, a girl will have her first menstrual period some time between the ages of 11 and 14, although menstruation will occasionally begin either earlier or later. Girls should certainly know about periods by the age of 10 so that initial menstruation does not come as a shock.

PROBLEMS AT PUBERTY

In some rare cases, puberty can fail to occur at all because of hormone imbalance. For most girls, however, the problems of puberty are usually psychological. Even such physical conditions as spots and blackheads, excessive weight gain, and heavy perspiration are usually more embarrassments than a sign of some abnormality.

As a result of psychological changes, the adolescent girl may appear aggressive and rebellious, and may challenge the authority of parents and teachers (and perhaps even the law).

Another common but temporary problem is lethargy. Its causes may be psychological; but the physical effects of hormones, the "growth spurt," or just too many late nights may be responsible.

PHYSICAL DEVELOPMENT

In girls, puberty begins at any time between the ages of 9 and 14, and ends between 14 and 18. (Boys generally mature later and more slowly than girls.) So some normal girls have completed puberty as others are just starting (especially as those who start early tend also to take less time over puberty). But on average, the changes start at about 11 and reach a peak at about 14. The order of events is also very variable, but changes in an average girl can be summarized as in diagrams below.

At pre-puberty, breasts are underdeveloped; there is no pubic or underarm hair, and body shape is boyish. By early puberty (11–13), the face becomes fuller; the pelvis starts to grow to allow future child bearing; fat begins to be deposited on hips; breasts start to develop and nipples stand out; pubic hair begins to grow in the genital area; internal and external genitals start to grow; vaginal walls thicken and

From girlhood to womanhood

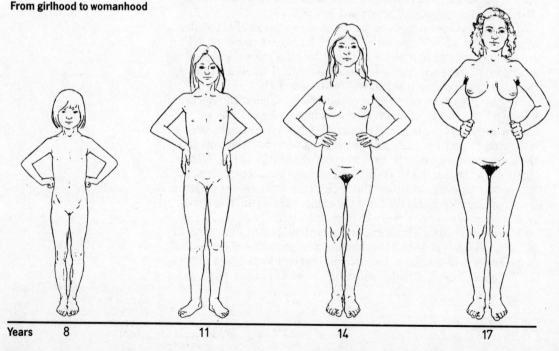

| Years | 8 | 11 | 14 | 17 |

menstruation may begin. By late puberty (14–16), breasts continue to grow; pubic hair thickens; underarm hair appears; and menstruation should be regular. At maturity (17–18), body shape is more rounded; growth of the skeleton ceases; genitals mature; and menstrual periods are now regular. At the same time, many other tissues of the body increase in size. The voice deepens slightly (though not as much as in boys) due to the growth of the larynx. Blood pressure, blood volume, and the number of red corpuscles all rise. The heart slows down; body temperature falls; breathing slows down but the lungs' capabilities increase. Bones grow harder, and also change in proportion. By about 18, the bulk of growth is over, so that a typical girl has usually reached her full height and almost her full weight.

THE AVERAGE HUMAN BEING

Adulthood

The average western woman is almost 5ft 3¾in (1.62m) tall; she weighs almost 135lb (61.2kg), her bust is 35½in (89cm), her waist 29½in (74cm), her hips 38in (96cm). The maximum weight she reaches is about 152lb (69kg), at between the ages of 55 and 64. The average man is just over 5ft 9in (1.75m) tall; he weighs almost 162lb (73.5kg), his chest is 38¾in (98cm), his waist 31¾in (81cm), his hips 37¾in (96cm). The maximum weight he reaches is about 172lb (78kg), between the ages of 35 and 54.

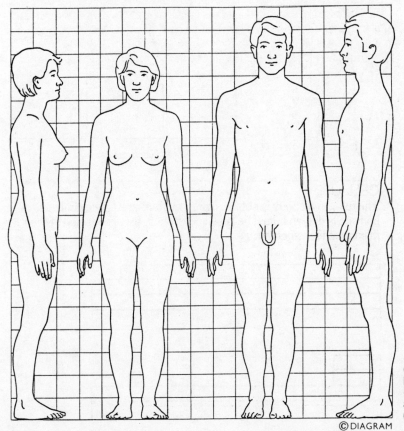

Comparative adult height and body shape, to scale
Each square represents approximately 4in (10cm) × 4in (10cm)

©DIAGRAM

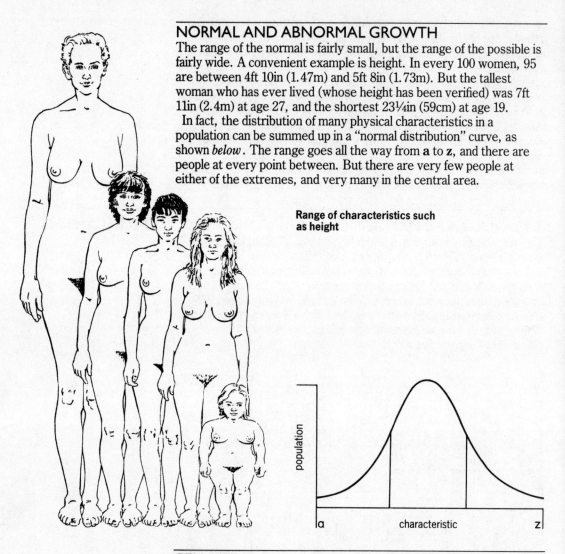

NORMAL AND ABNORMAL GROWTH

The range of the normal is fairly small, but the range of the possible is fairly wide. A convenient example is height. In every 100 women, 95 are between 4ft 10in (1.47m) and 5ft 8in (1.73m). But the tallest woman who has ever lived (whose height has been verified) was 7ft 11in (2.4m) at age 27, and the shortest 23¼in (59cm) at age 19.

In fact, the distribution of many physical characteristics in a population can be summed up in a "normal distribution" curve, as shown *below*. The range goes all the way from **a** to **z**, and there are people at every point between. But there are very few people at either of the extremes, and very many in the central area.

Range of characteristics such as height

population

a   characteristic   z

CELL LIFE

The full-grown body is still changing constantly: each day, millions of body cells die, and must be replaced. Below, we show some of their maximum life expectancies.

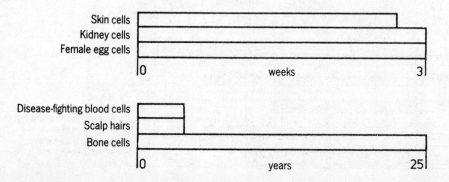

	0	weeks	3
Skin cells			
Kidney cells			
Female egg cells			

	0	years	25
Disease-fighting blood cells			
Scalp hairs			
Bone cells			

Male and female – the differences

Principal surface differences between an adult man and woman include:

a Different proportions between the shoulders, chest and hips

b Different patterns of body hair

c Greater surface prominence of the skeletal and muscular systems in a man due to less uniform skin fat

d Presence of the "Adam's apple" throat bulge, in a man

e Breast development and genital differences

Most of these differences are not obvious until puberty; but the basic difference in sexual organs is established within a few weeks of conception.

Physiology

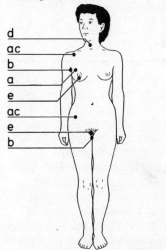
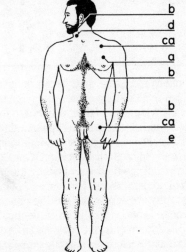

COMPARATIVE CHARACTERISTICS

The diagram below shows how some characteristics of the typical woman and man compare.

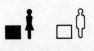

a Average brain weight
b Heart weight
c Quantity of blood
d Skin surface area
e Lung capacity (age 25)

©DIAGRAM

Reproductive systems

The male and female sexual and reproductive systems differ greatly in their structure and function. Nevertheless, they develop from the same original tissues in the embryo. So different parts of the final systems are comparable in origin and even partly in the role they play. The diagrams illustrate some examples of these "corresponding organs." For example, the same embryonic tissue that goes to form the outer vaginal lips in a female child forms the scrotum in a male.

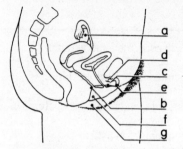 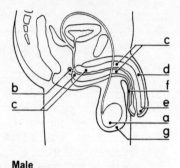

Type of organ
a Glands producing reproductive cells
b Minor fluid glands
c Erectile tissue
d Muscle tissue
e Sensory tissue
f Soft tissue
g Hair-bearing soft tissue

Female
a Ovaries
b Bartholin's glands
c Bulbs of vestibule
d Shaft of clitoris
e Head of clitoris
f Inner vaginal lips
g Outer vaginal lips

Male
a Testes
b Cowper's gland
c Bulb of penis/Spongy tissue of penis
d Shaft of penis
e Head of penis
f Underside of penis
g Scrotum

Intelligence and emotions

Most people would agree that there are observable differences in the way in which the majority of men and women think and behave, but opinions vary widely as to their cause. On the one hand, there are those who would claim that the apparent differences between the sexes are largely a result of social conditioning; and on the other, there are those who maintain that such differences are biologically determined from the moment of conception. But between these two extremes of opinion, there are many subtle theoretical variations.

However they are accounted for, the differences between male and female appear to be evident from earliest childhood. Girl babies, for instance, have been shown to respond more readily to the human face, voice and touch, while boys will pay more attention to their toys and to things around them. As toddlers and young children, girls develop more of an interest in people, and a natural reticence; while boys, who seem to be endowed with a greater share of aggression and daring, are far more interested in exploring the world around them and in finding out how things work. Of course, there are exceptions, but generally by the time they reach school age, girls are already demonstrating superior verbal skills, and they learn to read and write with greater ease and generally outperform their brothers in all academic areas until the age of puberty. At this point, boys come into their own, particularly in mathematical and scientific subjects, which demand a capacity for abstract thought, and a highly developed visuo-spatial sense.

Such mental and emotional differences are developed and refined in adulthood and may help explain (at least partly because social factors most certainly come into play) why more women than men are drawn toward the caring professions, while more men than women end up as computer experts, scientists, engineers and architects; why more men than women work in highly competitive jobs; and why men seem to be better at attaining and holding on to political and corporate power.

Some biologists maintain that the differences are physiological in origin. Recent research has shown, for example, that there are considerable differences in the ways in which men's and women's brains are organized. Many scientists would even say that these structural differences are unalterable, since they are caused by exposure to differing levels of male or female hormones while the brain is developing in the womb.

Men's brains are more specialized in function. In men, the left side of the brain is almost exclusively dedicated to verbal abilities, while the right side copes with visuo-spatial problems. In women, the same bias appears, but the distinctions are less clear cut. Within each hemisphere, the male brain has more areas reserved for specific functions, and there are fewer links between the two hemispheres in the male than in the female brain. It has even been suggested that this accounts for male single-mindedness, since men are less easily distracted by superfluous information when approaching a task. If asked to tackle the same problem, a man will typically go for the simplest solution, ignoring all that he considers irrelevant, while a woman may take longer to consider all the ramifications before she reaches her decision. Yet although the female brain is generally more diffuse in function than the male, it does have more areas reserved for verbal skills, which perhaps explains women's superiority in this field.

Differing hormonal patterns also play a part in the characteristic emotional behavior of each sex. Most people realize it is monthly hormonal fluctuations that often make women particularly prone to mood swings, but some scientists would say that our hormones are reponsible for the pattern of our entire emotional lives. It has been suggested, for example, that women find it easier to form intimate relationships than men because they lack the male hormones that encourage aggression and competition among peers.

However, any attempt to explain the complexities of human behavior in purely biological terms inevitably produces sexual stereotypes that border on caricature, and ignores the subtleties of society's pressures and expectations, as well as variations in individual character and culture. Comparisons between different cultures serve to underline the fact that the way men and women behave toward themselves and each other is socially, as well as biologically, determined. After all, the cult of "machismo," in which extreme displays of masculine behavior are applauded, is only prevalent in certain countries, and is counter-balanced by a tendency toward female emancipation and equality of the sexes in other parts of the world.

Nor is social organization static. The position of woman in the western world has undergone enormous changes over the last half a century; and although it is still true to say that men hold the balance of power in public life, it is not easy to predict whether or not this will necessarily always be the case.

Sport and endurance

Men tend to be larger, heavier and more muscular than women, and these differences contribute to variations in physical performance, as seen in a number of sports. Certain results have shown, for instance, that times for running are about 9 percent slower than men's (over 100 meters); and 12 percent, over 3000 meters. In freestyle swimming, the lag is about 12 percent, too, for 100 meters; 8 percent for 1500 meters. In high and long jumping, the female "shortfalls" are about 14 and 21 percent respectively. In discus throw and shot put, however, women's rewards are close to men's but with lighter missiles.

Differences in physical performance between the sexes explain why women compete separately from men in most events, and why few women take up "heavy" sports like wrestling or football. But because women's bodies are more flexible than men's, women are unrivaled in those gymnastic exercises that stress agility and grace.

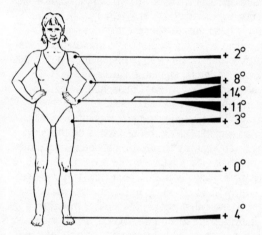

Flexibility
Women have far more body flexibility than men, as the chart shows. The number given for each indicated joint shows on average how many degrees more a woman can move that joint than can a man. Movement of the shoulder is backward; of the elbow is to bend and straighten; of the wrist is to raise to level (14°) and then bend; of the knee is to bend and stretch. Only the knee joint is as flexible in men as in women.

Strength
The graphs compare average muscle strength for men (**a**), actual average muscle strength for women (**b**), and the theoretical performance of women if they were the same size as men (**c**). The curves show the percentage of maximum strength at ages from 15 to 65.
Although women are about two-thirds as strong as men, their relative strength varies with different groups of muscles. Women's forearm flexors have only just over half the strength of men's. But hip flexors and extensors and lower leg flexors are four-fifths as strong as men's.

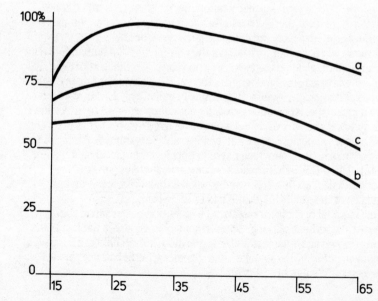

Worldwide, there are just over 100 women for every 100 men. But this ratio varies greatly from country to country. In most of Asia and the Middle East, and large parts of Africa, men predominate; in the United States and western Europe, women. But in some parts of the world, the lower status given to women may still mean that more effort is made to save a male child. Some less developed countries, though, show a female predominance.

A male predominance can also arise because of immigration. Men are usually the first to go to new countries in search of their fortune. But as standards rise, the numbers of women catch up. But Canada still has fewer women per 100 men than the United States.

THE AGE PATTERN

In most societies, fewer women than men are born. The ratio is generally about 100 female babies for every 105 male. But female life expectancy is longer in the USA and western European society. Parity between the sexes is usually reached between the ages of 30 and 40. After this, female predominance grows steadily until at 95, a man is outnumbered 4 to 1.

The female population

Female—male ratios
Parts of the world where women outnumber men

©DIAGRAM

Life expectancy

FEMALE LIFE EXPECTANCY AT BIRTH

The chart below shows life expectancy at birth for females born in various different countries, according to figures published in the World Health Statistics Annual 1988. As you can see, Japan scores highest with 82.1 years.

1	Japan	82.1	**9**	Austria	78.2	**20**	Argentina	75
2	Switzerland	81	**10**	UK	78.1	**21**	Bulgaria	74.7
3	Sweden	80.2	**11**	Denmark	77.8	**22**	Hungary	73.9
4	France	80	**12**	Israel	77	**23**	USSR	73.8
5	Canada	79.9	**13**	Costa Rica	76.6	**23**	Venezuala	73.8
5	Norway	79.9	**14**	Singapore	76.5	**24**	Australia	73
6	Holland	79.8	**15**	Ireland	76.4	**25**	Mauritius	72.3
6	Spain	79.8	**16**	Barbados	76.2	**26**	Guyana	71.9
7	Germany	78.9	**17**	Kuwait	75.8	**27**	Sri Lanka	71.6
7	Greece	78.9	**18**	Chile	75.4	**28**	Guatemala	64.6
8	USA	78.6	**19**	Poland	75.2			

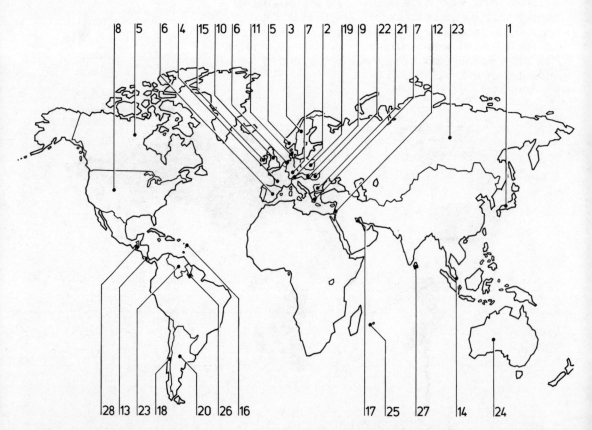

The chart below shows the chances per 1000 of a female dying from the listed causes. Figures are taken from the World Health Statistics Annual 1988. Note, for example, that Guatemala has the highest figure for infectious and parasitic diseases but the lowest for traffic accidents. (Highest figures for each cause are shown in bold, lowest in italics.)

Comparative statistics for likely causes of death

	Infectious/ Parasitic Diseases	Heart Disease	Traffic Accidents	Respiratory Disease	Malignant Neoplasms
Mauritius	14	336.8	3.3	90.1	88.4
Argentina	23.4	358.2	3.7	55.3	155.2
Barbados	23.2	218.4	2.1	43.3	176.2
Canada	6.1	336.5	7.7	81.1	214.8
Chile	28	188.3	2.2	121.3	183.7
Costa Rica	22.5	239.1	6.2	131.8	207.8
Guatemala	**165.1**	117.3	*0.6*	150.9	83.2
Guyana	18	158.4	*0.6*	68.4	67.3
USA	14.1	**387.4**	8.7	79.3	195.1
Venezuela	49.5	278.6	10.9	95.5	147.6
Sri Lanka	44.7	*73.5*	3.1	45.9	*46*
Austria	*2.3*	322.5	7.1	42.7	203.2
Bulgaria	4.4	301	5	60.7	112.2
Denmark	3.8	314.7	6.5	65.9	**238**
France	13.8	228.9	8.2	70.3	186.9
W Germany	6.2	330.2	5.3	48.1	216.7
Greece	5.2	302.8	7.8	56.6	137.5
Hungary	5.5	231.4	6.1	36.7	187
Ireland	5.9	320.3	4.4	146.1	196
Israel	21.8	330.6	5.6	69.9	165.5
Holland	6.1	296.4	5	73.9	219.4
Norway	6.9	303.7	5.2	103.7	198.7
Poland	5.0	188.9	5.1	*35.4*	152.1
Spain	8.2	261.2	6.2	79	155
Sweden	8.3	365.8	4.6	81.4	190.2
Switzerland	6.4	318.4	6.3	50.2	221.5
UK	4	293.6	4.5	102.6	222.3
Kuwait	34.7	181.3	**11.2**	72.5	101.7
Australia	4.7	358.3	9	55.1	196.2
Japan	11.3	231.4	5.6	105.2	172.9
Singapore	28	234.4	4.9	**186.6**	171.6

©DIAGRAM

Ethnic variations

No one now is very happy with the word "race"; it has been too much a part of humanity's inhumanity. But patterns of ethnic variation do, of course, exist and there are fairly consistent differences in the physical characteristics of different peoples.

Three great ethnic groups – Caucasoid, Mongoloid, and Negroid – account between them for almost all of the world's population. We have tried to illustrate their typical characteristics. But sometimes the differences within each group are as large as those between them. Taking, for example, skin color, Negroids range from near black to sallow; Mongoloids from yellowish to flat white to deep bronze; and Caucasoids from fair and pinkish to a tan shade. Another extreme variable is height.

Height relates partly to ethnic factors, but little to overall ethnic group. Average heights for a sample selection of peoples reveal a jumbled sequence of Negroids, Caucasoids, and Mongoloids (for example, Negroid peoples are both shortest and tallest). Even within a people, other genetic and environmental variations prevent too great a consistency. For example, the tallest pygmy is as tall as the shortest Sudanese negro.

Certain features, however, relate closely to origins. The extra melanin in dark skins, for example, gives added protection against the sun; and where the sun is no problem, pale skin allows better Vitamin D formation while olive or yellow skin contains a dense keratin layer that reflects light well in deserts or snow. Dark eye color also protects against sunlight; and so do thick, folded eyelids. Negroid hair protects against heat on the scalp, but allows sweat loss from the neck. Straight hair, grown long, protects against the cold. Typically, noses also vary with air humidity. In dry conditions, they are longer and narrower, so inhaled air is moistened. But the flat Mongoloid face developed as protection against the cold, and here the nose is not prominent and exposed. The Eskimo have taken this further, by developing facial fat.

Average weight is also greater the colder it is. For instance, the average Eskimo woman is considerably heavier than the average Spanish woman. Body area is larger, too, for weight, the hotter it is – a large area gives more skin from which to sweat and to radiate heat. Metabolic rate varies in the same way. A typical European has a "thermal equilibrium" of 79°F (25°C) – that is, with that temperature around her, naked, and standing still, she shows no tendency to get hotter or colder. The Eskimo's metabolic rate is 15 to 30% higher than the European's, giving her a lower thermal equilibrium, while an Indian's, Brazilian's, or Australian's metabolic rate is 10% lower than the European's.

Basic facial characteristics
a Caucasoid
b Mongoloid
c Negroid

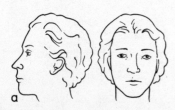
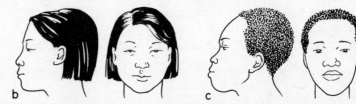

Women today represent more than half the world's population, yet nowhere in the world do they share the same status as men. The well-known United Nations quote from 1980, which describes the economic status of women, is still relevant: "Women constitute half the world's population, perform nearly two-thirds of its work hours, receive one-tenth of the world's income, and own less than one-hundreth of the world's property."

Women tend to work longer hours than men, have less economic and social power and still have primary responsibility for having and rearing children. They also continue to have primary responsibility for the sick and elderly and all aspects of domestic work, even where they also work outside the home – a common situation for the majority of women. Even in countries that have experienced considerable changes (such as the United States and Britain), women still earn on average 60 per cent of men's income and are more likely than men to be in unskilled, poorly paid employment. They also have considerably less political power.

In Britain, for instance, despite the fact that all adult women have had the vote since 1928, there are only about 44 women in Parliament out of a total of more than 600. The same imbalance can be found within professional work, and other positions of authority. Women are also, indeed, throughout the world, still subject to sexual abuse and harassment, rape, wife-battering, and the humiliations of pornography.

But the situation for today's women still varies enormously from country to country. In Afghanistan, only four percent of eligible girls are enrolled in secondary school: in Australia, it is 88 percent. In Belgium, 76 percent of adult women have access to contraceptives: in Angola it is fewer than one percent. Women in West Germany bear on average two children; in Ghana, it is six. In Jamaica, maternal mortality stands at 106 women per 100,000 live births, compared with 8 deaths per 100,000 live births in Norway.

The work of the 19th century feminists, and the great efforts of the international women's movement since the 1960s, have brought great changes. The right to vote has been won by the majority of the world's women – but in Surinam and various of the Middle Eastern nations women are still entirely excluded from full citizenship. (Only in 1971 did women in Switzerland get the vote.) Increasing numbers of women are also demanding their rights to be adequately paid. In the western world, and elsewhere, women are now entering all fields of employment, professional and otherwise, and are demanding increased facilities and training. A growing number of governments, too, are recognizing the need to legislate for women's rights and opportunities. It has always been campaigning by women that has produced equal opportunity legislation, abortion rights, improved healthcare, and work opportunities: no doubt future improvements will also be initiated and fought for by women.

Cultural and social comparisons

HEAD TO TOE

Greater understanding of how our bodies actually work is not only fascinating: it is also clearly of tremendous value when it comes to preventing certain physical conditions that are fairly readily avoidable. Read on to find out about both the inner and the outer woman. How does each of her systems function? What, in essence, makes her tick?

Chapter two

2.01 The inner woman
The structure and functions of the body's interior

The skeletal system

FUNCTIONS
The skeleton has several important functions: apart from supporting and protecting the internal organs, it also provides attachments for muscles to permit movement, stores minerals and makes blood cells. Although bone is often thought of as being rigid and inert, it is in fact a highly active part of the body, continually being repaired and maintained.

1 Names of bones
a Skull (29 bones)
b Clavicle
c Sternum
d Scapula
e Humerus
f Vertebral column
g Radius
h Ulna
i Pelvis
j Carpals
k Metacarpals
l Phalanges
m Phalanges
n Femur
o Patella
p Fibula
q Tibia
r Metatarsals
s Tarsals
t Phalanges

2 Types of vertebrae making up the spine
A Cervical vertebrae
B Thoracic vertebrae
C Lumbar vertebrae
D Sacral vertebrae
E Coccyx

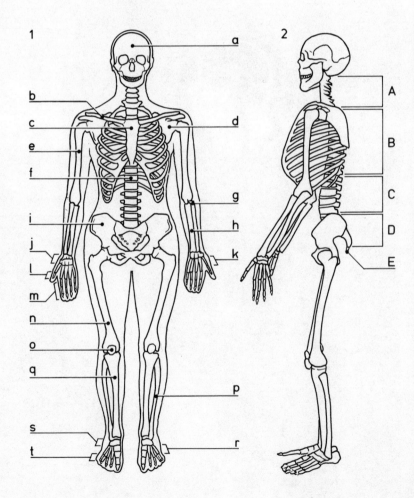

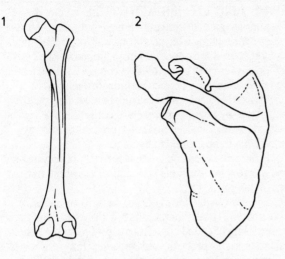

STRUCTURE

The shape and structure of each bone depend on its function and attachments to other bones or muscles, but bones are usually classified as long (e.g. the femur or thighbone), or flat (e.g. the sternum or breastbone). Flat bones generally have a protective role – for example, the skull bones shield the brain and eyes from injury. Long bones, with their extensive attachments to powerful muscles, act as levers for movement.

A typical long bone is composed of an outer layer of hard, dense bone and an inner layer of yellow marrow with honeycombs of spongy bone containing red marrow at the bulging ends. Flat bones consist of two layers of hard bone sandwiching spongy bone. The structure of healthy bone lends it great strength, with spongy bone organized along stress lines to augment the rigidity of the outer dense layer. Bone is usually covered by a membrane called the "periosteum" which contains blood vessels and nerve cells.

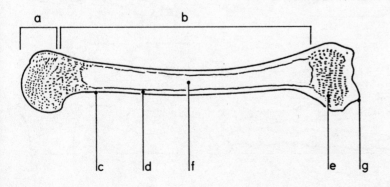

Section through a long bone
a Head
b Shaft
c Periosteum (thin coating)
d Hard, dense bone
e Soft, spongy bone
f Marrow cavity
g Cartilage

GROWTH, REPAIR AND OTHER ACTIVITIES

At birth, our bodies contain over 300 separate bones, but many of these fuse together as we grow resulting in an adult total of 206. In childhood, the growing ends of long bones are separated from the main shaft by plates of cartilage ("epiphyses"). When growth is complete, these plates are replaced by bone cells. If a bone is fractured, the broken ends secrete a substance that sets to become relatively hard and is gradually replaced with spongy bone by bone-making cells ("osteoblasts"). Bone-destroying cells ("osteoclasts") move in to remove the spongy bone and allow dense bone to be formed in its place.

Red bone marrow is the site of red and white blood cell production, and damage to the bone marrow (for example by toxins or radiation) may cause a severe form of anemia.

The skeleton acts as a storehouse for minerals, particularly calcium, magnesium and phosphate. These mineral salts are absorbed from the diet, incorporated into living cells and contribute hardness to the bone. Vitamin D is a vital factor in this process, and deficiency may lead to rickets (softening and deformity of bones). Lack of calcium in the diet or inability to make use of it may also be a factor in osteoporosis.

FUNCTIONS

Joints vary greatly in complexity and range of movement from a simple junction between two bones, as between skull bones, to the intricacy of, for example, the elbow. Some joints (known as "fibrous" or "cartilaginous" joints) are capable of very little movement – the joint at the pelvis front (the "pubic symphysis") is of this type and under normal circumstances does not move, although during pregnancy hormones have a softening effect which allows slight separation during childbirth.

1
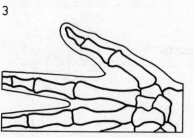

2
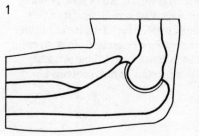

3
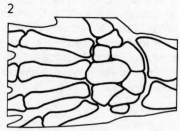

4
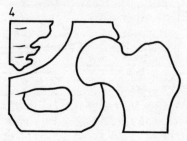

Types of joint
1 Hinge joint (e.g. elbow)
2 Gliding joint (e.g. wrist)
3 Saddle joint (e.g. finger)
4 Ball and socket joint (e.g. hip)

STRUCTURES

At its simplest a moving (or "synovial") joint consists of the two bone ends, each covered by a layer of smooth, hard cartilage, separated by a joint space containing lubricating fluid and surrounded by a capsule. However, this basic structure relies on the strong fibrous bands between the bones (ligaments) and the power of muscles and tendons to give it stability. Moving joints fall into four categories – hinge, gliding, saddle and ball-and-socket. The latter (e.g. the hip) have a wider range of movement than hinge joints (e.g. the elbow) but depend far more on muscles and ligaments to keep the joint stable and so prevent potentially harmful movements.

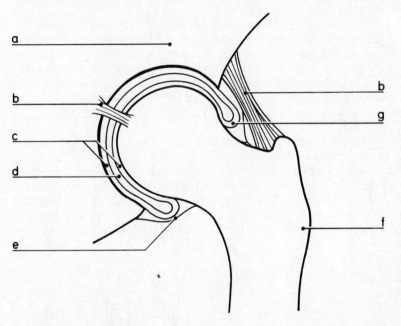

Section through the hip joint showing its structure
a Pelvis
b Ligament
c Cartilage
d Synovial (lubricating) fluid
e Capsule
f Femur
g Synovial membrane

JOINT DISORDERS

Not surprisingly, the complicated structure of moving joints makes them liable to many disorders, such as dislocation, sprains, torn ligaments and cartilages, injuries to tendons, and so on. Prolonged wear and tear cause **osteoarthritis**, while unaccustomed excessive use may result in inflammations such as tennis elbow. Even cartilaginous joints are not immune. The spine, for instance, a column of bony vertebrae separated by discs of cartilage, is heavily reliant on the strength of back muscles to maintain good posture and prevent backache and slipped disks.

The synovial or lubricating fluid allows joints free movement. But the membrane can sometimes become inflamed following overuse, causing a painful condition known as **tenosynovitis**, which can affect the wrists of typists, tennis players or rowers, for instance.

The muscular system

FUNCTIONS

Muscles are the body's motors. Not only do they move the limbs, they also push food through the intestines, drive blood through the body, and assist in the action of breathing. Some internal organs such as the uterus are largely composed of muscle, which in this case provides the power supply for pushing out the baby during labor.

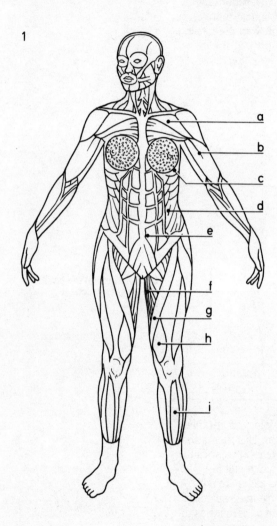

1

2

The body's muscles

1 Front view
a Pectoralis major (moves shoulder)
b Biceps (rotates and bends forearm)
c Serratus anterior (supports shoulder)
d External oblique (abdominal wall)
e Rectus abdominis (abdominal wall)
f Gracilis (bends and twists leg)
g Sartorius (bends leg)
h Quadriceps (straightens leg)
i Tibialis anterior (walking)

2 Rear view
j Trapezius (maintains shoulder position)
k Deltoid (moves shoulder)
l Latissimus dorsi (moves shoulder)
m Triceps (straightens arm)
n Gluteus medius (walking)
o Gluteus maximus (standing up)
p Gastrocnemius (walking)
q Achilles tendon

STRUCTURE

The body contains three different types of muscle: skeletal muscle (the kind which moves the limbs); cardiac muscle (which is only found in the heart); and smooth or involuntary muscle (found in the linings of blood vessels, intestines and many other organs). Skeletal and cardiac muscle are classified by anatomists as striated, a term describing the striped appearance of the bundles of muscle fibers when seen under a microscope, and both are regulated by their nerve supply although only skeletal muscle can be consciously controlled. Cardiac muscle contracts when it is stimulated by the heart's complex nerve "pacemaker." Smooth muscle is controlled by the autonomic nervous system (see p.54) and its associated hormones. It is not under conscious control but its actions are affected by stress.

Types of muscle
1 Skeletal muscle, which causes the skeleton to move
2 Cardiac muscle, from the heart
3 Smooth muscle, as found in the walls of the intestines

©DIAGRAM

HOW MUSCLES WORK

When muscle fiber bundles are stimulated by a nerve impulse, they shorten, causing contraction of the muscle. Skeletal muscles work in pairs, with one muscle contracting while the other relaxes. If one end of the muscle is attached to a bone on one side of a joint and the other end to another bone, the two bones are pulled toward each other so that the joint bends. This type of muscle is called a "flexor." Muscles which act to straighten a joint are termed "extensors." In the upper arm, the biceps is a flexor of the elbow and the triceps is an extensor. Some muscles, such as those that straighten the fingers, are found some distance away from the bones on which they act and are attached to them by long cord-like tendons.

Smooth muscle fibers, found in the walls of hollow internal organs, contract sequentially to propel the contents forward – for example, eating a fatty meal causes signals to be sent to the gall bladder where smooth muscle fibers contract and expel a quantity of bile into the duodenum to help digestion of fat.

Muscles require glucose, supplied by the blood vessels, as their energy source. As the glucose is consumed, lactic acid, water, carbon dioxide and heat build up, and these waste products must also be taken away in the bloodstream. The process of burning glucose and getting rid of the resulting waste is heavily reliant on oxygen, which is why strenuous exercise results in panting and a rapid heartbeat. Regular exercise improves the muscles' ability to clear lactic acid, giving greater endurance.

Muscles working in pairs
1 To bend the arm at the elbow, the triceps (**a**) relaxes and the biceps (**b**) contracts.
2 To straighten the arm at the elbow, the triceps (**a**) contracts and the biceps (**b**) relaxes.

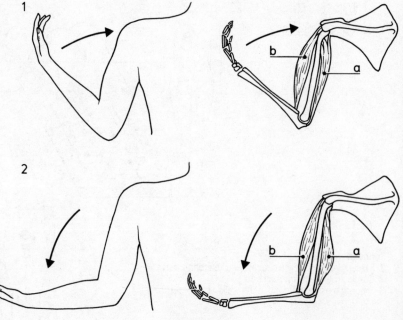

FUNCTIONS

The blood-filled system of pump (heart) and pipework (blood vessels) is the body's supply network. Each of the body's millions of cells require uninterrupted delivery of nutrients and oxygen and an equally reliable waste disposal service to take away the by-products of cell metabolism. Blood must be under pressure, to counteract the effect of gravity, and it must also have a complex delivery service to enable the substances it carries to reach every cell.

STRUCTURE

The heart is a highly muscular organ which weighs about 10oz (280g). The interior is divided into two parts by a thick wall or septum so that blood from the lungs containing oxygen in the left half is kept separate from deoxygenated blood from the rest of the body in the right half. Each half is further subdivided into two chambers, **atrium** and **ventricle**. The atria collect blood entering the heart from major blood vessels and, when valves into the ventricles open, propel it into the ventricles. They then contract to push the blood out, either into the **aorta** (from the left ventricle) or into the **pulmonary artery** (from the right ventricle). **Valves** made up of leaflets of tissue prevent backflow of blood between the chambers and at the exit points of the aorta and pulmonary arteries. The contraction sequence of the atria and ventricles is regulated by a nerve "pacemaker" in the wall of the right atrium and is controlled by the autonomic nervous system (see p.54).

The cardio-vascular system

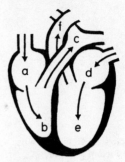

Bloodflow through the heart

a Deoxygenated blood enters right atrium by way of vena cava
b Deoxygenated blood goes from right atrium to right ventricle
c Deoxygenated blood goes to lungs via pulmonary artery
d Oxygenated blood from lungs goes by way of pulmonary vein to left atrium
e Oxygenated blood goes from left atrium to left ventricle
f Oxygenated blood leaves heart via aorta to travel around body

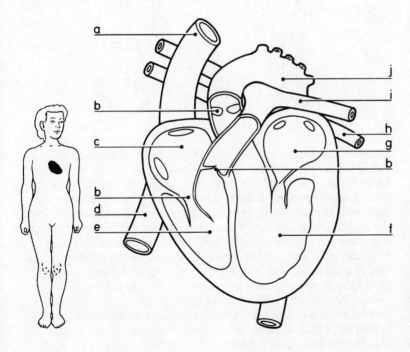

The heart and its blood vessels shown in section

a Superior vena cava
b Valve (prevents backflow of blood)
c Right atrium
d Inferior vena cava
e Right ventricle
f Left ventricle
g Left atrium
h Pulmonary vein
i Pulmonary artery
j Aorta

©DIAGRAM

BLOOD VESSELS

Principal arteries and veins
1 Important arteries
a Carotid (to head)
b Subclavian (to arm)
c Aorta (to rest of body)
d Pulmonary (to lung)
e Brachial (in arm)
f Hepatic (to liver)
g Gastric (to stomach)
h Renal (to kidney)
i Iliac (to leg)
j Femoral (in leg)

2 Important veins
k Jugular (from head)
l Subclavian (from arm)
m Pulmonary (from lung)
n Vena cava (from rest of body)
o Brachial (in arm)
p Renal (from kidney)
q Iliac (from leg)
r Hepatic portal (from intestines to liver)
s Femoral (in leg)
t Hepatic (from liver)

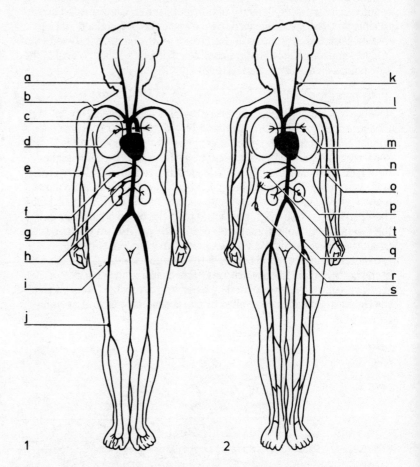

Blood vessel structure varies according to how much blood flows through them and whether they carry blood to or away from the heart. Large vessels carrying blood away from the heart, such as the aorta, are called **arteries** and have a relatively thick muscle component in their walls to maintain the pressure imparted by the pumping action of the heart. Arteries gradually divide into smaller **arterioles** carrying a lesser volume of blood but still maintaining pressure through their muscular tone. The smallest blood vessels are **capillaries** with walls only one cell thick. This is where the exchange of nutrients, waste products and gases takes place between the blood and the cells.

Blood, having collected carbon dioxide and given up oxygen, flows into **venules** and then into the larger **veins**, which have less muscle in their walls than arteries. Gravity helps to ensure good return of blood to the heart from the head and upper body, but in areas such as the lower leg there are valves to prevent backflow. Veins also partly depend on muscle action around them to help pump blood upward.

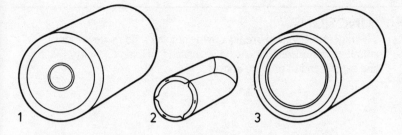

Blood vessels
1 Artery
2 Capillary
3 Vein

Blood itself has four main components: plasma, red cells, white cells and platelets. **Plasma** is a clear fluid containing mainly water, but also glucose and other nutrients, hormones, and salts. **Red cells**, manufactured in the bone marrow, contain hemoglobin (a pigment containing iron) which binds oxygen and transports it around the body. **White cells** are of several types: their function is to defend the body by recognizing and destroying foreign substances such as infective organisms. **Platelets** are very numerous small cells with a vital role in blood clotting. If a blood vessel is injured, platelets clump together to form a clot and prevent excessive blood loss.

Blood cells
Most healthy adults have about 8.8 pints or 10.6 U.S. pints (5 liters) of blood. It consists of an almost colorless fluid, called plasma, and three types of cells, all invisible to the naked eye.
a Red corpuscles
b Platelets (colorless, oval or irregularly shaped)
c White corpuscles (spherical with nuclei of different shapes)

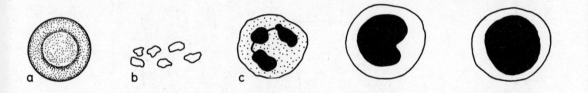

THE PULSE

This is a useful quick check of the state of both your heart's action and your arteries.

Every time your heart beats and drives blood into the aorta, a fluid muscular wave runs down the arteries and they swell momentarily. You can feel it where an artery is near the surface of the body – notably an inch (2.5cm) or so above the inside of the wrist.

The pulse beats in rhythm with the heart – about seventy times a minute – though it is faster in childhood and slower in old age. Your pulse will be faster too if you have a fever or have exerted yourself. **To take your pulse**, you will need a clock or watch with a second hand in view. If you have a watch, wear it on your left wrist and place the tips of the left-hand fingers at the base of the right-hand thumb. You will quickly find the pulse. Count the beats for fifteen seconds and multiply by four for your pulse rate per minute.

BLOOD PRESSURE

Measurement of the pressure that has to be applied to an artery to stop the pulse beyond the point of pressure is normally taken with a "sphygmomanometer" – an inflatable rubber bag strapped to your upper arm. Unusually high blood pressure may indicate disease of the arteries or kidneys, or stress. Low blood pressure is only rarely problematic.

©DIAGRAM

The digestive system

FUNCTIONS
The digestive system breaks down complex food molecules into simpler substances that can be absorbed and used for body building and repair, and to provide energy.

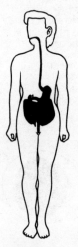

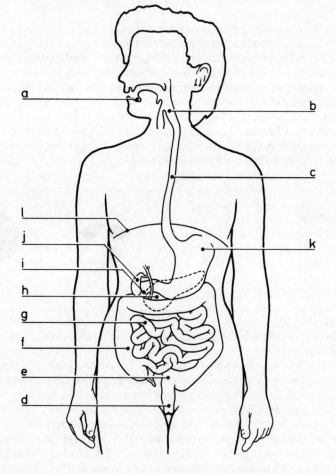

The digestive system
a Mouth
b Pharynx
c Esophagus
d Anus
e Rectum
f Large intestine
g Small intestine
h Pancreas
i Duodenum
j Gall bladder
k Stomach
l Diaphragm

STRUCTURE
The digestive tract forms a tube over 30ft (9.1m) long, beginning in the mouth and ending in the anus. Between them, it includes the **esophagus** (gullet), **stomach, small intestine,** and **large intestine.** In the mouth, food is chewed into smaller pieces, mixed with saliva, and formed into a rounded ball known as a "bolus." On swallowing, the bolus passes down the esophagus into the stomach.

The **stomach** varies in shape and size according to its contents. Its maximum capacity is about 2½ pints or 3.38 U.S. pints (1.6 liters). Here food is churned into even smaller pieces, and mixed with gastric juices, including hydrochloric acid. Fat is melted by the heat.

Food passes from the stomach into the small intestine. In the first 12in (0.3m) of this (the **duodenum**), the food is mixed with pancreatic and intestinal juices and with bile from the gall bladder. Then here, and along the remaining 21ft (6.4m) of small intestine, most of the useful elements in food are absorbed through the intestinal walls into the blood and lymph streams. In the 6ft (1.83m) long large intestine, water is absorbed into the body, turning the waste products into a soft solid (feces), a mixture of indigestible remnants, unabsorbed water, and millions of bacteria. Finally, the feces pass out of the body via the anus.

DIGESTION AND ABSORPTION

Food takes from 15 hours upward to pass through the whole system. It usually stays in the stomach for 3–5 hours, in the small intestine for 4½ hours, and in the large intestine (where the sequence of meals may get jumbled) for 5–25 hours or more.

Carbohydrate digestion begins in the mouth. It continues in the stomach, but the stomach usually empties itself before this is completed. In the duodenum, pancreatic juices break down the carbohydrates into **monosaccharides**, which are then absorbed into the bloodstream. But some forms of carbohydrate (e.g. **cellulose**) cannot be digested, while some sugars begin to be absorbed even in the mouth.

Fat digestion begins in the stomach, where naturally emulsified fats are converted into fatty acids and glycerol. (Unconverted fat causes food to be retained longer in the stomach.) In the small intestine, **bile** emulsifies the unemulsified fats, and **pancreatic juice** converts them into fatty acids. These are absorbed into the lymph vessels (70%) or the bloodstream (30%). Fat-soluble vitamins are absorbed at the same time.

Protein digestion begins in the stomach, where proteins are broken down into **peptides** In the small intestine, the pancreatic and intestinal juices break down the peptides into amino acids and these are absorbed into the bloodstream.

Water is absorbed in the large intestine, into the lymph vessels and bloodstream. It is not digested before absorption.

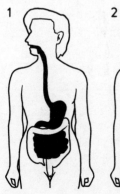
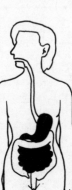
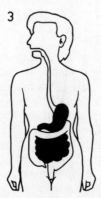
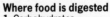

Where food is digested
1 Carbohydrates
2 Fats, fat-soluble vitamins
3 Proteins
4 Water, water-soluble vitamins

The urinary system

FUNCTIONS

All the body's activities produce waste products which are taken by the blood to the kidneys where they are filtered out. The resulting waste fluid, or urine, can then be removed from the body. The urinary system also makes sure that the body's water and salt levels stay the same.

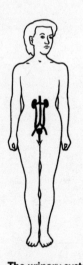

The urinary system
a Vena cava
b Aorta
c Kidney
d Ureter
e Bladder
f Urethra
g Urethral opening

STRUCTURE

The kidneys are located on either side of the spine. Each of the two is bean-shaped, and about 4in (10cm) long, 2½in (6cm) wide, and 1½in (3.8cm) thick. The kidneys are chemical processing plants. In them, waste material in the blood is filtered off under pressure, through more than two million tiny filtering units called "nephrons." The resulting waste fluid is known as urine.

The ureters are muscular tubes, each one about 10in (25cm) long, leading from each kidney to the bladder. Urine passes down the ureter at a rate of one drop every 30 seconds.

The bladder is a balloon-like, muscular bag that acts as a reservoir for the urine. When full, it holds about 1 pint or 1.2 US pints (0.57 liters) of urine. The desire to urinate is usually felt when the bladder is half-full. A muscle ring or **sphincter** surrounds the exit to the urethra. When contracted, it prevents leakages; while relaxed, it releases the urine to the outside.

The urethra is a tube, about 1½in (3.8cm) long through which urine leaves the body during urination.

Urine consists of 96% water and 4% dissolved solids. Only 60% of the water taken into the body is normally eliminated as urine: the rest is lost as sweat, in feces, and through the lungs. Urine is normally straw- or amber-colored. In 24 hours, an adult normally passes 1¼–2½ pints or 1½–3 US pints (0.8–1.4 liters), spread over 4 to 6 occasions which generally do not interrupt the period of sleep.

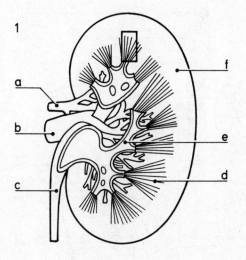

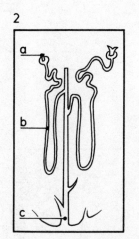

1 A section through one kidney
a Renal artery
b Renal vein
c Ureter
d Medulla
e Pelvis
f Cortex

2 The filtering unit or nephron
a Capillary network
b Kidney tubule
c Pelvis of kidney

The respiratory system

FUNCTIONS

The body's most urgent need is oxygen – deprived of this vital gas we die within minutes. An adult breathes in over 3,170 gallons (12,000 liters) of air every day in order to obtain the 634 gallons (2,400 liters) of oxygen contained in it. All this air must be warmed, filtered and moistened en route to the lungs where respiration takes place. Oxygen is not the only gas involved in breathing; carbon dioxide, formed by the body's cells as they use oxygen and burn fuel, must be got rid of in a two-way exchange within the lungs as oxygen is absorbed and carbon dioxide eliminated.

STRUCTURE

The term "respiratory system" includes all tissues involved in breathing, from the nasal cavity through the larynx and windpipe to the lungs and diaphragm.

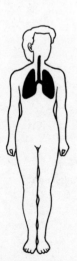

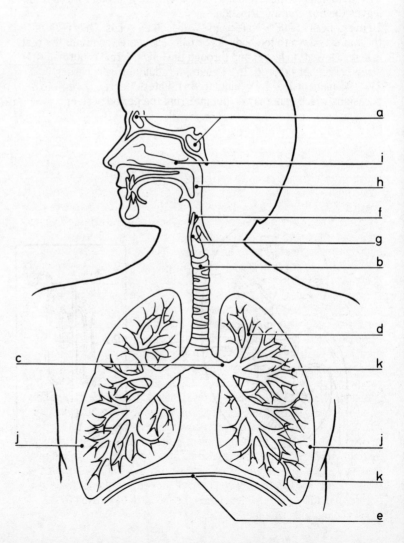

The respiratory system
a Sinuses
b Trachea
c Bronchi
d Bronchiole
e Diaphragm
f Epiglottis
g Larynx
h Pharynx
i Nasal passage
j Lungs
k Alveoli (at end of bronchioles)

BREATHING

The lungs and chest operate very much as a bellows mechanism, expanding to pull air in and releasing to expel it again. A powerful muscular sheet – the **diaphragm** – lives beneath the lungs and, as it contracts, it flattens and pulls downward while the muscles between the ribs contract and pull upward. These combined movements increase the chest cavity's volume and draw air inward. When the diaphragm releases, it moves upward, decreasing air space in the lungs and pushing air out.

Breathing is governed by sensors in the brain which monitor the amount of carbon dioxide in the blood and then send nerve signals to the breathing muscles.

How we breath in and out
1 Breathing in
a Ribcage pulled up and out
b Diaphragm contracts and flattens

2 Breathing out
a Ribcage sinks
b Diaphragm relaxes and becomes dome-shaped

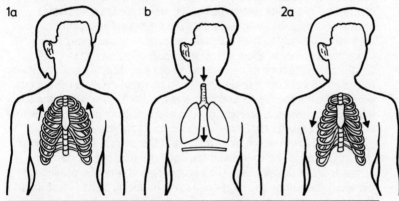
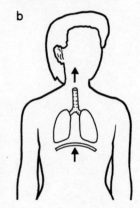

FROM NOSE TO LUNGS

Air warmed and moistened in the nose and **pharynx** passes over the **epiglottis** and **vocal cords** and into the windpipe (**trachea**).

The nose is an effective filtering device for breathed-in (inspired) air, being lined with a specialized membrane covered in tiny hair-like **cilia**. This membrane also exudes mucus to which dust and other particles stick and are pushed by swaying movements of the cilia toward the back of the nasal cavity and throat. The function of the **tonsils** and **adenoids** is to react to organisms invading through the respiratory tract and form antibodies to combat the infection. In children, whose immunity is gradually built up, these patches of tissue are relatively large indicating their high level of activity. Later in childhood, the tonsils and adenoids shrink as their role becomes less important.

Like the nasal cavity, the windpipe is also lined with a mucous membrane that traps dirt, dust and other irritating particles. In this case, the mucus is pushed upward, away from the lungs, to be coughed out.

Deep in the chest, the windpipe divides into two **bronchial tubes** – one **bronchus** leading to each lung where the tube then subdivides into an extensive branching structure of progressively smaller **bronchioles**. The final destination of inspired air is one of the minute multilobed chambers termed **alveoli**. This is where the exchange of gases takes place between blood and air, through thin membranes with a rich blood supply. Carbon dioxide moves into the air to be breathed out as oxygen diffuses into the blood to be carried to the heart and pumped round the body.

© DIAGRAM

The reproductive system

FUNCTIONS

Every month, one of the two ovaries releases an egg into a Fallopian tube. If the egg is fertilized, it will embed itself in the uterus and develop into a baby. If not fertilized, the egg will be removed with the lining of the uterus during **menstruation**.

STRUCTURE

A woman's reproductive organs consist of the vagina, uterus, Fallopian tubes, and ovaries.

The **vagina** is a muscular passage, lying between the bladder and the rectum. It leads from the vulva upward, and at an angle to the uterus. It is about 3–4 in (7.5–9cm) long and capable of great distension. Normally the vaginal walls, which are lined with folds or ridges of skin, lie close together. During sexual intercourse, they stretch easily to take the male penis and extend considerably more during labor to allow a child to be born. The vagina is usually moist, though moistness increases with sexual excitement and may also vary at different times of the menstrual cycle. A continuous secretion from the cervix and vagina of dead cells mixed with fluid lubricates the vagina, keeping it clean and free from infection. It is this self-cleaning quality that makes vaginal douching unnecessary.

The **cervix** is the neck or lower part of the uterus. It projects into the upper end of the vagina and can quite often be felt by sliding a finger as far as possible into the vagina. This may not be possible at certain times during the menstrual cycle or during sexual excitement if the uterus changes position.

The **os** is a tiny opening through the cervix, and is the entrance to the uterus. It varies in shape and size depending on whether a woman has had children, but remains very small. It cannot be penetrated by a finger, tampon, or the penis.

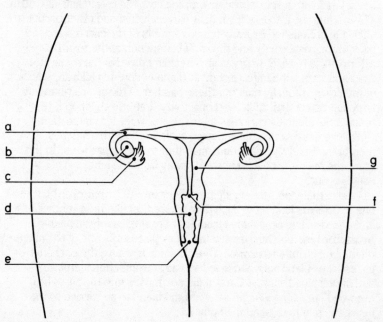

Section through a front view of the female reproductive system
a Fallopian tube
b Ovary
c Funnel of Fallopian tube
d Vagina
e Vaginal opening
f Cervix
g Uterus

The **uterus** is a hollow, muscular, pear-shaped organ, about the size of a lemon in its non-pregnant state. Seen from the front, the uterine cavity is triangular in shape and it is here that the fetus develops during pregnancy, pushing back the muscular walls in a surprising manner. During labor, the fetus moves from the uterine cavity through the cervix and vagina to be delivered through the vaginal opening. (For a full description of pregnancy and birth, see pp. 294–343.)

The Fallopian tubes extend outward and back from either side of the upper end of the uterus. They are about 4in (10cm) in length and reach toward the ovaries.

The **ovaries** produce the female sex cells (the eggs or "ova") and also the female sex hormones, estrogen and progesterone. (This makes them the female equivalent of the male testes.) Once a month, an **ovum** (egg) is released which floats into the funnel-shaped end of a Fallopian tube.

The **clitoris** is a small protrusion at the front of the vulva which is usually sensitive to sexual stimulation.

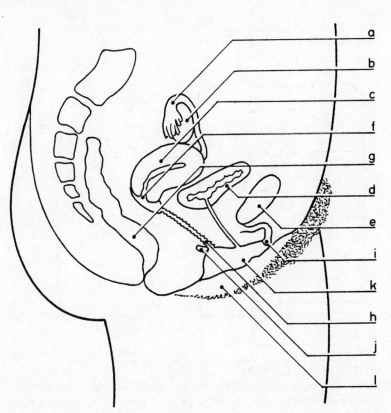

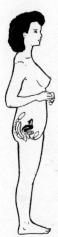

Section through a side view of the female reproductive and urinary system
a Fallopian tube
b Ovary
c Uterus and endometrium
d Bladder
e Pubic bone
f Cervix and os
g Rectum
h Vagina
i Clitoris
j Bartholin's glands
k Labia minora
l Labia majora

©DIAGRAM

Menstruation

THE MENSTRUAL CYCLE

Around every 28th day, from about the age of 12 to about the age of 47, a woman has a discharge of blood and mucus from the vagina. The discharge lasts from 2–8 days (4–6 is most usual) and may be preceded or accompanied by various unpleasant symptoms such as headaches and nausea. This is menstruation, or the "period" – the outward sign of the routine cycle of egg production and hormone change in a woman's body. It is a process that requires the wearing of pads or tampons (absorbent tubes placed in the vagina), if the menstruating woman is to avoid soiling her clothes.

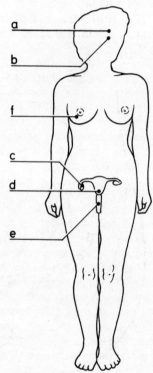

The control of menstruation
a Hypothalamus
b Pituitary gland
c Ovary
d Uterus
e Vagina
f Breast
g Releasing factors
h Follicle-stimulating hormone
i Luteinizing hormone
j Follicle
k Corpus luteum
l Ovum
m Estrogen
n Progesterone and estrogen

EGG PRODUCTION

Each ovary contains groups of cells called follicles, which themselves contain immature eggs (ova). When a girl is about 12, these eggs begin to mature at the rate of one every 28 days or so – usually in alternate ovaries. At birth, a female child's ovaries contain perhaps 350,000 immature eggs: but between puberty and menopause, only about 375 ever mature. As each egg matures, it bursts from the ovary – a process called "ovulation" – and passes into the Fallopian tube leading down from that ovary to the uterus.

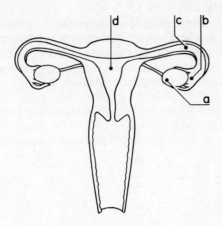

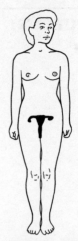

Position of the egg on various days of the cycle
a Day 3
b Day 14
c Day 16
d Day 21

If the egg is not fertilized by a sperm, it begins to degenerate 24–48 hours after leaving the ovary, and eventually passes unnoticed out of the body in the normal flow of fluid from the vagina. But meanwhile, the uterus has been preparing to receive a fertilized egg. Hormones have caused the lining of the uterus to thicken, and to secrete a fluid so that the fertilized egg could be nourished while implanting itself. When no fertilization occurs, further hormone stimulation causes the thickened lining to crumble, and to be discharged along with blood through the vagina.

MYTHS ABOUT MENSTRUATION

Throughout history, almost all societies have surrounded the menstrual process with myth and ritual. Even today, in some primitive cultures, the menstruating woman is thought to turn milk sour, turn food bad, damage crops, and even cause animals to abort! Elsewhere she may be completely isolated from the rest of the community in a special building. Modern western society still preserves some old myths about menstruation, all of which can be ignored. It is perfectly safe for the menstruating woman to bathe, shower, swim, wash her hair, and take part in any other activity she wishes although sexual intercourse during menstruation is taboo in some cultures and also currently advised against where there may be risk of infection with the AIDS virus.

SANITARY PROTECTION

The world over, women have always needed to prevent soiling during menstruation, and have resorted to many methods. Today, most use sanitary towels or tampons, both of which need to be changed at least 3–4 times daily when flow is at its peak. The latter should not be used between periods, however, and have at times been indicated as a cause of toxic shock syndrome (see p.180)

Some women are now using natural sponges to collect menstrual flow, but as yet no trials have been carried out as to any effects of these. The diaphragm or cap is also sometimes used to collect menstrual flow.

©DIAGRAM

The nervous system

FUNCTIONS

The nervous system controls our unconscious body functions, such as digestion and breathing, as well as conscious body functions, such as movement and thought. The brain and spinal cord make up the central nervous system, and the peripheral nervous system links this central nervous system with other parts of the body.

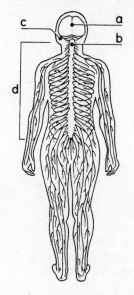

The nervous system
a Brain
b Spinal cord
c Cranial nerves
d Spinal nerves

CENTRAL NERVOUS SYSTEM

The brain is the seat of consciousness. Emotions, creativity, logical thought, and coordination of body movement all take place in this mass of nerve tissue, cushioned within the skull by the cerebrospinal fluid and protected by the three layers of membrane (the "meninges").

The millions of nerve cells ("neurons") and nerve pathways generate the infinite number of communications which produce individual intelligence and creativity.

The largest part of the brain is the **cerebrum**, consisting of the two **cerebral hemispheres** with deeply infolded surfaces. Its activities are complex but it can be considered to be the home of intelligence and memory. Motor and sensory areas are also located here, the left hemisphere controlling the right side of the body and vice versa. Signals pass between the two hemispheres through a mass of linking fibers called the "corpus callosum."

Below the corpus callosum lies the **hypothalamus**. Many functions not under conscious control – appetite, sleep, the menstrual cycle, and body temperature – are regulated by the hypothalamus, together with the pituitary gland, through the endocrine system (see p.55).

The **cerebellum**, at the base and rear of the brain, is the center for balance and fine tuning of muscle movements.

The **brain stem** connects the brain to the spinal cord and contains the **medulla** which controls body maintenance systems such as heartbeat, breathing and digestion through the autonomic nervous system (see p.54).

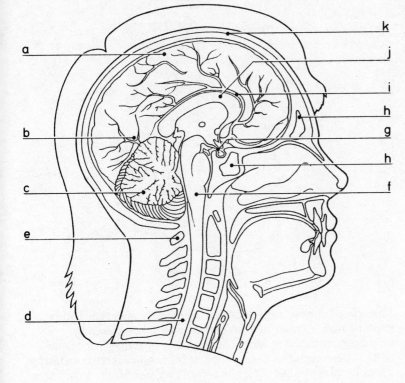

Section through the head
a Cerebral hemisphere
b Posterior cerebral artery
c Cerebellum
d Spinal cord
e Cervical vertebra
f Brain stem
g Pituitary gland
h Sinuses
i Anterior cerebral artery
j Corpus callosum
k Skull

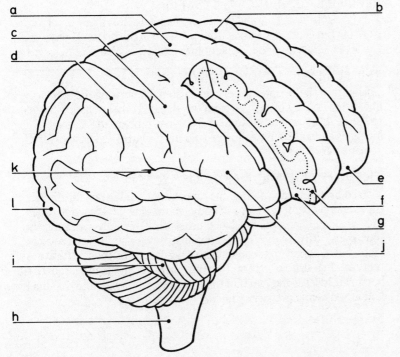

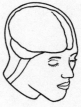

The brain
a Right cerebral hemisphere
b Left cerebral hemisphere
c Motor cortex (voluntary movement)
d Sensory cortex (bodily sensations)
e Frontal lobe (personality)
f Gray matter (nerve cells)
g White matter (nerve trunks)
h Brain stem
i Cerebellum (balance and position)
j Speech center
k Hearing center
l Occipital lobe (vision)

© DIAGRAM

53

Part of the spinal cord
a Spinal cord
b Peripheral nerve
c Vertebra
d Intervertebral disk
e White matter
f Gray matter

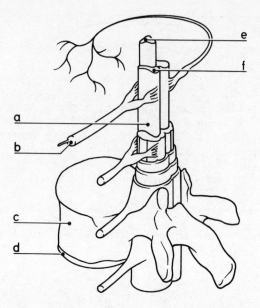

The spinal cord is made up of bundles of nerve fibers and extends from the brain stem to the base of the spine. It is enclosed by vertebrae and the same kind of meningeal membranes found in the brain. Where vertebrae meet, a pair of nerves leaves the cord taking motor impulses to, and receiving sensory impulses from, a particular part of the body.

PERIPHERAL NERVOUS SYSTEM
This controls voluntary and involuntary actions. It is made up of 12 pairs of cranial nerves arising from the base of the brain, 31 pairs of spinal nerves, and all the smaller nerves that branch off.

THE SOMATIC NERVOUS SYSTEM
That part of the peripheral nervous system comprising the sensory fibers that convey messages from the skin and other sensory organs to the central nervous system, and the motor fibers that carry impulses to those muscles under voluntary control, is known as the somatic nervous system.

THE AUTONOMIC NERVOUS SYSTEM
Two counterpoised systems, the sympathetic and parasympathetic, act as a kind of autopilot for the body, controlling vital functions such as heartbeat, digestion, and blood pressure. Generally speaking, the **parasympathetic system** predominates when we are in a relaxed state; blood supply to the intestine is increased and the heart rate is reduced. In a state of stress, the **sympathetic system** increases the heart rate, dilates the pupils of the eyes and sends blood to the brain, lungs, and heart, preparing the body for exertion.

The endocrine system

FUNCTIONS

The body has two types of gland, endocrine and exocrine. **Exocrine glands,** which include sweat, sebaceous and digestive glands, secrete into ducts. The **endocrine glands,** however – which include the pituitary, hypothalamus, thyroid, parathyroid, adrenals, and ovaries (in the female) or testes (in the male) – are ductless and their secretions are chemical messengers (called "hormones") that are distributed around the body through the bloodstream. Different **hormones** play different roles in the control of growth, reproduction and the body's internal chemistry by affecting specific target organs or other endocrine glands.

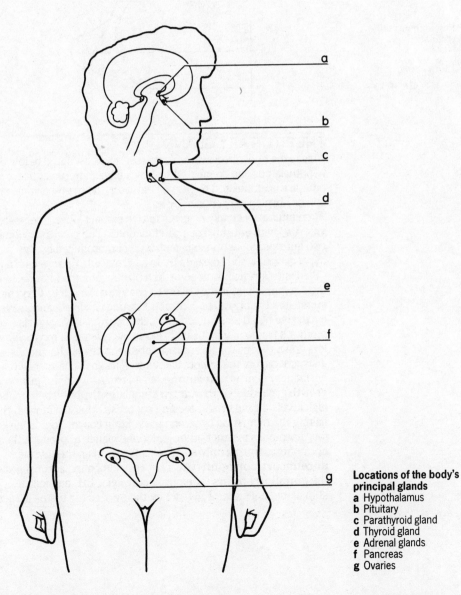

Locations of the body's principal glands
a Hypothalamus
b Pituitary
c Parathyroid gland
d Thyroid gland
e Adrenal glands
f Pancreas
g Ovaries

© DIAGRAM

THE HYPOTHALAMUS

This gland, which is situated at the base of that part of the brain governing instinct and bodily control, provides the essential link between the nervous and endocrine systems. It houses centers that govern sleep, appetite, temperature and sexual function, and also produces hormones which stimulate the pituitary.

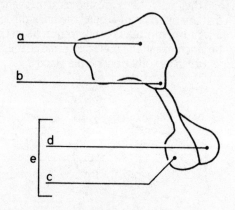

The hypothalamus and pituitary glands
a Hypothalamus
b Pituitary stalk
c Posterior lobe of pituitary
d Anterior lobe of pituitary
e Pituitary

THE PITUITARY GLAND

This is the endocrine system's master gland. Situated below the hypothalamus and connected to it by a stalk of nervous tissue, the pituitary is stimulated by nerve centers in the hypothalamus and stores hormones produced by it.

The pituitary actually consists of two distinct lobes, the posterior and anterior, with entirely separate functions. The posterior lobe stores two hormones, vasopressin and oxytocin, produced by the hypothalamus, and releases them as required. **Vasopressin** (also called antidiuretic hormone or ADH) acts upon the kidneys to regulate the amount of water they allow to pass into the urine. **Oxytocin** stimulates the uterus to contract, starting childbirth and preventing excessive blood loss immediately afterward. Nerve signals from the mother's nipple being suckled also cause release of oxytocin, which lets down the milk. The anterior lobe secretes six hormones upon instruction from the hypothalamus which sends out special releasing hormones. **Growth hormone**, as its name suggests, promotes growth in childhood. **Prolactin** stimulates the breasts to make milk; high levels during breast-feeding suppress other hormones, thereby halting the menstrual cycle and preventing conception. The remaining four hormones instruct other endocrine glands to produce their own hormones: **thyrotrophin** (TSH) is targeted on the thyroid; **adrenocorticotrophin** (ACTH) works upon the adrenal glands; and the **gonadotrophins** (luteinizing hormone, LH, and follicle-stimulating hormone, FSH) act on the ovaries (or testes in men).

THE THYROID GLAND

Under stimulation from TSH, the thyroid secretes **thyroxine**, a hormone regulating the body's rate of metabolism and growth. Amounts of TSH and thyroxine in the blood are normally balanced to maintain a steady metabolic rate. The thyroid needs iodine from the diet in order to produce its hormone – iodine deficiency may therefore have a dramatic effect with symptoms of personality change, fluid retention, puffy skin, delay in the onset of menstruation, or heavy periods and resulting anemia. Over-secretion, on the other hand, can result in **goiter** or enlargement of the gland, characterized by protruding eyeballs, rapid pulse, sweating and weight loss. The thyroid also produces calcitonin, which stores calcium in the bones.

1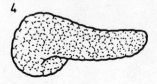

THE PARATHYROID GLANDS

These four tiny glands secrete **parathormone** to maintain calcium levels in the blood by withdrawing calcium from the skeletal stores.

2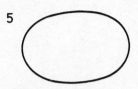

THE ADRENAL GLANDS

These two glands form a cap on top of each kidney. Strictly speaking, only the outer part (**adrenal cortex**) is an endocrine gland. The inner part (the **medulla**) is controlled by the autonomic nervous system and produces **adrenalin**, the hormone which prepares the body to face danger by increasing heart rate and blood sugar levels.

The adrenal cortex produces several "steroid" hormones, the most important of which is **cortisol**. The body needs cortisol to cope with stresses such as infections and injuries. Normally, ACTH blood levels from the pituitary and cortisol are balanced, but steroid drugs such as cortisone suppress the adrenal gland's cortisol-producing activity. The dosage must be tapered off gradually to allow sufficient time for cortisol secretion to recover.

3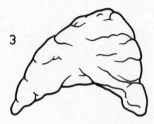

THE PANCREAS

Most of the pancreas' cells produce enzymes for breaking down foodstuffs in the digestive tract, but the remaining clumps of cells (2% or so) secrete **insulin**, a hormone controlling the ability of the body's cells to utilize sugar in the blood. Failure of insulin production causes the relatively common condition **diabetes**.

4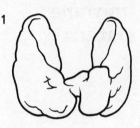

THE OVARIES

Until a girl is aged about 11 the ovaries are inactive, although they have contained hundreds of thousands of eggs from birth. Puberty is initiated by the hypothalamus sending its LH and FSH releasing hormones to the pituitary. (The resulting bodily development and menstrual cycle are described more fully on pp.50–51.) At any one time, only a tiny part of one ovary (the egg-containing follicle) is involved in the production of the hormones estrogen and progesterone. **Estrogen** helps to regulate menstruation and has an important part to play in the development of secondary sexual characteristics, while **progesterone** (also produced in tiny amounts by the adrenal glands) helps build up the lining of the uterus after ovulation and raises body temperature so that it is possible to tell when ovulation has occurred.

5

Some principal endocrine glands (not to scale)
1 Thyroid gland
2 Parathyroid gland
3 Adrenal glands
4 Pancreas
5 Ovary

© DIAGRAM

Immune system

FUNCTIONS

The body has effective first-line defense mechanisms: the skin forms an outer protective coating of hard dead cells, nasal membranes pour out mucus to carry away dirt and irritants; and sweat, saliva and tears are antibacterial lubricating fluids. But if invading organisms get past these defenses and into the tissues or bloodstream, the immune system must enter the fray to prevent overwhelming infection.

Recognition of material foreign to the body – viruses, bacteria, faulty or cancerous cells – is a task performed by white blood cells called **lymphocytes**. These cells, produced in the lymph nodes, circulate in the lymphatic system, tissues, and bloodstream. Upon encountering a bacteria or virus, some lymphocytes act as memory banks, "remembering" any previous encounter and triggering other cells to produce **antibodies** – custom-built molecules which bind to one specific organism. Once the invader has been "labeled" with antibodies and covered in complement (proteins found in the blood), other white cells are able to engulf (phagocytose) the organism and inactivate it. These other white cells, **neutrophils** and **macrophages**, are produced in the bone marrow by special stem cells.

Classic signs of infection – heat, swelling and the formation of pus – derive from an increased blood supply to the infected area and the accumulation of dead cells. A small number of bacteria or a weakened virus may produce only slight symptoms of illness so the body is given a good opportunity to mobilize its defenses: this is the rationale for immunization.

IMMUNIZATION

Highly effective immunization can be given to babies and children against a number of diseases. The chart shows typical ages at which vaccinations may be given, but schedules do vary. Be sure to check with your doctor whether there could be any contraindications.

Age	Disease	Method
3–6 months	Diphtheria, whooping cough, tetanus	Combined injection
3–6 months	Poliomyelitis	By mouth
4–8 months	Diphtheria, whooping cough, tetanus	Combined injection
4–8 months	Poliomyelitis	By mouth
8–14 months	Diphtheria, whooping cough, tetanus	Combined injection
8–14 months	Poliomyelitis	By mouth
15 months	Measles, mumps, rubella (MMR)	Injection
5 years	Diphtheria, tetanus	Combined injection
5 years	Poliomyelitis	By mouth
10–13 years	Tuberculosis	Injection
13–14 years	Rubella (girls only) if MMR not given earlier	Injection
15–19 years	Tetanus	Injection
15–19 years	Poliomyelitis	By mouth

THE LYMPHATIC SYSTEM

As blood is pumped around the body, clear fluid containing lymphocytes leaves through the blood vessel walls and enters the tissues. The fluid (**lymph**) then enters a branching system of channels (the lymphatic system) in which it is squeezed along by the action of surrounding muscles and arteries. The channels gradually merge until lymph is collected into one large duct that drains into the bloodstream of the upper chest. Situated at various points along the lymphatic channels are lymph nodes. These lumps of lymphoid tissue act as filtering points to arrest the spread of infection and also produce some lymphocytes. Lymph nodes are usually small and hard to detect, but if there is an infection in the area they drain they become much larger and can be felt easily, particularly in the armpit or groin.

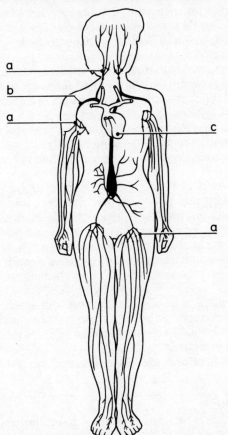

The lymphatic system
a Lymph node
b Lymph vessel
c Heart

THE THYMUS

The thymus gland is found in the chest, behind the breastbone. Like the tonsils and adenoids, it forms part of the body's immune system and is much larger and more active in childhood, while the immune system is learning to recognize and combat unfamiliar infections. Though its functions are complex and not well understood, it is vital for the "conditioning" of some white blood cells known as **T-lymphocytes**.

© DIAGRAM

2.02 The outer woman

The structure, functions and care of the body's exterior

The skin

FUNCTIONS

The skin is the largest organ of the body. It covers an area of about 17sq ft (1.6sq m) in the average adult woman – compared with 20sq ft (1.9sq m) in the average man. It accounts for about 16% of the total body weight. Skin thickness over most of the body is about ½₀in (1.2mm) – compared with ¼₈in (0.5mm) on the eyelids and ³⁄₁₆in–¼in (4–6mm) on the palms and soles.

The skin is attached to the underlying tissues by elastic fibers, which give it relative flexibility to allow for free joint movement. In old age the body bulk shrinks and the skin loses its elasticity, causing bagginess and wrinkles.

The skin is a versatile organ with a variety of essential functions. Most importantly, it protects the more delicate internal organs, acting as a barrier against physical damage, harmful sun rays, and bacterial infection.

The skin also acts as a sensory organ, being more richly supplied with nerve endings than any other part of the body. Sensations of touch, pain, heat and cold from the skin provide the brain with a continuous flow of information about the body's surroundings. Also very important is the skin's role in the regulation of body temperature: 85% of body heat loss is through the skin. During exposure to heat, blood vessels near the skin surface dilate so that more blood flows near the surface to lose its heat. When it is cold, these blood vessels constrict to reduce blood flow near the skin's surface.

Body heat is also reduced by the evaporation of perspiration on the skin, while perspiration's chemical content indicates the skin's function as an organ of excretion.

Finally, the skin helps make Vitamin D in sunlight, and even some antibodies.

STRUCTURE

The skin consists of two distinct layers – the **epidermis**, or outer layer, and the **dermis**, or inner layer. The epidermis is covered by a thin layer of **keratin** – the horny protein material also found in hair and nails.

Deep in the dermis, just above the subcutaneous fatty layer, lie the sweat glands which secrete sweat through ducts, or pores, to the skin surface. Also found in the dermis are nerves, and the blood capillaries which nourish the epidermal cells. Hairs are produced by specialized epidermal cells and grow from hair follicles that extend down into the dermal layer. Each hair has its own erector muscle, and a sebaceous gland which secretes grease, or sebum, to keep the skin supple.

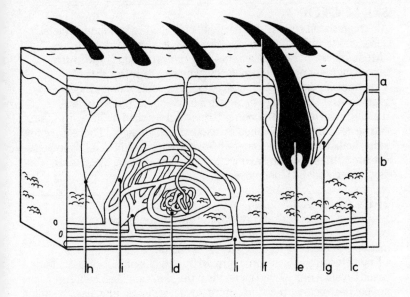

Cross-section of the skin
a Epidermis
b Dermis
c Subcutaneous fat
d Sweat gland
e Hair follicle
f Hair shaft
g Erector muscle
h Nerve
i Blood capillaries

PERSPIRATION

Perspiration means both the fluid produced by the sweat glands (sweat), and the process of sweating.

Sweat contains over 99% water, together with small amounts of salts, urea, and other waste products. An average person produces about 1½ pints (·75 liters) of sweat a day in temperate conditions. The process of perspiration helps keep body temperature down because heat is lost when sweat evaporates. Some sweating occurs even when the body is cool and the skin dry. In some areas of the body, perspiration is increased by exercise or mental anxiety.

BODY ODOR

Fresh perspiration produces very little smell in a healthy person. But stale perspiration results in body odor because bacteria that live on the skin act on the sweat to produce substances that smell. Body odor problems are commonly associated with the underarm and genital areas, where perspiration contains fats attractive to bacteria. Here, too, body shape and clothing cause a build up of perspiration by slowing down the rate of evaporation. Foot odor is another common problem caused by perspiring into a constricted area. Regular washing and changes of clothing help counteract body odor problems.

Most people also use a deodorant and/or antiperspirant. Chemicals in deodorants and some soaps slow down bacteria growth. With soaps, any lasting effect comes only from soap that remains in the pores after washing. Deodorants are more effective because they dry on the skin and can be concentrated where needed. Antiperspirants reduce perspiration in areas where they are applied, although perspiration over the body as a whole is not reduced. They work by blocking the pores, or by swelling the surrounding area to shrink the pore size. Manufactured sprays, sticks, roll-ons and creams usually contain both deodorant and antiperspirant.

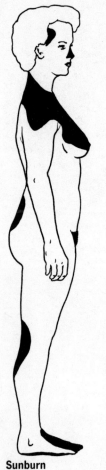

Sunburn

■ Sunburn danger areas

SKIN COLOR

A person's skin color is due partly to color pigments found in the skin cells, and partly to tiny blood vessels being near the skin surface.

Most important of the pigments that color the skin is **melanin** – a brown pigment present in skin cells known as **melanoblasts**.

The melanoblasts of dark-skinned people contain more melanin granules than those of people with fairer skins. The concentration of melanin in an individual's skin is largely determined by heredity – but can be considerably modified by exposure to sunlight. There are a few individuals whose bodies contain no melanin pigment at all. Known as **albinos**, these people have white hair, light-colored eyes, and a pale skin tinted pink by blood vessels.

SKIN AND SUN

Exposure to the sun's ultraviolet rays produces an increased concentration of melanin in the skin. In fair-skinned people this increase in melanin produces freckles and tanning.

Freckles are brown spots formed by patches of melanin. A suntan results from a more even increase in the skin's melanin content. Many people believe that they look more attractive when they have a suntan – and lying in the sun is a popular holiday pastime. Certainly the sun often improves skin conditions such as acne and sunbathing can produce feelings of relaxation and general well-being. If you are unused to the sun or have a very fair skin, it is essential to sunbathe with moderation. Painful sunburn (*left*) – or even sunstroke – may be the price of over-zealous exposure to the sun's rays. Long-term and repeated sunburn leads to skin peeling, wrinkling, and in some cases skin cancer. Gradual building up of sunbathing time and the use of sunblocks with a protective factor adequate for your skin type are simple precautions that are well worth the trouble.

SKIN CHANGES AND THE PILL

Freckles, irritation, oiliness, nodules under the skin, sensitivity to sunlight or acne are all known reactions to various types of contraceptive pill which usually disappear after switching to another pill or different method of contraception.

BIRTHMARKS

Birthmarks are various types of skin blemish present at birth.

Strawberry marks are red, slightly raised and spongy areas of skin containing enlarged blood vessels. They are usually fairly small and almost always disappears without treatment. It is rarely necessary to shrink a strawberry mark by injections or to remove it surgically.

Port wine stains are dark red in flat areas of skin containing enlarged blood vessels. They tend to be extensive and often occur on the neck and face. Surgical removal may not be recommended because of the risk of unsightly scarring. Various treatments have been developed by dermatologists to make the mark less noticeable, and special cosmetics provide reasonable concealment.

Vitiligo can be present at birth. This is a condition in which an area of skin always remains white whatever the color of the skin around it. It can be concealed, but there is no treatment.

MOLES

Moles are raised brown skin blemishes comprising a mass of cells with a high concentration of melanin. They are sometimes present at birth or may develop later – pregnancy often causes an increase in their size or number. Some moles have a growth of hair which should not be plucked because of the risk of infection. If removal of a mole is considered, it is important to consult your doctor. Most moles are harmless, but occasionally a mole may become malignant. Medical advice should be sought if a mole enlarges, ulcerates, or bleeds.

DERMATITIS (ECZEMA)

Dermatitis is a general term for inflammation of the skin. It is usually caused by exposure to a particular substance, but may also be of nervous origin or there may be an inherited tendency.

Some substances usually have an irritative effect on the skin: others affect only those people who are hypersensitive, or "allergic" to them. Frequent culprits include cosmetics, paints, detergents, insecticides, metals, textiles, rubber, and some plants. After contact with the offending substance, the blood vessels dilate and become porous. This allows fluid from the cells to collect in the skin and form blisters, which eventually burst. Later, the fluid dries out and the area becomes encrusted. The skin thickens around the sores and flakes off in scales. There is a serious risk of infection if the affected area is scratched or left untreated. Recurrence can be prevented by identifying the condition's cause and then avoiding or protecting against it.

Some eczema can also be exacerbated by emotional upheaval, particularly where it affects the elbows and knees.

BOILS

Boils are painful, pus-filled lumps caused by bacterial infection of a hair follicle, a sebaceous or sweat gland, a cut, or some other break in the skin. They occur most commonly around sites of friction with clothing, such as the neck or wrists, and may be an indication that a person is run down. Only after the dead skin that forms the boil's core has been released will the boil disappear. Most boils require no more than a protective dressing. Consult a doctor if a boil is particularly painful, if several occur, or if the sufferer is very young or old.

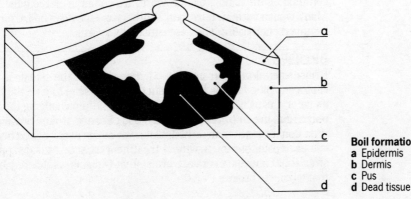

Boil formation
a Epidermis
b Dermis
c Pus
d Dead tissue

©DIAGRAM

ACNE

Acne is an infection of the sebaceous glands resulting in pimples, blackheads, whiteheads, and sometimes boils and cysts. It characteristically develops in adolescence, when the sebaceous glands become more active. Face, neck, shoulders, chest, and back may all be affected. Most cases clear up if attention is paid to diet, hygiene, and choice of cosmetics. Treatments include lotions and creams to reduce the spread of infection, make the skin peel, and unblock the pores. Antibiotics may be needed in severe cases. Exposure to sunlight or ultraviolet rays can also help make the skin peel, and through tanning, hide the spots. It is now thought that the underlying problem is excess androgen (male hormone), normally produced in small amounts in girls after puberty.

BLACKHEADS AND WHITEHEADS

A blackhead or whitehead appears when a skin pore becomes blocked by dust, dirt, or sebum. The waxy plug that blocks the pore is called a "comedone." This forms a blackhead when it is exposed to the air: oxidation turns the head of the comedone black. If it is not open to the air, a whitehead is formed. A pore may be cleansed by gently pressing out its contents but, unless this is done soon after the plug is formed, the spot is probably best left to take its own course. When cleaning out pores it is important to avoid damaging the skin or spreading infection. A preliminary wash with warm water will loosen the plugs.

PSORIASIS

Psoriasis is a chronic skin complaint characterized by red spots and patches covered with loose, silvery scales. The skin of the elbows, forearms, knees, legs, and scalp is most usually affected. The condition results from large-scale production of an abnormal type of keratin. It takes 28 days for normal skin to produce a mature keratin cell, but only 4 days for a person with psoriasis. The cause is unknown but there may be a genetic link. Psoriasis is not infectious and does not affect general health. The condition comes and goes intermittently but there is no cure. Various types of treatment bring some relief.

WARTS

Warts are small benign tumors of the skin. As well as the type common on the hands, plantar warts are common on the genitals. Many vanish without treatment – otherwise they can be frozen or removed chemically. They are caused by a virus.

BRUISES

Bruises develop when small blood vessels under the skin are ruptured. Blood seeps into the surrounding tissue to give the bruise its color – usually bluish or blackish at first, often changing through purple and green to yellow as the blood cells are broken down and their constituents reabsorbed. Cold wet compresses speed healing and ease pain, but even without treatment most bruises disappear after about a week. A severe bruise that remains painful may be a sign that a bone is broken.

HOW A CUT HEALS

1 If the skin is cut, the process of healing begins at once. Blood vessels constrict to stop the flow of blood and prevent the entry of bacteria. Then, clotting substances from the blood vessels form fine threads which knit together the sides of the wound.

2 During the first day, white blood cells enter the wound to break down and later absorb any foreign particles. At the same time the epidermal cells begin to multiply.

3 By the second day, a scab has formed over the wound. Beneath the scab, epidermal cells on each side of the wound join up to form a continuous layer.

4 About one week later, the scab comes away, revealing the new epidermis.

Healing
1 New cut
2 After 1 day
3 After 2 days
4 Healed skin
a Epidermis
b Dermis
c Blood vessels
d Blood cells
e Scab

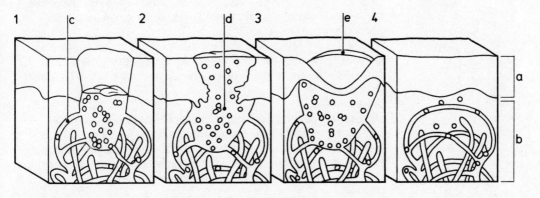

1   c   2   d   3   e   4   a   b

SKIN TYPE

Before embarking on a program of skin care, it is important to identify your skin type.

Normal skin is smooth, without any enlarged pores or flaking cells. Spots and blemishes are rarely troublesome.

Greasy skin is coarse in texture with open pores around the nose and on the chin. A tissue held against the face will be slightly greasy when it is removed. Greasy skin is very prone to spots and even acne.

Dry skin is flaky in texture and it tends to become lined early in life. It may become sore and red in cold weather, but spots are rare.

PLASTIC SURGERY

Plastic surgery is used to correct or improve minor disfigurements which are either congenital or caused by illness or injury.

The branch of plastic surgery which alters facial characteristics or disfiguring due to aging is often called **cosmetic surgery**. It can be used to remove the deep folds of skin or fat found as a double chin, sagging cheeks, or bags beneath the eyes. Cosmetic surgery can also be used to rid the face of wrinkles.

All cosmetic surgery is very costly and all evidence of it can take a long time to vanish. For many women, however, cosmetic surgery is invaluable since it can relieve extreme anxiety and restore undermined confidence.

© DIAGRAM

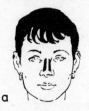

a

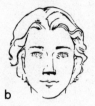

b

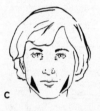

c

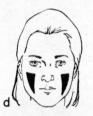

d

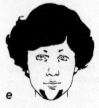

e

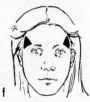

f

Make-up tricks to disguise
a Broad nose
b Long nose
c Broad jaw
d Wide cheeks
e Round chin
f Broad forehead
⬛ Darker shade

HOME BEAUTY TREATMENTS

Many beauty preparations can be made quite simply at home. Cucumber slices placed over each eye will refresh tired eyes. Pounded cucumber flesh mixed with milk makes a good toning lotion for normal or greasy skin. Mashed avocado flesh mixed with a little glycerin or lanolin makes a moisturizing mask for dry skin. Oatmeal mixed with orange juice makes a face mask for greasy skin. Raw egg white can be used to tighten the skin and to iron out temporarily any tiny wrinkles. Rose water diluted with mineral water makes a good toning lotion for dry skin.

SKIN CARE

Normal skin

Cleanse every night with a light cleansing cream. Remove the cream with a tissue and repeat. Wash with mild, unperfumed soap in the morning (or use cream again).
Tone with a mild skin tonic after cleansing. Apply with a cotton pad. Moisturize morning and night using a liquid moisturizing lotion.
Apply with the fingertips. Women over 25 may want to dab on a cream around the eyes.

Greasy skin

Cleanse with a medicated liquid cleanser at least twice a day. Pay particular attention to the extra-oily parts: chin, forehead, sides of nose. Remove the cleanser with a tissue and repeat. If the skin is blemished, medicated soap and water can be used after the cleanser. Moisturize once a day with a light liquid moisturizer.

Dry skin

Cleanse with a rich cream night and morning. Massage the cream in thoroughly, and remove with a tissue. Repeat. If you like to wash your face, use a mild, creamy soap, or a special creamy face-wash product. Tone with a gentle toner, preferably rosewater-based.
Moisturize in the morning with a light cream and at night with a rich, heavier cream.

CHOOSING COSMETICS

It is unnecessary to spend a lot of money on skin care and make-up products, though it is probably wise to avoid highly perfumed preparations or heavy, sticky creams, and to concentrate on simpler preparations containing natural ingredients rather than chemicals. Special hypoallergenic products made without perfume are useful for hypersensitive skins.

USING MAKE-UP

Make-up can accentuate the face's good points and disguise its bad ones. Always choose a basic foundation which suits your skin type and matches its natural color. By the skillful use of a darker shade of foundation or a blusher on top of the basic foundation, you can make the shape of your face look different.

The illustrations suggest simple make-up tricks that can help you do this.

The hair

FUNCTIONS

Hair has two major functions: it acts as a protective barrier, and it conserves heat.

The eyelashes protect the eyes, and the hairs in the nose and ears prevent the entry of foreign bodies. The eyebrows prevent sweat from dripping into the eyes.

Air trapped between hairs on the body insulates the skin and reduces heat loss. In the cold, or in danger, a tiny erector muscle attached to each hair follicle contracts to make the hair stand on end. The resulting "goose flesh" means that more air can be trapped, reducing even further the heat loss. Hair on the head is a particularly effective insulation.

Besides fulfilling these roles, hair is often considered an attractive bodily feature and it can play a part in sexual attraction.

Hair is found over the whole human body except the palms of the hands, soles of the feet, and parts of the genitals.

There are three types of hair: scalp hair, body hair, and sexual hair. Scalp hair resembles the body hair of other mammals. Human body hair is usually fine and light in color. Sexual hair develops around the genitals, the armpits and (in men) the face. Its growth is dependent on the male sex hormone testosterone produced by both sexes at puberty.

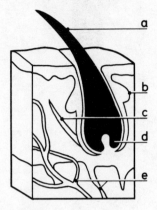

Hair shaft
a Shaft
b Sebaceous gland
c Muscle
d Follicle
e Capillaries

STRUCTURE

Each hair, properly called a hair shaft, grows from its own individual follicle, and each follicle has its own sebaceous (oil) gland, and tiny muscle. Capillaries supply nutrients from the blood stream.
A cross-section through the hair shaft (*right*) shows a hollow core (medulla) surrounded by an outer cortex, and covered by a thin coating of keratin – a shaft of horny cells which overlap one another. This coating is called the cuticle.

HAIR GROWTH

Hair on the scalp grows at the rate of about ½in (1.25cm) per month. (This means that the end of a hair measuring 18in (45cm) is about 3 years old!)

The root is the only live part of the hair: it grows and pushes the dead shaft out above the skin. Hair growth is cyclical with a growth phase followed by a rest phase in which the hair is loosened. The loosened hair is then pushed out by a new hair growing in its place. In this way, up to 100 hairs are lost each day from a normal head of hair.
Thickness of hair growth depends on the number of hair follicles. The follicles are established before birth and no new ones are formed later in life. The thickness of individual hairs is influenced by hereditary factors.

Illness and stress can both affect hair growth, making it thinner and more liable to split, and perhaps even causing a rest phase in a great number of hairs simultaneously so that a temporary sparse or bald patch may result.

Hair structure
a Medulla
b Cortex
c Cuticle

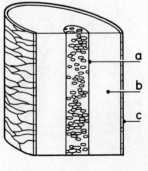

©DIAGRAM

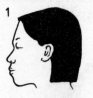

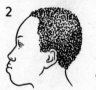

Types of hair
1 Mongoloid
2 Negroid
3 Caucasian

Hair colour
1 White hair
  Cortex contains
  transparent cells
2 Normal hair
  Cortex contains
  pigmented cells

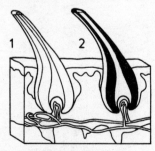

STRAIGHT OR CURLY?

The degree of curliness of the hair depends on the shape of the follicle from which it grows.

Straight hair grows from a more or less round follicle and is round in cross-section. This hair shape is characteristic of Mongoloids. Curly hair is oval in cross-section. It grows from a very curved follicle which forces the growing hair into curls. This hair shape is characteristic of Negroes. Wavy hair is kidney-shaped in cross-section. Curl extent depends on the curve of the follicle. This hair shape is characteristic of Caucasians.

HAIR CARE

a Wash your hair regularly. For normal Caucasian hair, this means every 5–7 days (Negroid hair requires less frequent washing), but if you have greasy hair (caused by overactive sebaceous glands) you will need to wash it more often. Remember, however, that washing can actually stimulate the glands through rubbing the scalp. Also detergent in shampoo can strip the hair of its natural oil and cause the glands to work overtime to replace it.

b Always choose a mild shampoo. Lots of lather feels good but it is caused by detergents. Use an appropriate shampoo for your hair type: lemon-based for greasy hair and cream for dry hair.

c Stick to a sensible diet.

d Choose a good quality brush and comb. Sharp teeth or bristles can damage hair.

e Unclean brushes and combs spread infection and bacteria. Keep them clean and do not lend them to anyone else.

f Do not tug at tangles as this will break your hair. Take a small strand at a time and beginning near the end, comb downward. Continue working toward the scalp, gently easing out the tangles as you go. Take special care when the hair is wet as it is then more prone to pull and split.

g Rubber bands should be avoided because they break the hair. There are special fabric-covered rubber bands for holding hair.

h Do not sleep in rollers. They will cause the hair to split or break.

i Be careful to wind your hair carefully around rollers. Hastily rolled hair causes knots when the rollers are removed.

j Remember that the condition of your hair reflects your state of health and general well-being. A balanced diet, plenty of sleep and regular trimming will do more to make your hair look good than anything else.

HAIR COLOR

The color of the hair is decided by heredity. Special pigment cells at the base of the hair follicle give a hair its color (*left*). These cells inject colored granules of black, brown, or yellow into the hair. If the cells receive no pigment, the cortex of each hair becomes transparent and the hair appears white.

"Gray" hair stems from a mixture of dark and white hairs.

DIET

Protein, vitamins of the B complex, and certain minerals are all essential for strong, healthy hair. The best sources of protein are meat, fish, milk, cheese and eggs. Vitamin B, obtained from liver and from brewer's yeast, is easily available in pill form. Iron, copper, and iodine are probably the most important minerals for healthy hair. Iron and copper are readily available in everyday foods like meat and green vegetables, and iodine is present in fish and shellfish. Women with greasy hair should avoid fried and fatty foods, and concentrate on meat, fresh fish, salads, fruits, vegetables, eggs and cheese. They should also drink plenty of water. Women with dry hair should include vegetable oils in their diet.

SCALP MASSAGE

Massaging the scalp with the fingertips increases the blood flow to the massaged area. This stimulates the follicles and can aid hair growth. It also means that the scalp is kept more healthy, with a greater supply of nutrients and speedier removal of waste products.

In scalp massage, it is important that the fingers do not slide over the scalp. This exerts pressure on the hair and can damage it. Massage can go from the neck up to the crown (as shown *right*), and then again from the temples back to the crown, thus covering the whole scalp.

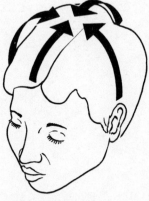

Scalp massage

SUDDEN HAIR GROWTH

This is usually due to a hormonal imbalance and can occur when the contraceptive pill is first taken or discontinued, during pregnancy or the menopause. Tufts of hair on either side of the chin or a fine down on the upper lip may appear.

Very often these will disappear once hormonal balance restores itself. However, if the growth is unusually marked and distressing, other hormones can sometimes be given to help adjust the balance – although correcting hormonal imbalance is a very complex and delicate process.

HAIR LICE

Two species of lice affect humans: *Phthirus pubis*, found in the pubic hair and *Pediculus humanus*, found in head hair. The latter can be acquired not only by contact with an infected person, but also via objects such as combs and hats.

The infestation causes severe itching. It is most easily diagnosed by examining the scalp for the tiny eggs ("nits") attached to the hair shafts. The lice themselves are more difficult to find. Suitable treatment should be obtained from a doctor or pharmacist: it will include a special shampoo and often also a scalp emulsion.

Pubic lice are transmitted by sexual contact and also by infested bedding or clothes. They, too, cause intense itching but scratching may only spread them. The treatment your doctor will usually recommend involves a cream, lotion or shampoo containing carbaryl.

©DIAGRAM

DANDRUFF

There are two kinds of dandruff. The first, affecting about 60% of the population to a mild degree, takes the form of fine, dry scales which fall from the scalp. The second kind, which is rarer, takes the form of thick, greasy scales adhering to the scalp.

The cause of both types is unknown and there is no real cure for dandruff, but it can be controlled. Washing the hair with ordinary shampoo may not help, so a medicated shampoo can be used instead to remove the scales and delay the recurrence. Some medicated shampoos have a simple antiseptic and others contain stronger chemicals. The most effective contain zinc pyrothionate, "ZP11".

LOSING YOUR HAIR

A number of hairs are lost from the scalp every day. These are usually replaced by new head hairs, but if they are replaced by fine, downy, hairs of the kind found on the face or arms, a thinning of the general growth of head hair results.

Only in very exceptional cases do women lose all their hair, though many notice a general thinning, particularly as they grow older. This condition is known as diffuse **alopecia** and is caused by an increase of male sex hormones in the body. If this hormonal imbalance is corrected, the full head of hair is usually restored. Stress can also cause hair loss because it interferes with the production of the hormones that stimulate hair growth. When the period of stress is over, normal hair growth is resumed.

After childbirth, many women notice an acute loss of hair. This too is a hormonal problem, but the hair soon returns to normal.

Some women also experience hair loss when they begin taking an oral contraceptive; others notice it when they stop taking the Pill. Again, it is possibly due to hormone levels. Anemia and an underactive thyroid may also be the cause.

HAIR REMOVAL

Superfluous hair can be removed in several ways. The different methods suitable for different parts of the body are shown *left*.

a Shaving: armpits; pubic hair, legs; toes
Hairs tend to regrow as prickly stubble.

b Plucking: eyebrows; chin
Not suitable for a large area.

c Waxing: armpits; legs
The skin is left silky smooth after a professional treatment.

d Bleaching: upper lip; arms; legs; toes
Try a test patch first in case the cream or liquid irritates your skin.

e Depilatory creams: chin; armpits; pubic hair; legs
Test a patch of skin before you try it over an extended area in case you are allergic to one of its ingredients.

f Electrolysis: upper lip; chin; breasts; legs; abdomen; pubic hair
Coarse hairs may require several treatments before removal is permanent, but growth should be weakened.

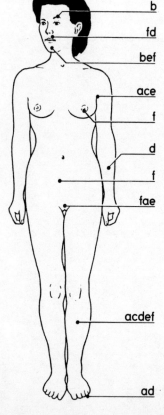

b
fd
bef
ace
f
d
f
fae
acdef
ad

PERMANENT WAVES AND STRAIGHTENING

A "perm" or "permanent" is a two-stage chemical process which causes each hair to alter the cell chain in its cortex. (The process is not literally permanent as the artificially created waves grow out as the hair grows.) After washing, the first solution is applied to the wet hair. This is an alkaline-based solution designed to soften the hair by breaking the cell chain. The hair is then wound around small curlers and the second solution applied. This is an oxidizing lotion that halts the softening process and causes the cells to coalesce again, but this time under the stress of the roller which gives the hair its "permanent" wave. The hair is then rinsed and wound around larger rollers for drying. A similar method can be used to straighten hair.

Some women are allergic to the chemicals involved, so it is important to make a test curl first to check for hypersensitivity. Dyed or bleached hair is particularly sensitive to the chemicals and it is essential to leave an interval of about 4 weeks between a "permanent" and a change of hair color.

CHANGING YOUR HAIR COLOR

The color of your hair can be changed by applying chemical or natural colorants. The color change can be permanent (not literally, because the effects grow out as the hair grows), semipermanent, or temporary. Although a change of hair color can give your whole appearance a "lift," too drastic a color change will not suit your natural coloring. Try on a wig in your chosen color before making the decision.

Permanent colorants

The application of a permanent colorant is a job for a hairdresser. A chemical compound of peroxide and ammonia is applied to the hair to "burn" away the color pigment. When the bleach has been rinsed off, the hair is porous and ready to receive the new color. The dye is applied and it is this synthetic pigment that gives hair its new color.

As the hair grows, the new growth near the scalp must be retouched to match the rest of the hair.

Semipermanent colorants

These colorants, designed to last through about 6 shampoos, can be applied at home. They do not contain bleach and the chemicals simply coat the hair shaft with color. A semipermanent colorant can also add body or bounce to thin or lank hair.

Color rinses

The effect of a rinse is only temporary. It simply colors the hair superficially rather like a watercolor paint, and washes out.

Natural colorants

Henna, mixed to a paste with hot water and applied directly to the hair, will dye hair a reddish color. An infusion of camomile, used as a rinse after shampooing, may lighten mousy hair.

Streaking and highlighting

This is an effective way of making the hair appear lighter by pulling a few strands only through a perforated plastic cap and dyeing these only, or by wrapping certain sections of hair to which bleach or other coloring has been added in strips of foil. The same process can be used to give lowlights if a darker colorant than the natural shade is used.

©DIAGRAM

The eyes

FUNCTIONS
The eyes – the organs of sight – lie in deep hollows in the skull, on either side of the nose.

They enable us to find out what is going on around us by use of light, to distinguish color and, since there are two of them with fields of vision that overlap, to estimate size and distance, and to perceive in 3-D.

STRUCTURE
The principal components of the eyes are as follows:

The conjunctiva is the membrane covering the front of the eyeball and the inside of the eyelids. It has a rich supply of blood vessels and is extremely sensitive.

The cornea is the clear part of the eyeball which lets in the light.

The iris controls the amount of light entering the eyeball. By constricting, it reduces the size of the pupil (the hole through which the light enters). The iris gives the eye its "color."

The lens has a firm center, surrounded by a softer substance contained in a fibrous capsule. By being stretched or thickened, it focuses light on the back of the eyeball.

The suspensory ligaments are attached at one end to the lens and at the other to the ciliary body. They hold the lens in place.

The eyeball
a Conjunctiva
b Cornea
c Iris
d Lens
e Suspensory ligaments
f Ciliary body
g Anterior chamber
h Sclera
i Choroid
j Retina
k Fovea
l Optic nerve
m Vitreous body
n Blind spot

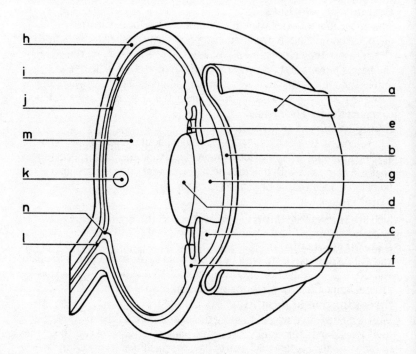

The ciliary body muscles control the lens shape. If they contract, the lens is stretched and light rays from long distances are focused on the retina. If they relax, the lens thickens, and close objects are focused. The process of thickening and increasing the curvature of the lens is known as "accommodation." Both lens and iris are controlled by the autonomic nervous system, and cannot be controlled at will.

The anterior chamber lies in front of the lens and is filled with a watery fluid called the **aqueous humor**.

The sclera or sclerotic coat is a layer of dense white tissue. It completely surrounds the eyeball, except where the optic nerve enters at the rear, and where it is modified at the front to form the transparent cornea. The sclera forms the "whites" of the eyes.

The choroid tissue lies beneath more than two-thirds of the sclera. It is colored brown or black, and contains blood vessels. The ciliary body and the retina are formed from the choroid. Its color absorbs excess light within the eyeball, making for clearer vision.

The retina is a thin layer of light-sensitive cells which lines the inside of the eyeball. It has a rich blood supply.

The fovea lies on the visual axis of the eyeball. It is a small depression in the retina, at which vision is sharpest. It contains only "cone" cells.

The optic nerve is a direct extension of the brain that enters the eyeball at the rear. Its head is called the optic disc and forms a blind spot in the vision, as there are no light-sensitive cells there.

The vitreous body occupies the space behind the lens with a transparent jelly-like substance that fills out the eyeball, giving it its shape. It contains small specks which are often seen when looking at white surfaces.

RODS AND CONES

Two types of light-sensitive cells exist in the retina. Classified by shape as rods and cones, they are connected by nerve fibers to the optic nerve.

Rods number about 125 million in each eyeball. They are sensitive to low intensity light, and are used mainly in night vision. Rods are not sensitive to color, and therefore give only a monochrome image (black, white, and shades of gray). Less than one four-hundredth of an inch in length and one-thousandth of an inch thick, they contain a purple pigment called rhodopsin. Light bleaches the rod as the pigment breaks down. This sets off electrical charges in the rods, which are transmitted down the optic nerve to the brain as nervous impulses.

Cones are shorter and thicker, for most of their length, than the rods. They are used for high intensity light, such as daylight, and give color vision.

The actual process of color vision is not known, but it is thought that there are three different classes of cones, each containing a different pigment. Each pigment would be sensitive to a different color: blue, green, or red. Other colors would be combinations of these. It is thought that the nerve messages are produced by bleaching, as in the rods.

Response to Light

When a light-cell pigment has been broken down, and an impulse has been passed, the pigment must re-form before another impulse is possible. This takes about one-eighth of a second. The eye is therefore like a cinema screen. It does not give a continual picture, but successive "stills" at intervals of one-eighth of a second. These seem continuous because they run together.

PROTECTING THE EYES

The eyes are protected in various ways.

Eyebrows prevent moisture and solid particles from running down into the eye from above.

Eyelids are folds of skin which, when closed, cover and protect the eyes. Each eyelid's inner membrane continues the conjunctiva covering the front of the eyeball.

Eyelashes are hairs that protrude from the eyelids. They prevent foreign bodies from entering the eye, and trigger off the protective blinking mechanism when touched unexpectedly.

Lacrimal glands produce a watery, salty fluid that cleans the eyeball front and also lubricates the eyelid's movement over the eyeball. When stimulated by strong emotion or irritants, the glands produce excess fluid.

Lacrimal ducts drain the fluid from the eyeballs into the lacrimal sacs which lead into the nasal passage. When the ducts cannot clear the fluid fast enough, it overflows and runs down the face as tears.

Blinking is a protective action of the eyelids which spreads the lacrimal fluid over, and cleans, the eyeball front. Blinking is controlled by the brain. It occurs every 2–10 seconds, and the rate increases under stress, in dusty surroundings, or when tired, and decreases during periods of concentration.

Protective structures
1 Eyebrows
2 Eyelids
3 Eyelashes
4 Lacrimal glands
5 Eyelashes
6 Lacrimal ducts
7 Lacrimal sacs

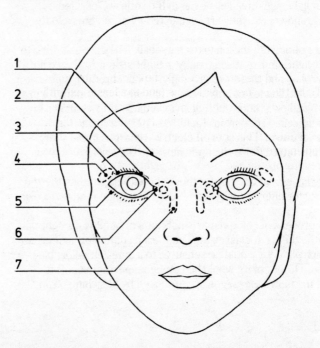

EYE MOVEMENT

Eyeball movement is controlled by six muscles attached to the outside of the sclera (as shown *below*).

Eyeball movement

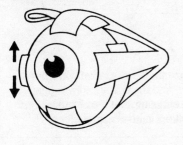
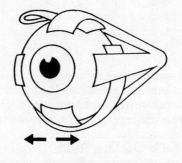
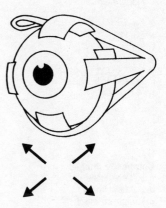

THE BLIND SPOT

To find your blind spot, hold the book at arm's length, and shut your left eye. Then look at the cross with your right eye, while slowly moving the book toward you. At one point the dot will disappear.

SIGHT

When the light rays from an object enter the eye they are bent ("refracted") by the cornea and the lens (and to a lesser extent by the aqueous humor and vitreous body). Because of this refraction, the rays are focused on the retina (though the image is upside down). The action of light on the retina cells triggers off an impulse that travels down the optic nerve to the visual centers of the brain. Here the impulses are interpreted and "seen" the right way up.

Refraction
The eye's lens changes shape to focus on objects at different distances

©DIAGRAM

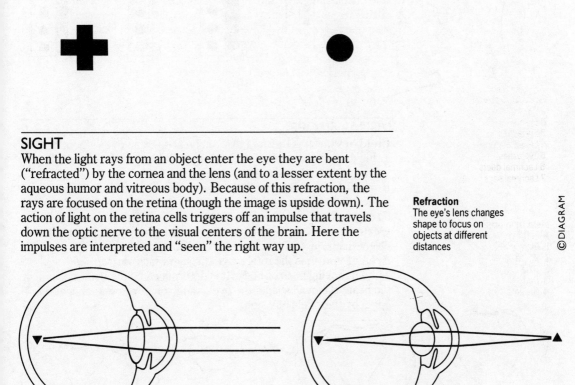

The eye compared with a camera
1 Camera
a Lens
b Closed shutter
c Stop
d Plate or film

2 Eye
e Eyelid
f Iris
g Lens
h Front of eye (transparent)
i Light-sensitive layer
j To the brain

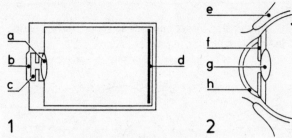

1   **2**

In many ways, the structure of the eye can be compared with that of a camera. The eyelids are like a shutter, and the cornea admits light. The iris regulates the amount of light entering; the lens focuses; and the retina receives the image, much like a light-sensitive plate.

COMPOSITE IMAGES

Composite images
a Left eye image
b Right eye image
c Composite image

Each eye sees a slightly different view of the same object. The images received in the two visual centers (at the rear of the cerebral hemispheres) are composite images from both eyes, mixed 50:50. The further away the object is, the less the discrepancy between the two views. This, plus the amount of tension needed to focus and the amount of blurring, forms the basis of judgment of distance.

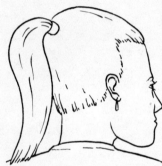

VISUAL SCOPE

Field of vision is the area that can be seen by an eye without moving it. Field size varies with different colors. White has the largest, then yellow, blue, red, and green.

Range of movement of the eyeball, with the head still, is also limited. The human eyeball can tilt 35 degrees up, 50 degrees down, 50 degrees in (i.e. toward the other eye), and 45 degrees out. The greater angle available when turning in allows an eye to focus on an object that is just within the other eye's outer range.

Area of vision is the total range through which we can see without moving head or body. It is determined by the eyes' position in the head; the head shape; the eyes' range of movement; and, at the edge, by their field of vision.

Field of vision
a Left eye
b Right eye
1 White
2 Blue
3 Red
4 Green

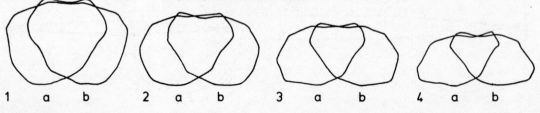

1   a   b   2   a   b   3   a   b   4   a   b

PERCEPTION

The ability to perceive objects, colors, and distances is learned by experience. To the newborn child, the images received are meaningless and confused. It takes time to learn to use the eyes and correlate past with present information to bring about recognition.

This dependence of perception on the brain's judgments can be shown by presenting the eye with trick pictures, ones that allow alternative interpretation, or that give evidence that seems contradictory. Our perception will then shift or struggle between the alternative interpretations. The same process can be observed when waking up in unfamiliar surroundings – a series of alternative pictures flash through the brain, as it tries to make familiar sense of the data it is receiving. In other cases, though, the brain accepts deceptive information unquestioningly.

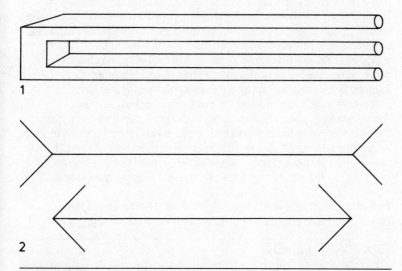

Optical illusions
1 Impossible solid
2 Lines of equal length do not seem so

EYE CARE

Injuries to the eye and the immediately surrounding area should receive expert medical attention. Infection is a danger even if there is no significant damage. The eyes are tough but should be treated with care.

Small foreign bodies that get stuck in the eye can usually be removed by blinking. If this fails, then pull the upper lid outward and downward over the lower lid. When the upper lid is released, the particle may be dislodged. A particle can also be removed with the corner of a clean handkerchief or by blowing it toward the edge. If none of this succeeds, get help and, if necessary, medical attention.

Black eyes are bruises of the eyelids and tissues around the eyes. They can be treated by applying a cold compress. If a black eye appears after a blow elsewhere on the head, see a doctor.

A **sty** is an inflamed sebaceous gland around an eyelash, caused by bacterial infection. It is most often found in young people. A large part of the eyelid may become affected. To treat a sty, remove the relevant eyelash and bathe the eye with **warm** water. Antibiotics should only be used in extreme cases.

Conjunctivitis is inflammation of the conjuctiva because of infection or allergy. If due to bacterial or viral infection, it needs the appropriate antibiotic eyedrops; if due to irritation, the irritant (e.g. an ingrowing eyelash) is removed. Bathing the eye with warm water and lotions is soothing and is all that is needed in mild cases. Bandages or pads encourage the growth of bacteria, but dark glasses or eyeshades protect the eye from light and wind. Conjunctivitis is not very serious in itself (except for the form found in the tropics), but can sometimes cause serious complications such as ulceration of the cornea.

CORRECTIVE LENSES

Spectacles (or contact lenses) are used because of faulty focusing in the eye. The artificial lens corrects the defective working part of one or both eyes.

Nearsightedness (myopia) is due to the eye's refractive power being too strong (e.g. the lens may be too thick) or to the eyeball being too long. In both cases, the light rays are focused in front of the retina, giving a blurred image. Concave corrective lenses are needed to focus on distant objects.

Farsightedness (hypermetropia) is due to the eye's refractive power being too weak or the eyeball too short. The light rays are focused behind the retina, again giving a blurred image. Convex corrective lenses are needed for close work such as reading.

Astigmatism means that the cornea does not curve correctly, and the person cannot focus on both vertical and horizontal objects at the same time. A special spectacle lens is needed that only affects the light rays on one of these planes. Alternatively, a hard contact lens can be used, as the fluid layer between eye and lens compensates for the cornea.

Presbyopia occurs in old age and involves a hardening of the eye's lens. Corrective convex lenses may be needed for reading.

CONTACT LENSES

Contact lenses are thin round disks of plastic that rest directly on the surface of the eye. They are increasingly used instead of spectacles, as they do not affect the appearance, often give better vision, and counteract many year-to-year changes in the eyesight. However, not everyone can wear contact lenses successfully, and some people find that they can wear them only part of the day. They also require more care because of their smallness and fragility, and because of the effect a damaged lens can have on the eye. They need to be cleaned and stored in special fluid when out of the eye, and it is wise to insure them against destruction or loss.

Types of lens

Contact lenses can be "hard" or "soft." Hard lenses are either "scleral" lenses – covering the whole of the visible part of the eye – or "corneal" lenses, which rest on the center of the eye, floating on a film of tear fluid.

Soft lenses are the most popular of all contact lenses, but scleral lenses are useful for very active sports. Soft lenses differ because they absorb water from the tear fluid.

Comparing hard and soft lenses

Soft lenses are immediately more comfortable, easier to get used to, can generally be worn for longer periods, can be left off for several days and then worn again without discomfort, can be alternated more easily with spectacles, and can be worn with less discomfort in dirty atmospheres.

Hard lenses are much less easy to damage, much cheaper, last perhaps 6 to 8 years (compared with 2 to 3 years for soft lenses with routine wear and tear, and often under a year if damage occurs), are more suitable for most eye prescriptions, often give clearer vision, are easier to keep free from bacteria, and are much easier for the optician to adjust if difficulty arises.

BLINDNESS

Obstruction of light occurs when areas of the eye's naturally transparent part become opaque, and light rays are prevented from reaching the retina. Opacity of the cornea can be caused by corneal ulcers, or by keratitis – that is, inflammation of the cornea. Lens opacity is commonly caused by its becoming hard and forming a **cataract**. Cataracts most often occur with aging, but can also be caused by wounds, heat, radiation, electric shock or diabetes. Blurred vision occurs in the affected eye or eyes. Today, removal of a cataract is in fact the most common of all eye operations and very effective.

Diseases affecting the retina

These are often caused by diseases elsewhere in the body, especially those involving the blood supply. Some of the most common include the following, and advances in surgical treatment – including use of lasers – continue apace.

Retinitis is inflammation of the retina with consequent loss of vision. It is associated with diabetes, leukemia, kidney disorders, and syphilis.

Retinopathy covers any disease of the retina that is not inflammatory. It is usually caused by blood vessel degeneration impairing the retina's structure and function. It can be due to high blood pressure, diabetes, kidney disorders and atherosclerosis.

Detachment of the retina in a primary form occurs if damage to the retina allows fluid from the vitreous body to leak through and lift the retina from the choroid. Treatment is possible. Secondary detachment occurs if the retina is pushed away from the choroid and damaged by underlying tumors, bleeding, or retinal disease. No treatment is possible.

Glaucoma may take two forms. When acute, it may occur in middle age and it is important it is treated as early as possible to avoid blindness. Simple or chronic glaucoma occurs with aging, and presents with very gradual loss of vision.

Symptoms of acute glaucoma include blurred vision, pain, hazy appearance of the cornea and perhaps vomiting.

Choroiditis is inflammation of the choroid due to infection (especially syphilis, allergy, or some other conditions, certain types of arthritis, for example.) The effects depend on the size and position of the inflammation: the nearer the fovea, the greater the vision loss. The inflammation can be treated, but damaged vision is seldom improved.

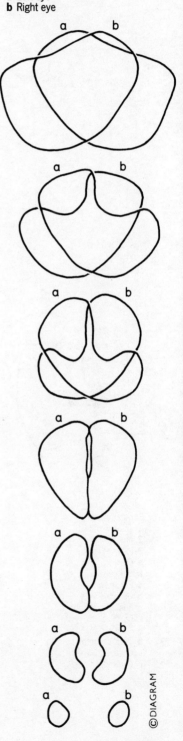

Declining field of vision in a case of progressive blindness in both eyes
a Left eye
b Right eye

©DIAGRAM

The ears

FUNCTIONS
The ears not only enable us to hear but also\contain the organ of balance which enables us to keep upright.

STRUCTURE
The ear comprises three parts.

The outer ear includes the external flap of cartilage (the "pinna" or "auricle"); and the ear canal (the "meatus").

The middle ear includes the eardrum (the "tympanic membrane)"; three small bones called the "ossicles," and known individually as the hammer ("malleus"), anvil ("incus"), and stirrup ("stapes"); and the eustachian tube, which opens into the back of the throat, and keeps the air pressure in the middle ear equal to that outside.

The inner ear includes the cochlea, a spiral filled with fluid and containing the "organ of corti"; the oval window; the round window; and the organs of balance.

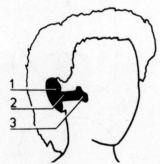

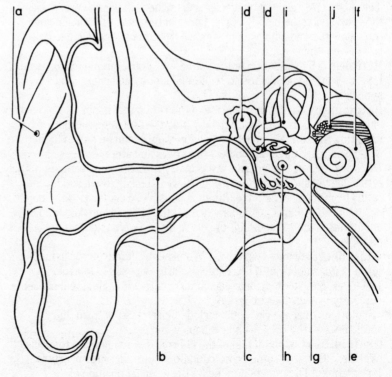

Ear structure
1 Outer ear
2 Middle ear
3 Inner ear
a Cartilage flap
b Ear canal
c Eardrum
d Ossicles
e Eustachian tube
f Cochlea
g Oval window
h Round window
i Organ of balance
j Auditory nerve

SOUND

When a solid object vibrates in air, it passes on this vibration to the surrounding air molecules. Sound waves are the vibration of air molecules.

Sound has three qualities:

Pitch is the highness or lowness of a sound, and depends on the "frequency" of the sound waves, or the number of vibrations per second. High pitched (piercing) sounds have a high frequency. Low pitched (deep) sounds have a low frequency.

Intensity is the loudness of a sound, and depends on the amount of energy in the sound waves, or how widely they vibrate. Intensity is measured in "decibels."

Timbre is the quality of a sound. Sounds with the same pitch and intensity can be distinguished by their timbre. Timbre is created by the subordinate tones that accompany the main sound.

HEARING

As part of the hearing process, sound waves are collected by the pinna and funneled into the ear canal. The eardrum vibrates in time with the sound waves. This vibration is passed on along the three ossicles to the oval window. The lever action of the ossicles increases the vibration's strength and allows the vibration to be passed from the air of the outer and middle ear to the fluid of the inner ear.

The vibration of the oval window makes the fluid in the cochlea of the inner ear vibrate. The pressure changes in the fluid are picked up by specialized cells in the organ of corti. This organ converts the vibration into nerve impulses, which pass along the auditory nerve to the brain. Meanwhile, the vibrations pass on through the cochlea and back to the round window, where they are lost in the air of the middle ear and eustachian tube.

SENSITIVITY

Loudness The human ear can hear sounds ranging in loudness from 10 decibels to 140 decibels (though the loudness becomes painful after 100 decibels). On the decibel scale, a ten unit increase means 10 times the loudness. Therefore, the quietest sound the human ear can hear is one 10 million millionth the loudness of the loudest. The volume of normal speech is 40–60 decibels.

Pitch Different frequencies stimulate different parts of the organ of corti. That is why we can distinguish one sound from another. The human ear can hear sound ranging in pitch from 20 cycles per second (low) to 20,000 cycles per second (high). Frequencies above this are called "ultrasounds," and can be heard by some animals but not humans.

Direction The slight distance between the ears means that there are minute differences in their perception of a given sound. The brain interprets these differences to tell from which direction the sound came. But if a sound comes from directly behind or in front of the listener, both ears receive the same message, and the listener must turn the head before pinpointing the location.

©DIAGRAM

BALANCE

The organ of balance is in the inner ear next to the cochlea. It consists of three U-shaped tubes ("semicircular canals"), at right angles to each other. They are filled with fluid which is set in motion when the person moves. Hairs at the base of each canal sense this movement and send messages to the brain, which are interpreted and used to maintain the person's balance. The organ also contains two other structures, the saccule and the utricle. These have gravity-sensitive specialized cells, and so keep a check on the body's position.

EAR CARE

The outer ear should be kept clean at all times, to prevent wax and bacteria from collecting in the ear canal and damaging the eardrum. But sharp objects should not be poked inside the ear when cleaning it.
Syringing of the outer ear cleans it, and washes out obstructions such as wax or foreign bodies. The doctor uses a large glass or metal syringe – one with a blunt point not more than 1in (2.5cm) long, so it cannot hurt the eardrum. The syringe is filled with warmish water containing, if necessary, an antiseptic and/or wax dissolving agent. The fluid is directed along the upper wall of the canal, and flows out along the lower wall.

SYMPTOMS OF DISORDER

Deafness can be temporary or permanent, caused by obstruction or disease.
The inner ear is tested by using a tuning fork. The fork should be heard clearly when it is held in front of the ear. If the tuning fork is heard more clearly when placed on the bone behind the ear, then either the outer ear is blocked with wax or, if not, the middle ear is faulty, since sound vibrations are being heard through the skull. If hearing is still poor when the fork is placed on the bone behind the ear, it is the inner ear or the auditory nerves that are at fault.
Earache is usually caused by infection and inflammation in the ear. In the outer ear, this can occur through physical damage, boils or eczema (a skin disorder). Large wax deposits can also cause earaches, in which case syringing may be necessary.
  Germs from throat infections may spread up the eustachian tube and cause middle ear inflammation (especially in children). This is common after tonsilitis, measles, flu or head colds, and can be very painful.
  Earache can also arise without any ear disorder, because of disturbances affecting the nerves it shares with other parts of the head. Tonsilitis, bad teeth, swollen glands and neuralgia can all cause earache in this way.
Ringing in the ears ("tinnitus") is usually associated with earache in the middle ear and/or high blood pressure. It is also caused by certain ear diseases.
Giddiness or vertigo can be caused by infection of the inner ear that affect the organs of balance.
Discharges can come from boils or other infections.

EAR DISORDERS

Otitis externa is infection and inflammation of the outer ear, due to physical damage, allergy, boils, or spread of inflammation from the middle ear. There is itching and often a discharge, which may cause temporary deafness if it blocks the ear canal. Treatment is by antiseptic syringing and use of soothing lotions. Hot poultices and aspirin may relieve the pain.

Otitis media is middle-ear infection, usually due to bacteria arriving via the eustachian tube. The eardrum becomes red and swollen, and may perforate. Pressure and pain increase as pus fills the middle ear. There is often temporary deafness and ringing, and sometimes fever. Treatment is with antibiotics. A form of otitis, in which a sticky substance is discharged in the middle ear is,common in children. The ossicles cannot function, and in severe cases deafness results.

Mastoiditis is a form of middle-ear infection that can spread to the mastoid bone – the part of the skull just behind the ear. Infection swells the bone painfully, and the patient is feverish. Treatment is by antibiotics or the surgical removal of the infected bone.

Ménière's disease affects the inner ear, and results in too much fluid in the labyrinths. Its cause is not known, but it tends to occur in middle age, usually affecting more men than women. The symptoms are attacks of giddiness and sickness, followed by deafness with accompanying ringing in the ears.

Treatment is with drugs and control of fluid intake – not more than 2 pints or 2½ (US) pts (1.2 liters) a day. In extreme cases the labyrinths or their nervous connections are destroyed.

Fungus infections can occur in the outer ear, but are more common in tropical climates. There is persistent irritation and discharge, which is treated with antibiotics and antiseptic cleansing of the ear canal.

Otosclerosis involves hearing loss due to overgrowth of spongy bone in parts of the middle ear (see p.84).

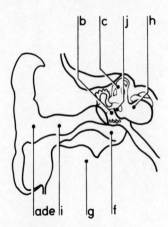

Possible sites of disorder in the ear.
a Blockage
b Ringing
c Vertigo
d Discharge
e Otitis externa
f Otitis media
g Mastoiditis
h Ménière's disease
i Fungus
j Otosclerosis

DEAFNESS

Conductive deafness refers to any failure in the parts of the ear which gather and pass on sound waves, e.g. blockage of the ear canal, eardrum damage, ossicle damage, etc. **Perceptive deafness** refers to any failure in that part of the ear which translates the sound waves into nerve impulses (the cochlea); or in the auditory nerves transmitting the impulses to the brain; or in the brain's auditory centers that receive the message. Perceptive deafness may not mean that the person can perceive no sound. It may be that sound is received, but so scrambled as to be unintelligible.

Some disorders of the ear can end in deafness. Any exposure to extremely loud noise, or continued exposure to moderately loud noise, can also damage the eardrum and middle ear, causing hearing decline and eventually deafness. The main victims are those who work in very noisy surroundings, and also the fans – and performers – of loud popular music. Continued use of personal stereo systems has also recently been blamed.

Congenital deafness at birth ranges from complete absence of the ears to minute mistakes in the internal structure. The latter can often be cured surgically. Congenital deafness can be due to inheritance of a genetic defect or can result from certain infections in the mother during the first few months of pregnancy, including German measles (rubella), and syphilis. If your baby's response to sounds gives rise to worry, consult your doctor.

Otosclerosis is a condition in which the stirrup becomes fixed within the oval window, due to deposits of new bone. About one person in every 250 suffers from this, and it is more common in women than men. Surgical treatment may give improvement, but there is no way of halting the process responsible (though it may stop spontaneously).

HEARING AIDS

Hearing aids work by amplifying sound. If the amplification is loud enough, it can overcome the blockage or damage that causes conductive deafness, and allow the sound to reach the inner ear. Amplification also seems to help in many cases of perceptive deafness. However, sometimes the aid does not allow speech to be distinguished: it only makes the person more aware of unintelligible noise.

The performance of a hearing aid depends on the frequency response (normal speech usually lies between 500 and 2000 cycles per second); the degree of amplification; and the maximum amount of sound that the aid can deliver. Too much sound can make speech unintelligible, and/or damage the ear mechanisms.

One common problem with hearing aids is "acoustic feedback" (the reamplification of sound vibrations that have already passed into the ear but have partly leaked out again).

Insert receivers are the most common type. They are molded to fit into the ear canal and form a perfect seal. No sound escapes, there is little or no acoustic feedback, and background noise is at a minimum. They can also be very small and, if transistorized, need no wires or attachments. A high degree of amplification is possible.

Flat receivers fit against the external ear cartilage, and are kept in place by a metal band. They are usually used only if there is a continuous discharge from the ear, or if there has been a serious mastoid operation. Because of the bad contact, many sounds escape, and acoustic feedback produces much background noise.

Bone conductors amplify the sound waves and send them through the bone of the head, not the air passages of the ear. They are uncomfortable and not very efficient, and are usually only used where some ear condition rules out an insert receiver.

At first, some people are reluctant to wear hearing aids because they do not want to admit they are not hearing too well – but having one expertly fitted can make all the difference to the hard-of-hearing, although gradual acclimatization may be required, together with careful adjustment.

The nose

FUNCTIONS
The nose is the opening to the respiratory system and is the organ of the sense of smell.

STRUCTURE
The outer nose consists of tissue and cartilage supported at the top by the nasal bones. The nasal cavity beneath is divided into two (left and right) by a wall of bone and cartilage called the nasal septum. Tiny hair-like nerve endings in the roof of the nasal cavity detect odorous molecules in the air, and transfer signals to the brain via olfactory bulbs and a set of nerve fibers called the olfactory tract.

Sense of smell
a Brain center for smell
b Olfactory tract
c Olfactory bulbs
d Olfactory hairs

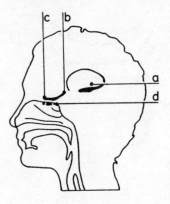

SENSE OF SMELL
The sense of smell is one of the keenest of all the human senses. It can for instance distinguish more odors than the ear can distinguish sounds. It is a vital part of the taste process – people who have lost their sense of smell cannot taste the full flavor of foods. The precise mechanism of smell remains a mystery. Similarly, attempts to classify different odors have mostly been unsuccessful. One theory has proposed four categories – fragrant, burnt, acid, and rancid – and suggested that every smell is a blend of these four basic odors.

NOSE DISORDERS
The common cold is a viral infection of the respiratory system resulting in a running nose, reduced sense of smell, and sometimes a cough.

Hay fever is an allergic reaction which causes the mucus membranes in the nose and eyes to become swollen and irritated. It may also cause a watery discharge or sneezing.

Nose bleeds are usually caused by a ruptured blood vessel inside the nose. The bleeding may result from a blow, violent exercise, or exposure to high altitudes, or may be a sign of high blood pressure. It can usually be relieved by pinching together the nostrils; but severe or persistent bleeding needs medical attention.

Polyps are benign tumors in the nasal passage that cause a permanently stuffy nose. Often the result of frequent colds, they are easily removed by simple surgery.

Rhinitis is inflammation of the nose's mucous membranes caused by colds or hay fever.

The sinuses
Sinuses are air cavities in the skull which open into the nasal passages. Sinus inflammation is called sinusitis and symptoms include headaches and pain in the cheek bones. Drugs are used to treat most cases; minor surgery can improve more severe ones.

◼ Sinuses

COSMETIC NOSE SURGERY
Surgery can correct the bridge line, shorten the nose, build a depressed nose, straighten a crooked one, or alter the shape of the tip. All involve shaving back or implanting extra bone or cartilage. The incisions are made inside the nose, and the new shape takes about 6 months to settle. Though such surgery is often performed at the patient's whim, in many cases it relieves very real distress.

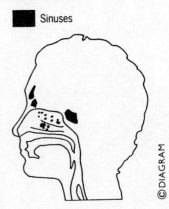

© DIAGRAM

The mouth

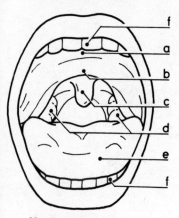

Mouth structure
a Hard palate
b Soft palate
c Uvula
d Tonsils
e Tongue
f Teeth

1 Taste
a Nasal cavity
b Food
c Nerves
d Salivary gland

2 Taste areas of the tongue
A Back
B Front
a Bitter
b Sour
c Salt
d Sweet

FUNCTIONS
The mouth is the entrance to the digestive system and one opening of the respiratory system. It also houses the tongue and therefore plays an important part in the taste process and voice production.

STRUCTURE
The mouth is completely surrounded by muscle except for the hard palate and lower jaw which are rigid. Behind the hard palate is the soft palate from which hangs the uvula, a projection of muscle tissue important in speech. On either side of the back of the mouth are the tonsils – oval masses of lymphoid tissue. The cavity is lined with mucous membrane. The mucus it secretes, along with saliva from the salivary glands, cleanses the mouth, and keeps it lubricated. The central part of the mouth contains the tongue, and the opening is bound by the lips.

THE TASTE PROCESS
Before it can be tasted, a piece of dry food must be moistened and partly dissolved in the mouth by saliva from the salivary glands. The saliva, containing the particles of food, stimulates the taste buds on the tongue. Different areas of the tongue register different tastes.
   The taste buds send signals to the brain which interprets these signals as tastes.
   The sense of smell is also part of the taste process. The food odors enter the nasal cavity and stimulate the olfactory system. This greatly heightens the sensation of taste.

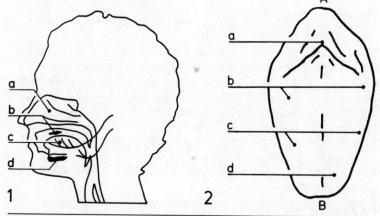

MOUTH DISORDERS
Very few serious disorders affect the mouth. A mixture of saliva, mucus, and secretion from the tonsils keep it moist and mostly germ-free. Any injuries seem to clear up more quickly than they do elsewhere, and there is considerable resistance to infection. The most common minor disorders are ulcers, cold sores and thrush.
Ulcers are inflamed sores in the mouth's mucous membrane usually caused by a scratch or similar injury. Most people suffer occasionally from small ulcers of this type which usually heal on their own, but mouth ulcers can also be signs of diseases such as diphtheria, leukemia, and cancer.

Cold sores (*Herpes simplex*) are small inflamed blisters that appear around the mouth. They are usually the result of a virus which many people carry around in their bodies all their lives. An eruption can be triggered by another infection, or by exposure to very hot or cold weather.

Thrush (*Moniliasis*) is a mucous membrane infection of the mouth, caused by a yeast-like fungus. It produces white patches inside the cheeks, but can sometimes signify a more serious underlying illness.

CONGENITAL DEFECTS

Cleft palate In the unborn baby, the palate develops in two halves which fuse. In some babies, the palate has not fused completely. This condition is known as cleft palate.

Harelip is the failure of the upper lip's three parts to join – a congenital defect usually associated with cleft palate.

Both defects can usually be corrected by plastic surgery in operations beginning soon after birth.

FUNCTIONS

Teeth are hard structures set in bony sockets in the upper and lower jaws. Their main function is to chew and prepare food for swallowing. They also help in the articulation of sounds in speech. In humans there are three main types of teeth.

Incisors are sharp, chisel-like teeth at the front of the mouth, used for cutting into food.

Canines are pointed teeth at the corners of the mouth, used for tearing and gripping food.

Molars and **premolars** are square teeth with small cusps, which grind food at the sides of the mouth.

STRUCTURE

A tooth consists of the root, embedded in the jaw; and the crown, projecting out of the jaw. Where the root and crown meet is called the neck. Each tooth is made up of enamel, dentine, pulp, and cementum.

Enamel is the hardest tissue in the body, and it protects the sensitive crown of the tooth.

Dentine is a slightly elastic material forming most of the tooth under the enamel. It is sensitive to heat and chemicals. **Pulp** is the soft tissue inside the dentine, and contains nerves and blood vessels, which enter the tooth's root by a small canal.

Cementum is a thin layer of material covering the tooth root and protecting the underlying dentine. It also helps attach fibers from the gum to the tooth.

The teeth

1 **Types of teeth**
a Molar
b Canine
c Incisor
2 **Parts of a tooth**
d Crown
e Neck
f Root
3 **Section through a tooth**
g Enamel
h Dentine
i Pulp
j Cementum
k Periodontal membrane

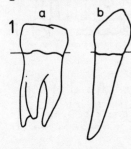

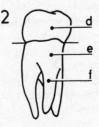

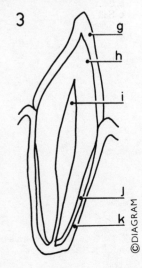

©DIAGRAM

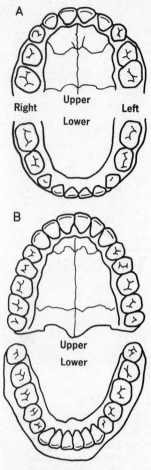

A

Upper

Right   Left

Lower

B

Upper

Lower

Looking into the mouth
A Primary or milk teeth
B Adult teeth

TWO SETS OF TEETH

In humans there are two successive sets of teeth. The primary or "milk" set arrive 6 to 24 months after birth. Later, they gradually fall out, from the age of 6 on, as the permanent teeth appear. Most of these materialize by the age of 13, but a "wisdom tooth" (at the back of the mouth) can erupt as late as the age of 25, or never.

Human teeth do not keep growing, but reach a certain size and then stop; and when the permanent teeth fall out, they are not replaced by a new set. But in some animals, such as the rabbit, the incisors keep growing, as they are worn down by use, while the shark grows set after set of teeth – to its great advantage!

Age of appearance

These are average figures only: actual dates vary greatly from child to child.

Primary or milk teeth

Central incisors	6–8 months
Lateral incisors	9–11 months
Eye teeth (canine)	18–20 months
First molars	12–17 months
Second molars	24–26 months

Adult teeth

First molars	6–7 years
Central incisors	6–7 years
Lateral incisors	7–9 years
Canines	10–11 years
First premolars	10–11 years
Second premolars	11–12 years
Second molars	11–16 years
Third molars	17–21 years

The final number of adult teeth is between 28 and 32, depending on how many wisdom teeth appear.

Sequence of appearance of adult teeth (upper jaw)

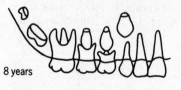

5 years

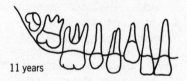

11 years

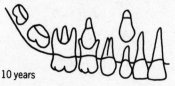

8 years

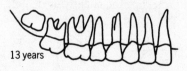

13 years

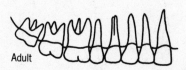

10 years

Adult

PREVENTING DENTAL TROUBLE

Diet At any age, the ideal diet for dental health should be well balanced and adequate, so general heath is maintained; chewable enough to stimulate the gums; and low in sugar content. Diet balance and adequacy is especially important for expectant mothers and growing children, so that strong teeth form.

Oral hygiene Teeth should be cleaned at least twice a day – after breakfast, and last thing at night. But it is better if they are cleaned after every meal. Cleaning polishes the teeth and removes stains and food debris.

Methods of cleaning vary from culture to culture. The toothbrush can be used ineffectively, and even cause damage (electric toothbrushes tend to be better). **Dental floss** is a fiber which will help remove plaque from areas between the teeth where a toothbrush cannot reach. Soft wood toothpicks are also valuable for dislodging food between the teeth. Highly effective techniques used elsewhere include the fibrous chewing stick used in Africa, and the Muslim tradition of rubbing the teeth and gums with a towel.

Dental inspections Regular visits to the dentist about every six months catch disease early and so avoid drastic measures later.

Fluoride is a tasteless, odorless, colorless mineral which, if added to drinking water in small amounts, reduces tooth decay in children under 14 (only) by 60%. (Excessive amounts can cause the enamel to become mottled.) Fluoride treatment as a preventive measure is now widely given to children. Some toothpastes also contain fluoride, and tablets can be bought to add to unfluoridated water. So far, no ill effects from fluoride use in these quantities have been established, but this remains a controversial area

CLEANING THE TEETH

Most people use scrubbing motions, backward and forward and up and down (see *right*). Backward and forward strokes with the brush length are good for the tops of the molars (**a**), and the back of the front teeth (**b**). But on the side teeth, use the brush sideways in a repeated stroke in one direction – upward on the bottom teeth (**c**), and downward on the top ones (**d**).

Use of **disclosure tablets** is sometimes recommended by dentists so that you can appreciate the extent to which you need to brush in order to remove harmful plaque. A tablet should be chewed and spread with saliva on to all tooth and gum surfaces. After rinsing your mouth with water, all areas of plaque will be stained red, but the coloring can be removed by adequate brushing.

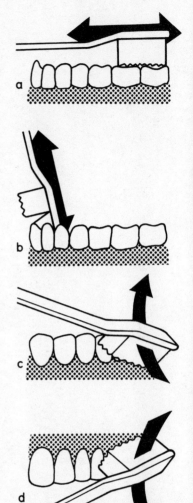

Correct brushing techniques
a Tops of molars (across)
b Backs of front teeth (up and down)
c Side bottom teeth (upward)
d Side top teeth (downward)

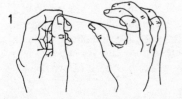

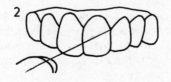

Use of dental floss
1 Break off a piece of fiber about 18in (45cm) long
2 Guide it between the teeth with a sawing action

©DIAGRAM

DENTAL DISORDERS

Tooth decay is the most universal of human diseases. It especially afflicts those who eat a highly refined diet which is overcooked, soft, sweet, and sticky. Bacteria in the mouth change carbohydrates in the food into acids strong enough to attack tooth enamel. Gradually, the enamel is broken down and bacteria invade the dentine, forming a "cavity." The pulp reacts by forming secondary dentine to ward off the bacteria, but without treatment the pulp becomes inflamed and painful toothache may result.

The infection may then pass down the root and cause an **abscess** – a painful collection of pus, affecting the gum and face tissues.

Periodontal disease denotes disorders in the teeth's supporting structures: the gums, cementum and other tissues. The commonest cause is overconsumption of soft food, which cannot stimulate and harden the gums. Other causes include sharp food that scratches the gums; inefficient brushing; badly contoured fillings; ill-fitting dentures; irregular teeth; and teeth deposits. General factors such as vitamin deficiencies, blood disorders and drug use may also be involved.

Periodontal disease can be painless but, if allowed to progress, the gum may become detached from the tooth. The socket enlarges, securing fibers are destroyed, and the tooth loosens. Many teeth can be lost in this way.

Painful periodontal disorders include abscesses in the gum and **periocoronitis**. The latter is inflammation around an erupting tooth (usually a "wisdom tooth"), caused by irritation, food stagnation, pressure, or infection. It may be accompanied by swollen lymph glands.

DENTAL TREATMENT

The dentist's intricate work has to be carried out in the confined, dark, wet, and sensitive environment of the mouth.

Filling cavities Tooth decay is dealt with by drilling out the decayed matter and filling up the resulting cavity. All decayed and weakened areas must be removed, otherwise decay will continue beneath the filling. The cavity must also be shaped so that the filling will stay in securely and withstand pressure from chewing. High-speed electric drills are now usual, and so is the use of injected local anesthetic to make the procedure painless.

A lining of chemical cement is put in the prepared cavity to protect the pulp from heat and chemicals. The filling, placed on top of this, is usually an amalgam of silver, tin, copper, zinc alloy, and mercury. Alternatively, translucent silicate cement is used, for its natural appearance – but since it can wear away, this cannot be used on grinding surfaces. When the filling has hardened, it is shaped, and any excess trimmed off.

Other restorative work can be prepared outside the mouth, and then cemented into place. **Inlays** are cast gold fillings, shaped to fit a cavity in the crown of a tooth. A wax impression of the cavity is made, and the resulting mold filled with molten gold. **Crowns** are extensive coverings to the crown of a tooth, made of porcelain or gold. All the tooth enamel is removed, an impression taken, and the crown made from a model.

Pulp and root canal treatment If the pulp or root canal is decayed, normal fillings are complicated. Part or all of the pulp may have to be removed. The root canal is sterilized and a silver pin sealed in place to fill it. The pulp cavity is then filled in.

Extraction is necessary if teeth are irretrievably decayed, or so broken that they cannot be replaced, or if new teeth are erupting and have no room. Forceps are used to grip the tooth at the neck, while the forceps blades are inserted under the gum. The tooth is then moved repeatedly to enlarge the socket, and finally can be pulled out. Local or general anesthetic, by injection or gas, usually makes extraction painless.

Treatment of gum disorders involves drainage of pus, antiseptic mouthwashes, antibiotics, and tooth extraction if necessary. Surgery may be needed to cut away the diseased gum. Long-term treatment aims at eliminating as many causes as possible, by improving oral hygiene, diet, and general health.

THE TEETH WE LOSE

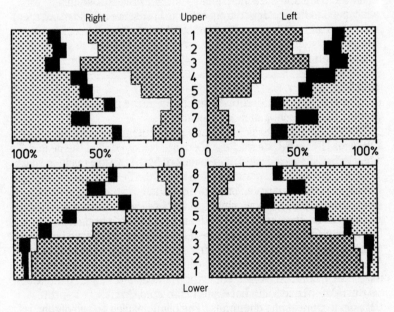

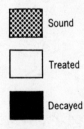

Here we chart the average fate of western teeth. For example, upper right 3 is sound in over 60% of adults, treated in over 10%, decayed in about 5%, and missing in the remainder. Upper right 6, in contrast, is missing in about 55%.

Sound

Treated

Decayed

Missing

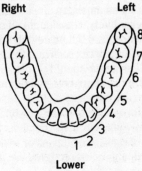

Right   Left

Upper

Right   Left

Lower

©DIAGRAM

ORTHODONTICS

This branch of dentistry deals with preventing and correcting teeth irregularities, e.g. variations in teeth numbers and abnormalities in their shape, size, position, and spacing. All these can cause defects in eating, swallowing, speech, and breathing. **Malocclusion** is the typical example: when the jaws are closed, teeth are not in the normal position, relative to those in the opposite jaw. Teeth may stick out or in, or there may be spaces between the biting surfaces due to uneven growth of teeth or jaws. Irregularities may be caused by dummies (pacifiers) and thumb-sucking; loss of teeth, non-appearance of teeth, and appearance of extra teeth; birth injuries and heredity; and disease and poor health.

Treatment may be long-term, but is needed if the mouth's health, function, and esthetic appearance are to be preserved. Methods include elimination of bad habits such as thumb-sucking; practice of exercises to strengthen certain muscles and improve mouth movements; relief of overcrowded teeth by extraction; or surgery on the soft tissues or bones to recontour the jaws.

But the commonest technique is to attach "braces" or similar appliances to the teeth, to apply continual pressure and so make them shift position. The braces, made of steel bands, wires, springs, or bands of elastic, may have to be worn for up to 2 years, or more. They are more effective in the young.

FALSE TEETH

Ideally, false teeth ("dentures") should preserve normal chewing and biting, clear speech, and facial appearance.

Types of dentures include full sets, partial dentures, and immediate dentures. For a **full set**, all the teeth are removed, and the healed bony ridge acts as a base. Impressions of both jaws are made in warm wax, to give the basic patterns from which the dentures are made up.

With **partial dentures**, the new teeth are attached to surviving natural ones to keep them anchored. Where the anchoring teeth are not alongside, they are linked to the false teeth by a bridge.

With **immediate dentures**, the false teeth are prepared before the teeth being lost have been removed. After extraction the empty sockets are immediately covered with the new dentures, and healing takes place beneath. A new set is then needed after about 6 months, as the ridge where teeth have been extracted shrinks.

Using dentures can sometimes be uncomfortable. To avoid gum soreness, new dentures should at first be used only with soft food chewed in small amounts. If soreness does occur, the dentist should be consulted. Dentures should not be left out for more than a day or two, or any remaining natural teeth may begin to shift position.

False teeth should be brushed after every meal, and detachable dentures should be soaked overnight in water containing salt or a denture cleaner.

Bonding is a technique which can be used for cosmetic reasons or to prevent decay. It involves use of a sealant, or attachment of plastic or porcelain to fill gaps or level off any chipping. (It may not be as strong as a crown, however, and usually needs renewal every few years.)

Types of denture
1 Tooth crown
2 Bridge
3 Partial denture

1

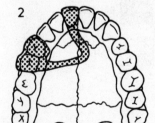

2

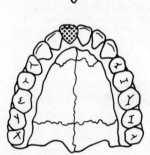

3

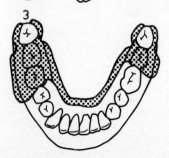

The hands

FUNCTIONS
The hand is remarkable for its flexibility. In particular the thumb's ability to move in opposition to the fingers enables the hand to grasp objects and perform other delicate tasks.

STRUCTURE
The hand contains 3 important sets of bones: **carpals** in the wrist, **metacarpals** in the hand itself, and **phalanges** in the fingers.

Finger movements are controlled by tendons attached to the forearm's muscles. The hand is very strong – even a tiny baby can exert a very powerful force.

HAND CARE
The following points will help to keep the hands in good condition.
1 Do not wash hands more than necessary – soap removes some of the oils that keep the skin pliable.
2 Use hand cream when necessary to prevent dryness and redness, e.g. if hands have constantly been in water, and in cold weather.
3 Wear rubber gloves for all heavy jobs and for washing up.
4 Avoid direct contact with detergents and scouring products – an allergic reaction may result.
5 Do not expose hands to extremes of temperature. Exposure to extreme cold, for example, causes chilblains.

HAND PROBLEMS
Only a few serious disorders affect the hands. **Rheumatoid arthritis** is probably the most severe of the common diseases affecting the hands. The lining of the finger joints becomes inflamed, causing the joints themselves to swell painfully. Treatment varies, but medical advice should be sought as early as possible.
Swollen fingers are very occasionally a symptom of heart disease, and need immediate medical attention.
Warts often appear on the hands and are a particular problem in childhood for some people.
Whitlows or felons are areas of inflamed tissue surrounding the nail. Pus often develops, and a poultice may be used to draw it out, and antiseptic creams applied to prevent the spread of infection. Alternatively, a whitlow may be lanced by the doctor.

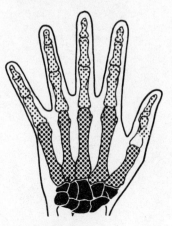

The three sets of bones in the hand

■ Carpals
▨ Metacarpals
▥ Phalanges

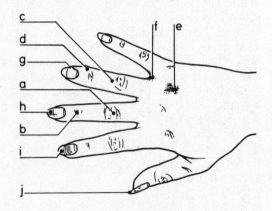

Hand and nail problems
a Rheumatoid arthritis
b Osteoarthritis
c Swollen fingers
d Warts
e Chapped skin
f Dermatitis
g Whitlows
h Weak nails
i Ridges
j White spots

©DIAGRAM

The nails

STRUCTURE

A nail consists of a small plate of dead cells. The horny, visible portion is made up of keratin – the substance found in skin and hair. The nail grows from a bed, or matrix, protected by a fold of skin at the base. The white crescent at the nail's base is the visible part of the nail bed. The nail rests on soft tissues which contain blood vessels to nourish the matrix. Nails grow about 1½in (3.8cm) a year, though the rate varies with the individual.

NAIL CARE

Nails are easily damaged and it can be a long time before the damage grows out. To keep the nails in good condition:

a Never use a steel file; it will tear the delicate keratin layers. Instead, use an emery board.

b Always file from each side of the nail toward the center – never a sawing, back-and-forth motion.

c Never file down the side of the nail as this will weaken growth.

d Do not shape nails to a point as this will encourage them to break.

e Use a nail conditioning cream on the base of the nail if necessary, to strengthen new nail growth.

f Clip away pieces of skin around the nail only if they are causing irritation. Regular use of hand cream will soften the skin and make it less likely to split.

NAIL PROBLEMS

Weak and brittle nails can be the result of incorrect filing, dietary deficiencies, nail biting, too frequent immersion in water, or general ill health. The nails can be strengthened by:

a the use of nail hardening preparations

b a diet rich in calcium

c careful filing.

"Doses" of gelatin in the form of jello cubes, and courses of iodine tablets, may also help.

Ridges across the nail are due to a deficiency caused by ill health. A course of Vitamin A, iodine, and calcium may help improve their condition. Ridges down the nail are a feature of old age and rheumatism, but vitamins and special nail cream can alleviate this condition.

White spots are common on weak nails and are usually caused by injury. This causes the nail cells to separate and allows air to filter between them. Over-acidity and lack of zinc may also be a cause of white spots.

Nail biting often begins in childhood, perhaps caused by stress of some kind, whether from a nervous disposition or a specific outside cause. It then develops into a habit difficult to break. Biting off the nail leaves it weak and rough, and the irritation caused by the ragged edge will encourage further biting. Use of evil-tasting chemical preparations painted on the nail is an effective deterrent, but it is also a good idea to try to pinpoint and remove any causes of stress. Adults anxious to break the habit may find it helpful to concentrate on allowing one nail at a time to grow longer.

FUNCTIONS

The legs, which enable us to move, have larger and stronger bones than the arms because they have body weight to bear.

STRUCTURE

The leg contains 3 important bones – the **femur** (thighbone) in the upper leg, and the **tibia** (shinbone) and **fibula** in the lower leg.

The upper femur meets the hip in a ball and socket joint (which allows free movement). The lower femur and upper tibia meet at the knee joint, a hinge joint allowing movement in one direction only. Here cartilage forms buffers between these bones, and the front and base of the lower femur abut the synovial membrane – a sac filled with lubricating fluid. The **patella** (kneecap) covers and protects the knee joint.

The thigh muscles are used to bend the knee, while the lower leg muscles move the feet and toes. The sciatic nerve – the longest and thickest in the body – provides the nervous system for most of the leg. Blood feeds into the thigh through the femoral artery, and back toward the heart through two systems of veins, one deep, one superficial.

LEG DISORDERS

Dislocated hip Hip dislocation may be present at birth or occur later. It causes delay in onset of walking, a lurching gait, backache in middle age, and sometimes osteoarthritis. Treatment varies with age, and may involve an operation.

Dislocated knee Slipping of the kneecap to the side may result from an injury, or the tendency may be present from birth. Doctors may recommend rest, or sometimes an operation.

Housemaid's knee Kneeling on hard surfaces for long periods may inflame the fluid-filled sac (bursa) that lies in front of the kneecap. Tissues at the knee joint swell, become tender, and make knee-bending painful. Poulticing or minor surgery may be needed.

Water on the knee is a collection of fluid beneath the kneecap. It may be due to infection, rheumatoid arthritis, or to a blow or strain. Rest usually brings recovery.

Rheumatoid arthritis Hips, knees, ankles, and feet can be badly affected. Painful joint swelling is sometimes followed by joint erosion and dislocation. Cortisone treatment is used, among other drugs, and hip and knee joints are sometimes replaced with metal or plastic devices.

Sciatica Inflammation of the sciatic nerve produces this form of neuritis. A slipped disk in the spine may press on a nerve, producing intense pain in the leg and lower back. Bed rest, heat applied to the painful area, physiotherapy, and special exercises may bring relief.

Swollen ankles Persistently swollen ankles may be a sign of a heart or kidney complaint. More usually, however, it is simply puffiness due to fluid retention and can be treated by your doctor with a diuretic to reduce the body fluid. It can also be a sign of toxemia in pregnancy. Some people find that their legs swell when they fly, but this generally subsides within a few hours.

Legs and feet

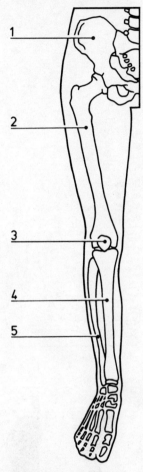

Principal bones of the lower limbs
1 Hipbone
2 Femur
3 Patella
4 Tibia
5 Fibula

© DIAGRAM

Varicose veins are swollen veins in the legs, which stand out above the surface and can be acutely painful. Their exposed position also makes them vulnerable to bleeding and ulceration. Varicose veins develop if the valves in the leg veins fail to prevent the back flow of blood. They are more likely in occupations involving long periods of standing – and also where there is a swelling of the abdomen, as in obesity, chronic constipation, and pregnancy. This last is why 1 in 2 women over 40 suffer from varicose veins, but only 1 in 4 men of the same age. Possible treatment include wearing pressure bandages and resting with the leg raised; courses of injections; and surgical tying or removal of the varicose veins.

Thrombophlebitis A blood clot in a deep vein produces intense pain and a swollen ankle, and can be very dangerous. A blood clot in a superficial vein produces tenderness and a red, cord-like formation beneath the skin. The patient may feel ill and have a high temperature. Medical aid must be sought in either case. Treatments include anticoagulants, supportive stockings, and resting of the leg.

THE FOOT

Each foot comprises 26 bones with 33 joints, linked by more than 100 ligaments. (Muscles, tendons and ligaments keep the foot in different positions.)

There are 3 sets of foot bones:

a 7 tarsal or ankle bones forming the ankle and the rear of the instep, and jointed for foot rotation;

b 5 metatarsal or instep bones forming the front of the instep; and

c 14 phalangeal or toe bones – 3 for each small toe and 2 for the big toe. (The ball of the foot is formed where the phalanges and undersides of the metatarsals meet.)

ARCHES

The normal foot has 2 important arches, one running lengthwise from the heel to the ball of the foot, the second running across the ball of the foot. These allow the spring needed for walking. In flat feet, the arches have fallen so that weight is borne on the sole.

ATHLETE'S FOOT

This common fungal disorder, is best avoided by keeping the foot clean, dry, and cool, and avoiding contact with infected people and with changing-room floors. It is caused by a fungus infection, and first appears in the toe clefts. There may be splits and flaking, or pieces of dead white skin. Treatment involves rubbing away the dead skin, applying a mixture of water and medicinal alcohol, and using a special dusting powder. A fungicidal ointment may be prescribed by the doctor. The feet should be exposed to the air as much as possible, and panti-hose or socks should be clean every day.

INGROWING TOENAILS

These can be very painful and may become infected. It will be best to see your doctor or chiropodist.

Bones in the foot
a Phalanges
b Metatarsals
c Tarsals

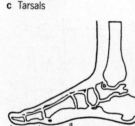

a   b   c

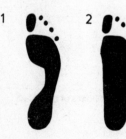

Arches
1 Print of normal arch
2 Print of fallen arch

COMMON FOOT DISORDERS

Calluses are areas of skin hardened to form protection for parts that suffer pressure or friction. To clear them, soak the foot in warm water, and remove the callus by rubbing with an emery board.

Corns are a type of callus usually caused by ill-fitting shoes. They have a cone-shaped core which causes pain when it presses on nerve endings. Corn pads may relieve pain but removal should be left to a chiropodist.

Plantar warts, or **verrucas**, are the result of a virus infection, and are often contracted at swimming pools. The warts grow into the skin and cause pain, and should be treated by a doctor.

BUNIONS AND HAMMER TOES

A **bunion** is a hard swelling at the base of the big toe. Ill-fitting shoes cause the big toe to bend in, forcing out the base of the toe in a bony outgrowth. A fluid-filled sac (bursa) may develop between the outgrowth and the skin.

A **hammer toe** is a toe bent up at the middle joint, where it presses on the shoe and causes a corn. Both these conditions can improve with exercise, manipulation, or well–fitting shoes, but severe cases may need surgery.

Foot problems
A Foot with bunion
1 Bony outgrowth
2 Bursa
3 Bone to be removed
B Foot after surgery
1 Bone regrowing
C Hammer toe
1 Bone to be removed
2 Corn
D Toe after surgery

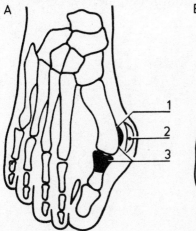

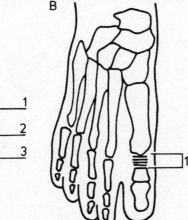

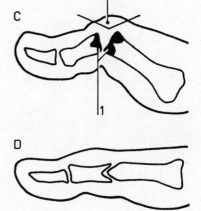

FOOT CARE

a Wash feet at least once a day. Soaking in cold, salt water or diluted cider vinegar refreshes the feet in hot weather.

b Cut toe nails straight across and not in at the edges.

c Wear comfortable, well-fitting shoes. Very high or very flat heels on shoes can force the body into an unnatural position, and cause considerable discomfort.

d Consult a chiropodist or your doctor whenever foot problems occur. Diabetics in particular need to take extra special care

e To prevent chilblains, try to avoid extreme cold.

© DIAGRAM

GOOD HEALTH

A total fitness program requires active full-time participation: there is no sitting back. But the road to good health – on both a physical and mental level – need not be a hard slog: rather, it can and should be part and parcel of a thoroughly enjoyable way of life.

Diet, exercise, sufficient sleep and relaxation, confidence-building and regular health-checks – complementary therapies, too – all help toward maintaining the body at maximum efficiency. Be well!

Chapter three

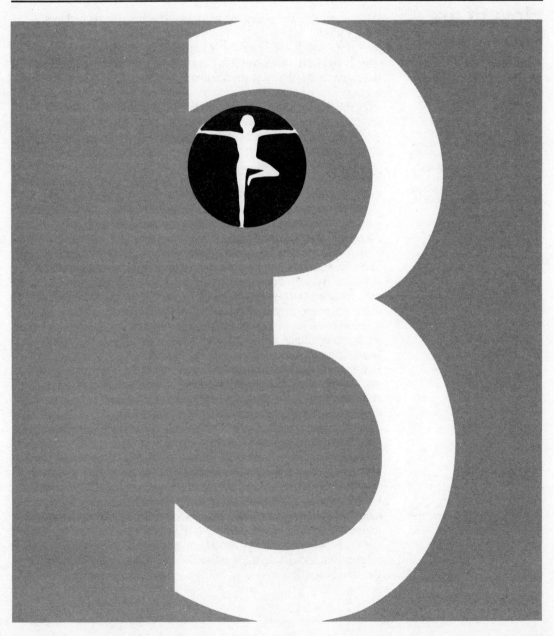

Measuring fitness

How fit are you?

Fitness tests
1 Run on the spot for 1 minute. Then measure your pulse. If it is still under 120 beats per minute, you are probably quite fit.
2 Using a bottom stair, which should be about 8in (20.5 cm) high, step on to it first with one foot and then the other. Then step down to the floor with each foot. Repeat 20 times, and then check your pulse rate. Again, if it is under 120 beats per minute, you are probably quite fit.
3 Pinch your skin at the waist. If you can grip more than 1in (2.5 cm) of fat, you are probably overweight. (Check your weight and height against the table on page 227, too.)
4 Breathe in deeply. Can you hold your breath for 30 seconds?

When you climb the stairs, do you feel out of breath? If you have to run for a train or bus, do you find yourself gasping? Do you always use the car instead of walking? Do you smoke? Is your job a sedentary one? If you have to answer "yes" to one or more of these questions, the chances are that you are not nearly as fit as you should be. And it may not be just a matter of age: you could well be neglecting yourself.

Try the tests suggested here. Stop, however, the moment you find any of them strenuous; and most certainly do not try them if you have a heart, joint or cartilage problem or suspect that they are way beyond your capabilities.

POSTURE

Your posture – how you stand, walk, and sit – can make all the difference to your appearance and also how fit you are. If you stand straight, walk tall, and sit comfortably, you will both feel good and look good. And if you normally have a tendency to slump, standing and walking tall will make you look inches thinner!

Bad posture is tiring: a person who stands and moves awkwardly wastes a great deal of energy. Once you fall into bad posture habits, your muscles will be pulled and stretched to cope with your body's unnatural movements. This can lead to joint damage and pain.

Be aware of your posture, of how you hold and use your body. Think what you are doing as you stand in a queue, walk along the road, carry heavy bags, or bend down to pick up something from the floor. Remember that your mood can affect your posture, but that in turn your posture can affect your mood. Next time you feel tired and start standing badly, try "pulling yourself together" – improve your posture and see how the tiredness lifts.

CHECKING YOUR PULSE

You can feel this in several places but the inside of the wrist is the most common checking point. Normally, it will be regular and quite strong; but if it seems very slow or fast, it is wise to see your doctor. Use the tips of your center three fingers to feel for it, and see how many beats you count in one minute when you are at rest. If you are under 40 and the count is below 80, this is very good; if it is up to 92, this is also fine; but if it is over 100, this should be investigated. Remember, though, that the pulse rate rises with exertion. With age, the safe range declines.

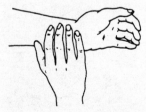

CHOOSING YOUR FORM OF EXERCISE

Exercise should be a pleasure, not a punishment! So try to choose a form of exercise that you enjoy if you would like to improve your fitness, or you will soon be finding an excuse to give it up!

Think about your personal needs and your lifestyle. Is there a particular part of your body you want to improve? What facilities for sports are there near you? How much time each week can you spend exercising? Would you prefer to exercise on your own or to work in a group? Consider your body type, too. Research has shown that certain body types are more suited to some sports and forms of exercise than to others.

Finally, remember that for total fitness your personal exercise plan should include three basic essentials: strength exercises, suppleness exercises, and stamina exercises. **Strength exercises** give shape to your body muscles, and prepare it to cope with any situations that need extra effort; **suppleness exercises** keep your body flexible, loosen stiff joints, and help you move gracefully; and **stamina exercises** improve the performance of your heart and lungs. Use the summary *below* to help you choose complementary exercises that will give you the best all-round results. (On pages 114-121, you will find a guide to all the principal benefits of improved physical fitness.)

Body types
Which are you?
a Ectomorph
The long bones and straight slim shape of the ectomorph are easily identifiable. Ectomorphs are naturally thin, usually long-legged, and have very little natural musculature. They may be lacking in energy and vitality. Ectomorphs never seem to put on weight, however much they eat, but may develop poor eating habits, such as a diet containing too much sugar and starch.
b Mesomorph
Mesomorphs may be tall or short, but all are naturally powerful and muscular. Their shape is like an inverted triangle, with slim boyish hips and well-developed shoulders. Mesomorphs have a great deal of energy and find exercising easy. They are unlikely to suffer from any real weight problems, provided they remain active.
c Endomorph
This type is naturally rounded, often plump, and not very tall. Endomorphs have wide hips and heavy bodies, but small and delicate hands and feet. Most endomorphs have a weight problem; they put on weight very easily, and have great difficulty in losing it again. Their body movements tend to be slow and deliberate.

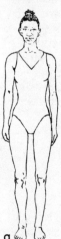
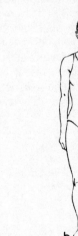
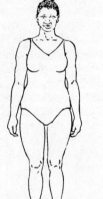

a   b   c

	Yoga	Stretching	Dancing	Weight training	Aerobics	Walking	Jogging	Jumping rope	Cycling	Racket sports	Swimming	Skiing	Martial arts
Ectomorph	●	●	●		●	●	●	●	●				
Mesomorph	●	●	●	●	●	●	●	●	●	●	●	●	●
Endomorph	●	●	●		●			●		●			
Strength			●	●	●					●	●	●	●
Suppleness	●	●	●		●					●	●	●	
Stamina			●		●	●	●	●	●	●	●	●	●

Examining your breasts

There is a simple test that all adult women should make each month for early signs of breast cancer. If the breasts are examined regularly in this way, it will be easier to spot any changes: and if you do notice something different, it can be dealt with promptly.

If you examine your breasts immediately after a period when they are at their softest, this will be best. (Older, post-menopausal women should choose a date they will remember easily.)

The diagrams *below* show the various stages in examining your breasts. Follow them carefully, while sitting or standing in front of a mirror. There is no need to be concerned if one breast is a bit larger than the other – this is the case with most women, in fact. But you are looking for a change in size as well as change in either nipple, bleeding or discharge from either nipple, unusual dimpling, or very prominent veins, as well as feeling for lumps or thickening.

1 Raise your arms above your head, and turn from side to side. Can you see any changes in appearance, including dimpling?

2 Squeeze each nipple very gently. Is there any unusual discharge or bleeding?

3 Lie down on the bed. Have a folded towel under each shoulder as you lean on it to examine the breast on the other side. Now examine each breast in turn, using the flat fingers of the opposite hand. (Have the hand you are not using under your head.) Start from above each breast, and use a circular movement, gently but firmly working in decreasing circles toward the nipple. Can you feel any lumps?

4 Next examine each armpit, again with flat fingers and a circular movement. Again, can you feel any lumps?

See your doctor if you sense there is a change. (Do not panic as it could be nothing at all or just a cyst or a benign – that is, noncancerous – growth but it is just as well to check.)

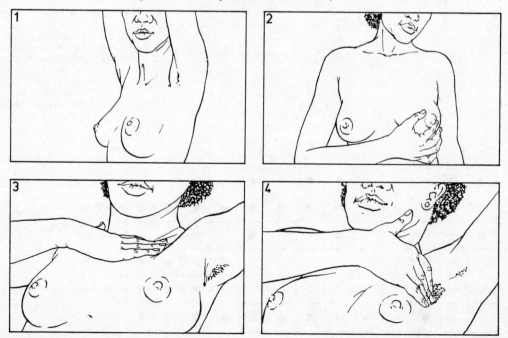

Pap (cervical smear) test

Also known as the Pap test (named after the doctor who invented it – George Papanicolaou), a cervical smear test involves the removal of some of the outer layer of cells lining the cervix. It only takes a minute or so and is usually quite painless.

Doctors now recommend that it should be a routine screening procedure every three years at least in order to detect early stages of cancer in all sexually active women under 40, and more frequently thereafter. (It can also be used to investigate certain infections and sexually transmitted diseases.)

Either your doctor or a gynecologist will carry out the test. When you make your appointment, see that it is not at a time when you are likely to have your period. You need only undress the lower half of your body, so it will be best to wear a top and skirt or trousers, rather than a dress. At the doctor's office, you will be asked to lie on your back, and your head will be raised slightly. Then you will be asked to draw up your feet slightly toward your buttocks and let your knees flop outwards. A warmed speculum is then used to separate the walls of the vagina. Once in place, it is opened so that the examiner can see the cervix. The surface of the cervix will be gently scraped with a spatula to collect a few cells with the secretions. The sample will be smeared onto a glass slide and then sent to the laboratory. The speculum is then closed and removed. When the examination is at an end, you will be able to dress and leave right away. The results should be sent to the gynecologist or doctor within a few weeks, and you will be advised if any further course of action is needed.

There are no known risks to a Pap test, and the nurse, gynecologist or doctor performing the vaginal examination takes the usual precautions to prevent infection. The benefits depend on how frequently a woman has a test. If a woman does have cervical cancer, or precancerous cells, the sooner these are detected, the simpler and more successful the treatment. The Pap test is a very valuable first line of defense.

There are several categories into which the results may be classified. If the result is completely negative, you will simply be asked to have another test after the recommended routine interval. If there is a mild abnormality found, it may just mean that you have an infection and so you will be asked to have the test more regularly. But even a positive result may not mean that there is necessarily a cancerous growth: investigations by colposcopy and biopsy will confirm this. **Colposcopy** involves viewing the cells of the cervix and vagina with a colposcope (a low-power microscope) in order to spot precancerous changes or the actual presence of cancer. If necessary, a tissue sample (**biopsy**) from the abnormal area will then be taken for examination in the laboratory. (A **cone biopsy** involves the removal of a cone-shaped piece of tissue from the cervix, and is carried out under general anesthesia in hospital but is less frequent today than colposcopy and a simple biopsy).

Cervical cancer is readily detectable and treatable in its early stages, yet each year thousands of women die unnecessarily because it was not recognized sufficiently early. All women – and this means those who have only ever had one partner, too – should be regularly screened.

Pap test
Position during procedure

A speculum holds the walls of the vagina open, while a spatula is used to collect cell samples.
a Spatula
b Speculum
c Cervix

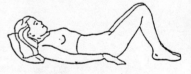

©DIAGRAM

Healthy intake

Food requirements

There are five different food groups that you need for health: **proteins, carbohydrates, fats, minerals,** and **vitamins**. You also need water, which is found in most foods. It is important to eat a varied diet, regularly including some foods from each group. But exactly how much of each you should eat daily is a contentious question, as the minimum requirements recommended by some experts may be six to eight times as great as those suggested by others.

Few foods actually belong entirely to just one food group. For example, wholewheat bread is 8% protein, 53% carbohydrate, and 39% water. But its main element is carbohydrate, and so it is grouped as a carbohydrate. But in recent years experts have pinpointed four factors in our western diet that seem to have a direct – and often adverse – effect on our health: too much salt, too much sugar, too much fat (especially saturated fat), and too little dietary fiber.

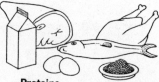

Proteins

PROTEINS
Proteins perform a number of functions in the body. They are needed to repair cells in the digestive system, skin, blood, liver, kidneys, heart, and bones, and also for the production of hormones and enzymes that control all the reactions that take place in the body.

Proteins are made up of chains of **amino-acids**. There are 20 amino-acids in human protein and they occur in a variety of combinations. The body can synthesize 10 of them; but the remaining ones, the so-called **essential amino-aids**, have to be obtained from your diet.

Food protein is classified as either complete or incomplete. **Complete protein** is protein that contains all eight essential amino-acids; **incomplete proteins** contain only some of them. Eggs and milk contain amino-acids more suitable to human needs than others. Meat is the next best, then pulses, peas and nuts. Proteins in cereal, bread, vegetables and fruit are of a lower quality.

The diet should ideally contain about 15% protein. But many of us in the West consume 2–3 times what we really need.

Complete animal proteins include meat (especially liver and kidneys), fish, eggs, milk and cheese. **Complete plant proteins** include brewer's yeast, cereal germ, and soybeans.

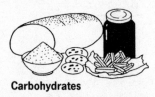

Carbohydrates

CARBOHYDRATES
The principal function of carbohydrates is to supply energy. They play a particularly important role in the healthy functioning of the central nervous system, the internal organs, the heart and muscles.

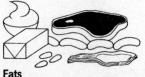

Fats

Carbohydrates should ideally make up 50–60% of the body's total daily calorie intake. After digestion and absorption as glucose into the bloodstream, carbohydrates may be used directly, temporarily stored in the muscles and liver as glycogen, or converted into fat and deposited in the adipose tissues of the body.

The most important of the dietary carbohydrates are **sugar, starch** and **fiber.** Sugar comes in various forms, including sucrose (table sugar), fructose (in fruit), maltose (in malt), and lactose (in milk). In the western world, there has been a marked shift away from starch and toward sugar as the main source of carbohydrate in the diet. At the beginning of the century, 75% of the average carbohydrate intake was starch; now it is only 50–60%, with the rest being eaten in the form of sugar. Sugar contains no vitamins or minerals, whereas starchy foods such as potatoes and corn contain vitamins and protein, and so are more valuable sources of carbohydrate.

Foods high in carbohydrates include sugar, rice, cornflakes, pasta, dates, cookies, chocolate, cake, bread, potato chips and beans.

FATS

Fats are also essential to the diet. During digestion, they are broken down into glycerin and fatty acids. The body can synthesize some fatty acids from other sources, but three essential ones are made only from fats.

Fats are important in relation to vitamins, too, since they act as carriers of the fat-soluble Vitamins A, D, E and K. These cannot be absorbed from the intestines into the blood without fat and bile. Fats stimulate bile production and that of the fat-digestive enzyme, lipase.

There are two different kinds of fats: **saturated fats**, and **unsaturated** – often known as **polyunsaturated** – **fats**. Saturated fats have been linked with high cholesterol levels and blood disease, and it is thought that eating unsaturated fats is healthier.

Many Americans and Europeans eat far too much fat. Only 30% of the total calorie intake should come from fats, but the average figure in the USA is nearer 40%. Food high in fats include cooking and salad oils, cooking fat and dripping, regular margarine, dried coconut, almonds, fried bacon, pork sausage, steak or lamb with fat, and cream.

VITAMINS

Vitamins are organic compounds that are found in food and are essential to health. They are known as co-enzymes, working with enzymes to bring about chemical changes in the body. There are about 40 known vitamins; some, such as Vitamins A, D, E, and K, are fat-soluble; while others, such as Vitamin C, are water-soluble. Of the 40, 12 are essential for health and must be included in your diet. Your body can make only one vitamin – Vitamin D, from sunlight. A deficiency of any of the 12 essential vitamins may lead to illness.

Those on a normal balanced diet will not usually require vitamin supplements of any kind; but there are occasions when your doctor may recommend them, as in pregnancy or during convalescence. Note, too, that excessive intake of Vitamins A, D, E and K may actually do harm.

Principal vitamins: their sources and function

VITAMIN A
Helps eyes adapt in dark, and maintains healthy skin: but in excess can cause liver damage. Best sources include fish-liver oils, animal liver, kidney, dairy produce and eggs.

VITAMIN B COMPLEX
There are 8 vitamins in this category.
Good sources include yeast extract, offal, green vegetables, eggs, milk and whole grains.

VITAMIN C
Helps absorption of iron, and maintains healthy skin and bones. You may need more when you have a cold. Note that the body cannot store it, and so daily intake is required. Found in citrus fruits, blackcurrants, strawberries and vegetables, which should be fresh and lightly cooked, if not eaten raw.

VITAMIN D
Helps absorption of calcium. Lack of this vitamin can cause bone weakness. Good sources include sunlight, cod-liver oil, herrings and eggs.

VITAMIN K
Essential for blood-clotting function. Found in many foods including green vegetables and fish-liver oils.

VITAMIN E
Thought to aid healthy skin. Sources include eggs and wheatgerm oil.

©DIAGRAM

MINERALS

As well as vitamins, the body needs 20 essential minerals. Minerals are inorganic substances present in food and water. They are needed to regulate body fluids and the balance of chemicals within the body. Mineral deficiencies can cause illness: too little iron in the diet, for instance, can cause anemia. Different minerals are needed by your body in different amounts. You need larger amounts of sodium, potassium, calcium, magnesium, phosphorus, and chlorine than you do of iron, zinc, copper, manganese, cobalt, iodine and sulfur. Very small amounts (traces) of chromium, nickel, vanadium, tin, molybdenum, selenium, and fluorine are also needed. The level of minerals present in food relate to the type of soil in which it was grown: mineral-rich soil produces mineral-rich foods.

Good sources of calcium include dairy products and green vegetables; of zinc – fish, meat, nuts and wholegrains; of magnesium – cereals and vegetables; of iodine – seafood and kelp (seaweed); of copper – liver, bread, and cereals; and of manganese – wheatgerm, bran, green vegetables and nuts.

DIETARY FIBER

In recent years, nutritionists have realized that fiber plays an important role as part of a balanced diet. It helps by maintaining the bulk and softness of the intestinal contents, so preventing constipation and straining. Eating foods high in fiber also makes us feel full and helps us to remain feeling satisfied, regulating food intake.

Fiber is best taken in the form of wholemeal bread, muesli, brown rice, pulses, nuts, and fruit and vegetables. (Buying organically-grown produce also ensures that the fiber-rich skins do not contain chemical residues.)

CHOLESTEROL

This is a fatty substance that is found in the blood. The body needs some cholesterol; but if the level becomes too high, fatty deposits can form on the walls of arteries, reducing their efficiency.

Reducing the amount of fat in your diet will help to reduce the level of cholesterol in your blood. Diets high in fat are also a major cause of overweight: keeping down the fat level will help you keep your weight down. As well as reducing the overall level of fat in your diet, experts recommend replacing saturated fats and foods high in saturated fats with unsaturated fats as far as possible.

SALT

Salt occurs naturally in many foods. It is essential to life, but the daily body requirement is very small – just over one hundredth of an ounce. It is widely thought that too much salt in the diet may be a contributory factor to hypertension, strokes, and coronary disease in general. A great deal of salt is still used in the canning and curing industries, so check the labels on all packets and cans before adding more salt to processed foods. In fact, if you add salt to your cooking, you may end up eating 30 times as much salt each day as your body actually needs.

SUGAR

Refined sugars (whether brown or white) and refined sugar products are unnecessary in a healthy diet. The body needs some sugar, but can easily obtain it from foods such as fresh fruit and vegetables. These unrefined sources can be used by the body to greater benefit than refined sugars, because they also contain vitamins, minerals and dietary fiber. But refined sugars are regarded as one of the principal causes of dental decay and obesity. If you find the thought of a diet that does not include sweet things intolerable and you are trying to lose weight, try switching to commercial brands of non-sugar sweeteners for use in drinks and cooking.

Although there are many different views on healthy eating, one point on which all experts tend to agree is that you need to eat a varied diet that includes all the different food types. They recommend that you cut down on sugar, other refined foods, and animal fats, replacing them with more fresh fruit and vegetables, wholegrain cereals, and unsaturated fats as far as possible.

Eating habits

ASSESSING YOUR EATING HABITS

Do you want to change to a healthier pattern of eating? In order to work out how you will need to change your present eating habits, make yourself a chart using the suggestions below as guidelines. Fill the chart in honestly for two weeks, and see if a pattern emerges. Each time you eat, ask yourself why you are eating: are you hungry, or is it just because it is the time when most people have a meal? Use the information you have collected to help you break your bad habits and plan your new eating pattern.

Know your food
This list shows the calorific changes that occur to a potato when it is cooked by different methods or processed commercially.

Frequency of eating
Time started
Time finished
What eaten
List what you have
eaten every time
you eat
Type of food
Convenience
Fresh
Cooking method
List how food was
cooked – raw, fried,
steamed, etc.
**Position in which
you eat**
Sitting
Standing
Walking
Running
Lying
Effects of eating
Repleteness
Hunger
Physical discomfort

FREQUENCY OF EATING		TIME		TYPE OF FOOD	COOKING METHOD
		STARTED	FINISHED		
Monday	BREAKFAST	8·20	8·35	FRESH	RAW
	LUNCH	12·05	12·20	CONVENIENCE	BOILED
	SUPPER	7·10	7·30	FRESH	STEAMED
Tuesday	BREAKFAST	8·15	8·30	FRESH	FRIED
	LUNCH	12·10	12·25	FRESH	STEAMED
Wednesday					
Thursday					
Friday					
Saturday					
Sunday					

150	Potato chips, 159 calories
	Instant mashed, 105 calories
100	
	French fries, 68 calories
50	
	Roast, 32 calories
	Raw, 23 calories
	Jacket baked, 23 calories
	Steamed, with skin on, 23 calories
	Boiled, without skin, 23 calories

©DIAGRAM

What do you eat?

Which of the two menus below most resembles your everyday eating pattern? Menu **A** is based on processed and fatty foods; Menu **B** relies more on unrefined and raw foods. Menu **B** is better for you, as the foods are unprocessed, and either raw cooked without added fat.

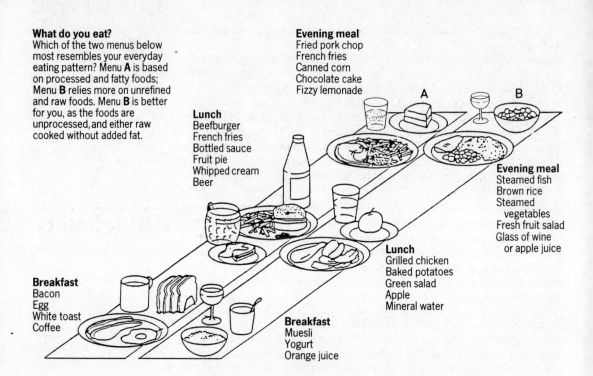

Evening meal
Fried pork chop
French fries
Canned corn
Chocolate cake
Fizzy lemonade

Lunch
Beefburger
French fries
Bottled sauce
Fruit pie
Whipped cream
Beer

Breakfast
Bacon
Egg
White toast
Coffee

Evening meal
Steamed fish
Brown rice
Steamed
  vegetables
Fresh fruit salad
Glass of wine
  or apple juice

Lunch
Grilled chicken
Baked potatoes
Green salad
Apple
Mineral water

Breakfast
Muesli
Yogurt
Orange juice

BUYING AND PREPARING YOUR FOOD

Always choose ingredients that look and smell fresh. Fruit and vegetables should not be wilted or discolored. Cracked or wilted vegetable leaves indicate a mineral deficiency in the plant: avoid them as they will not provide you with the necessary minerals. Cut down on red meat, eat white meat and fish instead. Choose brown rice, wholewheat bread, wholewheat flour, and wholewheat pasta in preference to their white equivalents. Whenever possible, eat fruit and vegetables raw. If you boil vegetables, a lot of the vitamins will be destroyed. Some of the valuable vitamin content will pass into the cooking liquid, so keep it to use as stock. Try to eat at least one salad a day. Steam fish instead of deep frying. Cook foods without adding fat whenever possible. This means boiling, baking, steaming or grilling (broiling) instead of frying. Replace foods high in fat with a low-fat alternative. (For instance, use plain yogurt instead of cream to top a fruit salad.)

DIGESTIVE PROBLEMS

Dyspepsia or indigestion is one of the most common digestive problems. Symptoms are nausea, heartburn, epigastric pain, discomfort or distension. The cause may be psychological or intolerance to a particular type of food, or it may be a sign of an organic disease. It can also be the result of overwork, overweight, bolting food and eating meals when excessively tired, or of smoking or drinking too much. If there is no organic disease, sufferers are usually advised to have a bland diet, avoiding spices, fried foods, excess sugar and rich heavy puddings. Regular meals at short intervals are recommended, too.

Malnutrition

Malnutrition should not be a problem in the West, but ignorance of what the body needs may put some people at risk. Food habits are acquired early in life and it is difficult to change them. Age, sex, lifestyle, pregnancy and illness are all factors that influence people's nutrition needs. But the average woman will be able to get all necessary nutrients, vitamins and minerals if her diet includes 2 servings of meat, fish, poultry, eggs, beans, peas or nuts per day; about ½ pint of milk or the equivalent in cheese or yogurt; 4 servings of fruit or vegetables (to include both) per day; 4 servings of cereal, bread, pasta or rice per day; and a little oil, lard, cream or sugar.

EFFECTS OF INADEQUATE NUTRITION
There are many theories about the link between diet and disease. Some of the most commonly known effects are listed here.
1 The hair may become dull and brittle, or it may fall out.
2 Headaches may be related to vitamin deficiency.
3 Nightblindness may arise from a lack of Vitamin A.
4 The tongue may become inflamed as a result of vitamin deficiencies.
5 Bleeding gums may be a sign of scurvy (Vitamin C deficiency).
6 Enlargement of the thyroid gland (goiter) may be linked to iodine deficiency.
7 Rashes, itching, soreness, scaliness and cracking of the skin may be the sign of a number of vitamin deficiencies.
8 Obese people often experience breathing difficulties.
9 Backache may occur as a result of obesity.
10 Too much food, particularly fat and carbohydrate, will lead to obesity. Too little food will cause wasting of the tissues and ultimately starvation. Failure to thrive in children may be a sign of marasmus or kwashiorkor (forms of malnutrition).
11 Heart disease can occur as a result of obesity, and heart failure may be a result of extreme anorexia nervosa.
12 Softening of the bones may be a sign of rickets (lack of Vitamin D).
13 Loss of motor function in the legs may be a sign of beriberi (lack of Vitamin B_1, or thiamine).
14 Lesions in the spinal cord may be a sign of Vitamin B_{12} deficiency.
15 There are a number of conditions affecting the stomach and digestive system as a result of diet. Symptoms may include diarrhea, nausea, vomiting, pain and cramps.
16 Stones may form in the kidneys as a result of insufficient fluid.
17 The formation of gallstones is associated with a fatty diet.
18 Too much alcohol may cause cirrhosis of the liver.
19 Insufficient iron will cause anemia.
20 Constipation can be caused by lack of fiber in the diet.
21 Piles (hemorrhoids) may also be a result of lack of fiber.
22 Painful feet may be a sign of Vitamin B_{12} deficiency.
23 Numbness in the toes may be a sign of vitamin deficiency; and attacks of gout are connected with rich food and alcohol.

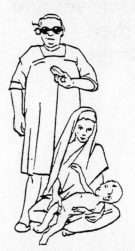

Western and Eastern diets
The West offers the most varied, cleanest and most readily available supply of food in the history of the world. But this brings its own problems including obesity, diabetes (associated in some cases with excessive carbohydrate intake) and digestive diseases associated with lack of fiber. However, 75% of the world's population lives mainly on a diet of one food, usually a cereal such as rice. Deficiency diseases and lack of food because of crop failure are common in undeveloped countries: yet in times of plenty these diets often provide more nutrients than the average western diet.

Food additives and other dangers

A food additive is any substance not normally consumed as food itself, which is added to food to preserve it, or to enhance its flavor, color or texture. The majority of packed foods contain additives, and there are around 3,500 of them currently in use worldwide. Some of these substances are found in nature – the pectin that is used to set jams, for example, is taken from plants. Other additives are made by food manufacturers – azodicarbonamide, which is added to flour to help bread dough hold together better, is one example.

A growing desire among the public for better information about what they are eating, coupled with concern about the effects that additives might have upon health, has recently led governments in several countries to pass legislation obliging food manufacturers to list all the ingredients in their products. In several countries, ingredients are now listed in descending order of weight: and usually in the ingredients list, additives must be listed by type and chemical name or by number, or both together.

Improved labeling has proved a great benefit to the consumer, who is now able to see exactly what goes into the food he or she is buying. This means we can avoid any additives we know may provoke an allergic reaction: for although most people do not have an obvious reaction to additives, there is a significant minority that does. Symptoms of additive intolerance are wide-ranging, and may include asthma, rashes, headaches and a general feeling of malaise. In children, such intolerance may also be an important contributing factor in behavioral problems. Research has pointed to the artificial azo dyes such as Tartrazine (E102), for instance, as a possible cause of hyperactivity. As a result, many doctors now recommend that the diet of a hyperactive child is modified to exclude all food and drink containing synthetic colorings and flavorings.

However, against the view that all additives are potentially harmful has to be ranged the argument that many are performing a vital function in preserving foods against bacteria, which are themselves injurious to health.

These very points are also being raised in defense of the process of irradiation – the practice of passing small quantities of radiation through food to render harmless the bacteria that cause deterioration. Irradiation is a contentious issue in certain countries, however. Some scientific organizations are worried that it may allow manufacturers to pass on inferior food which has lost its nutritional value to the public, since there will be no visible evidence of decay. They also feel that more research is needed into the possible long-term effects of irradiation, since it is not known how changing the molecular structure of the food we consume may ultimately affect our health.

In the meantime, there are other measures that we can take to ensure the safety of our food. Always check the 'best before' or 'sell by' dates when buying packaged foods, and take particular care to make sure that storage conditions in the kitchen are suitable and food preparation areas hygienically maintained. Recent concern over the safety of microwave cookers has highlighted the need to make sure that manufacturers' recommendations on cooking and standing time are scrupulously observed, so that harmful organisms are destroyed.

Dietary control

Your need for energy from food is measured in calories. Requirements vary from person to person, depending on a variety of different factors. Age, sex, size, physical activity, and climate all affect the number of calories that are needed.

Calories are used both to maintain body functions and to provide energy for exercise. But an increase in weight results if a person takes in as food more calories than are needed. If calorie intake is below requirements, however, fat stored in the body is converted to energy and weight is lost. A table showing the calorie content of a number of everyday foods can be found on p. 400.

USE OF CALORIES
Calories are needed to supply energy for every activity. Approximately 1400 calories a day – about 2/3 of her total daily requirement – are needed by a typical woman in order to maintain basic life processes such as heartbeat, breathing, and digestion. A further 600 to 800 calories a day should probably be plenty to provide the energy needed for other activities.

CALORIES IN CHILDBEARING
Women have higher daily calorie requirements during pregnancy and when breastfeeding. Estimates of these increased requirements vary, but the increases suggested below should be sufficient to meet the needs of most women today.

During the second half of pregnancy, an increase to 2250 calories per day is suggested. This estimate assumes some reduction in the level of exercise toward the end of pregnancy. A woman who is breastfeeding her child should allow 500 calories per day above her usual requirements.

CALORIES AND EXERCISE
People use up calories every minute of the day. This is true even when they are asleep or lying doing "nothing." When a person is resting, most of this calorie expenditure is used to maintain body functions. (A typical woman uses about 55 calories an hour when she is asleep.) Estimating the rate of calorie expenditure during different activities is more difficult – some people are naturally more energetic than others, even when doing the same thing. For example, if you walk quickly you use more calories than if you walk at half that rate.

Everyday activities and calorie expenditure
Standing: 90 calories per hour
Walking: 200 calories per hour
Running: 400 calories per hour
Walking upstairs: 800 calories per hour
Sitting: 75 calories per hour
Knitting: 90 calories per hour

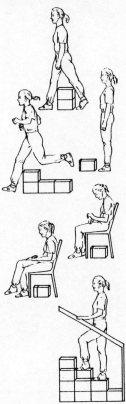

Every woman's daily calorie requirements

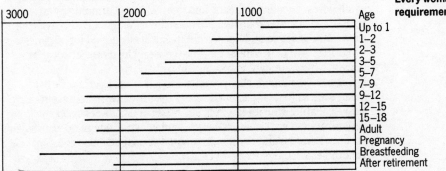

3000	2000	1000	Age
			Up to 1
			1–2
			2–3
			3–5
			5–7
			7–9
			9–12
			12–15
			15–18
			Adult
			Pregnancy
			Breastfeeding
			After retirement

© DIAGRAM

The vegetarian diet

A **vegetarian** is a person who does not eat the meat of any mammal, bird, or fish. There are two main types of vegetarian: **vegans**, who eat nothing at all of animal origins, and **lacto-ovo-vegetarians**, who do allow themselves some animal products such as milk, cheese, eggs, and honey. (Some people also call themselves vegetarians but do eat fish.)

Reasons for vegetarianism vary from society to society and individual to individual. It has been advocated for religious, philosophical, moral, economic, and health reasons, and also at times adopted as a necessity. Many primitive peoples, for example, have lived on a diet of fruit, nuts, and berries, with meat only when it could be obtained.

But perhaps the most powerful arguments for vegetarianism in modern society are the inefficiency of the animal food production chain in a largely underfed world; the relative cheapness of the ingredients of a vegetarian diet; and the possible unhealthiness of eating meat that contains crop pesticides, antibiotics and hormones given to the animals, and that has been processed in many ways that are not necessarily hygienic or beneficial. A great number of people, of course, also feel that the slaughter of animals is cruel and debasing, and that vegetarianism is part of a more peaceful and harmonious way of life.

Despite the claims of vegetarians, there is no established evidence that eating meat is unhealthy in itself: and despite some claims that vegetarians eat poorly, it is certainly as possible for them to be as healthy, strong, and long-lived as it is for a meat-eater.

A woman who chooses to give up meat must, however, be careful that her diet still provides enough of the right nutrients. There are no problems with unrefined carbohydrates (obtained from grains, cereal products, potatoes, fruits); fats (contained in vegetable oils, dairy products, nuts, margarine); and minerals and most vitamins (found in vegetables and fruits).

Obtaining an adequate supply of protein and certain vitamins can, however, be more problematic for vegetarians than for meat-eaters. Protein is readily available from eggs and dairy produce, nuts, soybeans, raisins, grains, and pulses. But a vegetarian should be sure to get a good selection of essential amino acids at each meal. This is not difficult where eggs or dairy produce are eaten: cereal and milk, bread and milk, and bread and eggs are all good amino acid combinations. But vegans must depend on soybeans, or on carefully planned vegetable combinations. These include lentil soup and hard wholewheat bread; and beans and rice. Vitamins requiring particular attention in a vegetarian diet are cobalamin (Vitamin B_{12}) – available from dairy produce and yeast, and, particularly useful for vegans, in synthetic form; and Vitamin D – also needed in synthetic form by vegans where sunlight is insufficient.

Iron and calcium are also sometimes lacking even in the diets of meat-eaters. In fact, there are many excellent vegetarian sources: raisins, lentils, wheatgerm, prunes, spinach and other leafy vegetables, as well as bread, eggs, and yeast. Calcium occurs in dairy produce, dried fruit, soybeans, sesame seeds, and also in leafy vegetables.

Nutritional medicine

Nutritional medicine, also known as nutrition therapy, is in some ways related to naturopathic healing techniques. Naturopathy's basic aim is to help the body to assert its own inbuilt powers of healing in the face of stress or disease, and nutritional medicine emphasizes the role of healthy eating habits as an essential part of this process. Many of the dietary principles propounded by naturopaths are in accord with traditional medical thinking: both agree on the harmfulness of eating large amounts of saturated fats and refined carbohydrates. Differences arise, however, in their view of how healthy an "average" western diet can be. Nutritional therapists think that many ailments are provoked by poisonous or allergy-producing substances in a normal diet, and they may recommend the use of supplements of vitamins, minerals, and other substances to restore the body's natural balance, along with a diet that includes plenty of raw vegetables, fruit, and whole grains. They think that average or recommended daily intakes of vitamins and minerals do not take into account the wide range of individual requirements, particularly in the face of biochemical imbalance caused by illness. Some traditionally trained physicians practice elements of nutritional medicine as part of a holistic approach; but treatment with supplements should always be under the guidance of a trained practitioner because of the dangers of creating greater imbalance through inappropriate self-medication.

Attention to diet has indeed been proved beneficial to all manner of ailments, among them skin complaints, diets, high blood pressure, digestive problems and cancers.

DETOXIFICATION AND CANCER DIETS

Good results have been claimed for strict diets which, by eliminating foods regarded as polluting, cleanse the body of toxins and enable it to fight back against diseases such as cancer. It is hard to evaluate the therapeutic effects of such diets in a truly objective manner: sceptics might state that a person determined enough to adhere to such a rigid diet has the type of personality which is often associated with a better outcome anyway. However, as diet has been shown to have important effects in the causation of many diseases, so it may be equally vital in maintaining remission or even curing them. One element of detoxification diets – fasting on fruit and vegetable juices – is not suitable for people with cancer, however: for them, a diet including beans (and beansprouts), seeds, legumes, vegetables, whole grains, fruits, and nuts is recommended. Salt, sugar, meat, saturated fats, alcohol, coffee, and tea are excluded. Organic produce is preferable; or if this is unavailable, fruits and vegetables should be washed in a basin of water to which vinegar has been added. Beneficial effects may take a while to appear, and it is not uncommon for patients following a naturopathic or detoxification diet to feel briefly unwell before beginning to respond. This sort of reaction is taken to indicate that the body is being effectively cleared of harmful toxins.

For further information about diet and cancer, see p. 195.

Physical fitness

Exercise benefits

Exercise is a basic need. The human body is built for use; and without, it will deteriorate. By denying yourself exercise, you are functioning below your possible best, and so are also denying yourself the chance of getting the most out of life. An unfit body is only about 27% efficient in its exploitation of the energy available for use, but this low rate of efficiency can be raised to over 56% with regular exercise. Such increased efficiency will be appreciated in every area of life. Your work and your leisure will become less tiring and more enjoyable as your capacity for activity increases. Improved organic efficiency also means that you will be less likely to succumb to illness; healthy, active life will therefore be extended, and the signs of aging delayed.

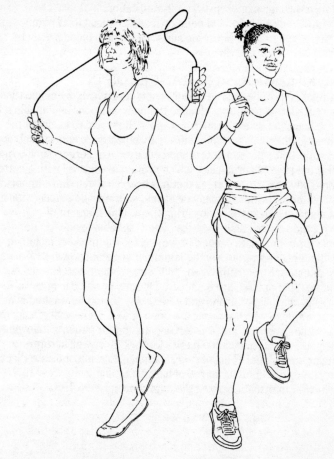

Benefits of regular exercise
Nervous system
Coordination and responses improve
Stress decreases
Heart
Blood volume per beat increases
Coronary circulation increases
Pulse rate decreases
Lungs
Capacity increases
Circulation increases
Efficiency increases
Muscles
Circulation increases
Size, strength and endurance increase
Oxygen debt capacity increases
Bones and ligaments
Strength increases
Joint tissues strengthen
Metabolism
Body fats decrease
Blood sugars decrease

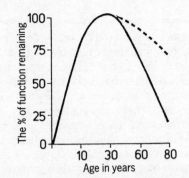

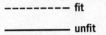

Decline of abilities
Functional abilities decline more slowly with age in a fit person than in an unfit person

- - - - - - - - - fit
——————— unfit

Physiologically, all your body systems will benefit from regular exercise. Depending upon the degree of exertion and the exercise performed, muscles may increase in size, strength, hardness, endurance and flexibility, with improved reflexes and coordination.

Regular exercise also greatly reduces the risk of heart disease by increasing the strength, endurance and efficiency of the heart. A fit heart pumps 25% more blood per minute during vigorous exercise than an unfit heart. A fit person's heart beats 60–70 times per minute (86,400–100,800 beats per day); an unfit person's heart beats 80–100 times per minute (115,200–144,000 beats per day). With exercise, the cardio-vascular system improves its carrying ability, too. More capillaries (small blood vessels) are formed in active tissues to improve the supply of food and oxygen, and exercise burns up excess fats in the system and checks the deposit of fats in the arteries, so reducing the risk of thrombosis.

Likewise, exercise increases the ability of the respiratory system. The lungs' vital capacity (the amount of air taken in at one time) and ventilation (the amount of air taken in over a period of time) are both increased, as is the efficiency of the exchange of gases that takes place in the lungs. The nervous system benefits, too, becoming more coordinated and responsive. (For some people, alertness and absence of tension are related to fitness, especially if it is achieved by rhythmic exercise or games that involve enjoyable competition.)

In addition to benefiting specific body systems, fitness brings other advantages. A fit person may take less time to recover from illness; can withstand fatigue longer; uses less energy for any given job; and is most likely to sleep well each night, have a good appearance and feel more healthy and positive than an unfit person. The positive effects of exercise can also help you to fight negative habits such as smoking and excessive eating and drinking, as well as showing you how much better you are without them.

Choose a time to exercise that suits your personal routine and body rhythm best. Be sure to allow yourself time for a recuperation period after you finish, too. Morning exercise necessitates a long warming-up period to arouse the body from sleep, but it can be an excellent way to wake up. It also has the advantage of leaving the rest of the day free. Noon exercise is good for city workers with nearby facilities. It breaks up the day, leaves the evening free, can prevent afternoon tiredness and boredom, and helps dieting. Exercising before a meal can also help you reduce, diverting blood from the digestive tract and so relieving feelings of hunger. But evening exercise is often said to be best of all as it rids the body of tensions and relaxes it for sleep.

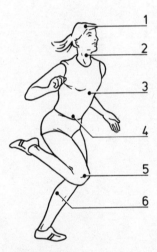

Warning signs
Stop exercising and see your doctor if you experience any of the following:
1 Dizziness, lightheadedness, loss of coordination, confusion, cold sweat, glassy stare, pallor, blueness, fainting
2 Irregular or racing pulse, very slow pulse after training, fluttering, pumping or palpitations in the chest, pain or pressure in the arm or throat
Rest if you suffer from any of the following, and see your doctor if they persist:
3 Rapid heart rate some time after exercise, extreme breathlessness, nausea or vomiting after exercise, prolonged fatigue
4 Side stitch (cramp of the diaphragm)
5 Pain in the joints
6 Muscle strain

©DIAGRAM

Keeping fit

A daily exercise program – even a gentle one – can work wonders for almost everyone. Labor-saving equipment has made our lives easier in many respects, but by reducing general levels of physical exercise, it has helped produce a population that is chronically unfit. A body that is short of exercise is stale, sluggish, and generally inefficient. But the situation can be remedied – easily, and even enjoyably. There is no need to embark at once on an intensely vigorous exercise program – indeed, such a course of action would be positively unwise. Exercising *regularly* is the real key to improving fitness levels. A few simple exercises – such as those described here – can prove dramatically effective if they are carried out every day.

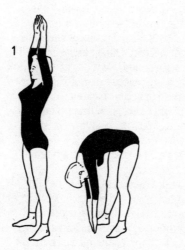

1 Stand with your feet apart and raise your arms above your head. Bend and touch the ground between your feet
2 Stand with your feet together. Grasp a raised leg by knee and shin. Repeat with the other leg
3 Stand with your feet apart, hands to your sides. Bend to the left. Repeat, but bend to the right
4 Make large circles with your left arm, forward then back. Repeat using your right arm

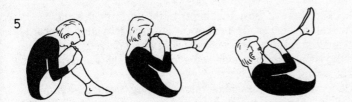

5 **5** Sit on the floor, grasping your knees. Bring them toward your chin and rock back. Hold for 5 seconds

6 Lie face down with your arms by your sides, and legs together. Raise the upper body and legs into the position shown

7 Lie on your back, with knees bent, feet on the floor and arms back. Swing your arms forward to sit and touch your toes

8 Lie on your side in the position shown. Raise one leg and then lower it. Roll onto your other side and repeat

9 Lie face down with your hands under your shoulders. Push your body off the floor, keeping your knees on the floor

10 Lie on your back, with legs together and arms by your sides, palms down. Raise one leg and then lower it. Repeat with the other leg

6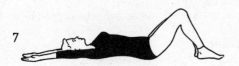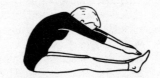

7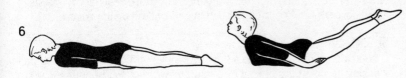

8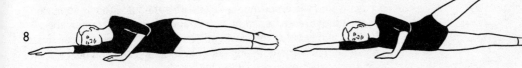

9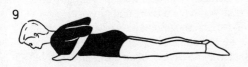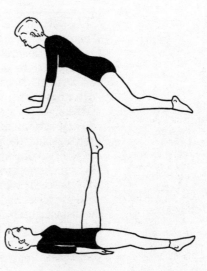

10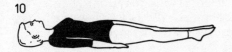

Aerobic exercises

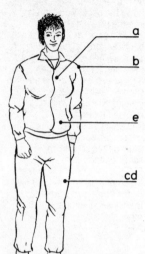

Aerobic exercises are those that improve the performance and endurance of the heart and lungs, or cardiovascular system. Mobility and strength exercises alone will have little effect on your overall bodily fitness unless you include some form of aerobic exercise in your fitness program.

Whether your lifestyle is completely sedentary or whether you engage in a lot of active sports and pastimes, your system will benefit from an improvement in the cardiovascular system; your heart and lungs will work more efficiently and become more resistant to disease and disorders, and your circulation in general will be improved.

SIGNS OF UNFITNESS

If you suffer from any of the following problems, your body will not be working at maximum efficiency – in other words you are unfit and your body would benefit greatly from an aerobic exercise program.

a Breathlessness and a pounding heart after even very short bursts of exercise such as running for a bus or lifting a trash can.

b Bad posture caused by weak muscles or laziness

c General aches and pains, expecially in the back and legs, caused by weak muscles.

d Aching muscles after mild exercise.

e Excess weight caused by lack of exercise or overeating.

AEROBIC TESTS

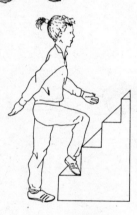

You can judge the condition of your circulatory and respiratory systems by your performance in simple tests such as these. If you are very unfit, you will find even these tests strenuous: stop as soon as you feel out of breath or if your heart begins to race uncomfortably.

1 Walk up and down an average staircase at normal speed three times. Can you do this without feeling out of breath, and can you hold a normal conversation immediately without gasping?

2 Can you easily walk for one mile (or 1 km or thereabouts) at your normal speed?

3 Can you run for 50 yards (45m)?

GENTLE AEROBIC ACTIVITIES

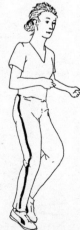

If you are very unfit, and cannot perform even the simplest aerobic tests well, then your body will need to be eased very gradually into exercise. We recommend that you have a thorough physical examination before you embark on any kind of exercise. Once your doctor has given the go-ahead, try some of these activities.

1 Walking is perhaps the best way to ease your system into aerobic exercise. On your first day, walk as far as you can without excessive tiredness, and then increase the distance gradually each day. Once you can walk several miles, increase the speed of your walking so that your fitness improves.

2 Cycling will probably make you out of breath very quickly, but it is good exercise. Start with a gentle ride on level ground, and increase the distance each day: try uphill terrain when you are ready.

3 Jogging can be started as part of your walk: jog for a few yards every 5 or 10 minutes, and make the jogging stretches gradually longer as your fitness improves.

RUNNING AND JUMPING

Running and jumping rope (skipping) provide very good aerobic exercise for people who are fit.

Jogging will improve your circulatory-respiratory system considerably as both your heart and your lungs are working hard. But some experts now say that brisk walking is preferable.

Sprinting requires short bursts of energy, and will tax your lungs and your heart with the extra oxygen required and the speed at which your heart needs to pump the blood around your body.

Orienteering and cross-country running with friends are also pleasant ways of getting aerobic exercise.

Running in place is an indoor alternative to ordinary running in bad weather; or you could use a running machine that measures the number of steps you have taken and converts them into distance equivalents.

Jumping rope (skipping) provides very vigorous aerobic exercise if it is done strenuously. Try turning the rope backward for variety, or turn the rope extra fast so that it passes under your feet twice before you land back on the ground.

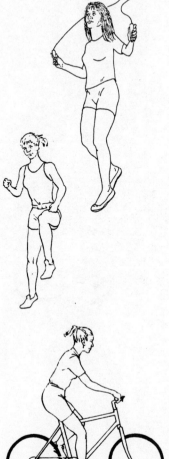

STRENUOUS AEROBIC ACTIVITIES

When you have gradually built up your fitness and capabilities through walking, jogging or cycling, for example, you will find that the following activities provide more strenuous aerobic exercise.

Racket sports provide good exercise because of the amount of running that they entail. The same is true of most ball games such as hockey, basketball and volleyball. Many Sports such as canoeing, rowing, skiing, swimming, hurdling, skating and cycling also tend to provide aerobic exercise but they are not recommended for people with heart trouble or for those past middle age.

Hill-walking, or walking over any rough terrain, will provide good aerobic exercise if you keep up a brisk walking pace and cover several miles or more.

Vigorous repetition of many exercise movements, as in a step test, will provide aerobic exercise if the movement is repeated many times in succession.

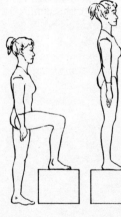

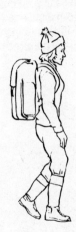

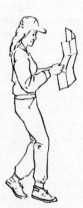

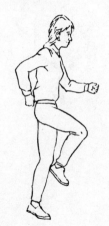

Sports

Taking part in a sport you enjoy can provide all the incentive you need to keep you exercising regularly. But you will need to develop a reasonable level of skill before you can really consider your chosen sport as part of your fitness program. For example, you will get very little exercise if you spend most of your tennis matches retrieving the ball from the back of the court!

For most sports, developing the necessary skills will mean going to classes or coaching sessions. These sessions often include training exercises: practiced regularly, these exercises will not only help you improve your performance in a sport but will also make you fitter. Whichever sport you choose, you will get the greatest fitness benefits if you aim for at least three energetic 30-minute sessions each week. The sports described here are particularly useful as part of an exercise program. Remember that different sports make different demands on your body, and that some will need supplementing with other types of exercise for all-round fitness.

SWIMMING

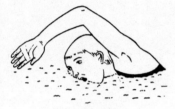

Swimming helps strengthen muscles, increases suppleness, and improves stamina. The water resists your movements, and it is working against this resistance that makes swimming such a very effective form of exercise. It is particularly useful for anyone who is overweight, or who has back or leg problems. Because the water supports your weight, it is possible to exercise energetically without risking muscle or joint damage.

Swimming can only be useful as exercise if you swim vigorously. Aim to complete one length of an average pool in about 1½ minutes, and to keep up this rate for 15–20 minutes. Vary strokes for the best results. Front crawl is best for increasing stamina and for improving your body shape; breaststroke strengthens your upper body; backstroke is good for your abdomen, legs and upper arms; and butterfly stroke exercises your chest, arms, thighs, and shoulders.

MARTIAL ARTS

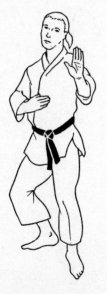

The oriental martial arts range from the non-combative tai chi to the highly aggressive karate. All of them are excellent for developing your suppleness and strength, providing that you have learned them properly from a qualified instructor. The more aggressive martial arts will also help you to develop your stamina, as classes usually include 15-20 minutes of sustained exercises.

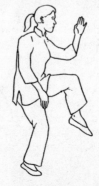

RACKET SPORTS

Squash is far are more physically demanding than tennis and
badminton, but any of the racket sports will help you improve your
stamina if you play them regularly, energetically, and at a reasonable
level of skill. The twisting and turning involved will help you improve
your suppleness, but may also put you at risk of damaging your joints
and ligaments if you are not fairly flexible already. Watch out too for
uneven muscle development: because your racket arm is doing most
of the work, it may become stronger than your other arm.

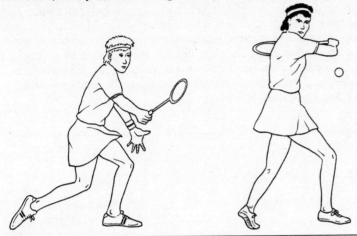

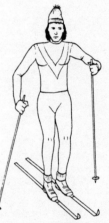

SKIING

There are two main types of skiing – downhill (also called Alpine
skiing) and cross-country (also called Nordic skiing or langlauf).
  Because downhill skiing alternates short bursts of strenuous activity
with rests and rides on ski-lifts, it does not usually provide enough
steady sustained exercise to help you improve your stamina.
However, you can use it as a stamina exercise if you can develop
enough skill to be able to tackle runs that need 15–20 minutes of
continuous skiing. Downhill skiing is very useful for developing
strength and suppleness in your legs, especially if you practice pre-ski
exercises regularly.
  Cross-country skiing is one of the best and most demanding forms of
all-round exercise. It exercises nearly all the major muscle groups in
your body; and because you can ski continuously for long periods, it is
also an excellent stamina exercise.

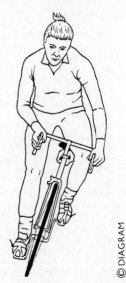

CYCLING

Cycling will help you improve your stamina and strengthen your leg
muscles providing you cycle at a minimum speed of 9 miles per hour
(16–24km/h) and keep up this pace for at least 15–20 minutes. For
best results, pedal up hills instead of dismounting and walking up, or
cycle along the flat using a gear that offers plenty of resistance for
your muscles to work against. For all-round fitness, supplement
cycling with strength exercises for the upper part of your body and
with a full program of suppleness exercises. Cycling is not
recommended for anyone with back problems as the riding position
can make them worse.

Massage

Massage is a very effective way to reduce stress and tension. It stretches and relaxes the fiber of the muscles, making them more supple and increasing the blood flow to the area which in turn helps to remove waste products and impurities that collect in stiff muscles. And because it makes you feel physically relaxed, a good massage will leave you feeling mentally relaxed as well.

You have several choices when it comes to massage. You can go to a professional for treatment, ask a friend to massage you (and then massage him or her in exchange), or even massage yourself. And you can choose from several different types of massage – **reflexology**, for example, in which only the feet are massaged, or **shiatsu**, a Japanese form of massage performed almost entirely with the pad of the thumb (see pp. 156 and 150). The most usual type of massage for relaxation is described here. It is based on Swedish massage, and uses a wide variety of strokes made with different parts of the hands and with different amounts of pressure.

Massage strokes

If you have a professional massage you will find that a number of different manipulative techniques, called strokes, are used. In the basic stroke, the hands glide over your skin. The masseur or masseuse will fit his or her hands to the contours of your muscles and then move them over your skin with differing amounts of pressure, depending on how tense you are.

Kneading movements, in which the muscles are gently lifted, wrung, and squeezed, are used to stimulate the blood supply. Friction – massaging in small circles using the pads of the fingers, the thumb, or the head of the hand – is used where work is needed on "knots" in the deep tissues. Percussion movements (including hacking, tapping, slapping, and pinching) are used to stimulate, rather than relax, the system.

1 Stroking movements
2 Kneading movements
3 Friction
4 Percussion movements

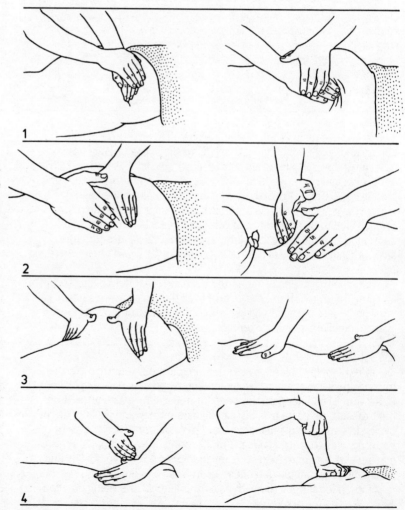

HOME MASSAGE

You need very little equipment for a home massage. If you have a large, sturdy table, cover it with towels or a blanket, and use it as a massage table. If not, spread out your towels or blanket on the floor. Don't use a bed for massage: however hard the bed, it will still be too soft for the massage to be effective.

Make sure that the room is warm and that the lighting is soft. Try to avoid being disturbed, and switch off the telephone. If you are giving the massage, make sure that your nails are short and that your hands are warm. You will need some oil to use as a lubricant to avoid friction. Special perfumed massage oils are available, but a bland vegetable oil will be just as effective.

Never pour the oil directly onto the skin of the person you are massaging. Warm it first by pouring it into your hands and rubbing it between your palms. The person who is being massaged should preferably be naked. Use a towel or blanket to cover the parts of the body that are not being worked on to prevent them getting cold.

Massage should always be done gently. Use even pressure, and take care when you are working on the less protected parts of the body, such as the abdomen and the kidney area. Once you have started a massage, try to keep at least one hand in contact with the person being massaged until you have finished. And use your own body carefully when you are giving a massage: make sure that you do not strain your back.

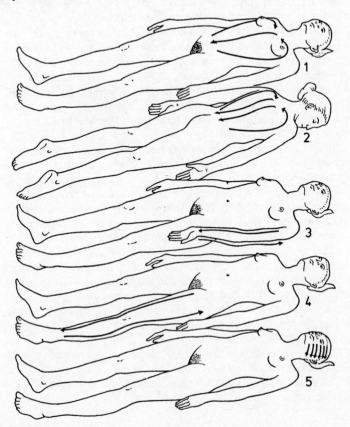

Full body massage
This is a simple program of massage for the whole body, using the basic stroking movement.
1 With your hands parallel to each other, stroke down the front of the body and up the sides.
2 Place your hands parallel to each other on either side of the spine. Stroke downward to the buttocks and then upward round the sides of the body.
3 Starting at the shoulder, stroke down the front of the arm, then up the back of it.
4 Starting at the thigh, stroke down the front of the leg, then up the back of it.
5 Place the palms of the hands over the eyes, covering the face. Stroke outward with both hands at the same time.

©DIAGRAM

Women and doctors

The relationship between a woman and her doctor is an important one. Women visit doctors more than men, take more medication than men, and are responsible for the health of others to a far greater degree than men. And yet, many women are reluctant themselves to visit the doctor, or remain silently dissatisfied with the treatment they receive.

Research shows that many women patients feel intimidated or vulnerable in a doctor's surgery and believe that they have little control over the situation. In particular, female patients often complain that their doctor does not take them seriously, does not allow time for consultation, and is not prepared to discuss their anxieties. In fact, many women feel dismissed by their doctors.

There are various reasons for this. Even today most doctors are men: and it has been argued that, for centuries, a male-dominated medical profession has undermined and trivialized women's problems. But there is much that women can do to improve their relationship with their doctors and to ensure a satisfactory level of health care. Most important is for a woman to inform herself about her body, and state of health, and not to rely on doctors as the source of all knowledge. Today, a vast amount of literature is available on all aspects of women's health, from pregnancy through to sexually transmitted diseases: and many women find that they can meet their doctors on an equal basis if they have taken the time to inform themselves in advance.

Choosing a doctor is a personal matter. Some women feel more comfortable with a woman doctor, particularly if they have gynecological problems. Others are less concerned. No matter what a woman decides, she has the right to meet a prospective doctor before registering, and the right to find out the doctor's views on matters of importance such as abortion, contraception, the menopause, depression, and other possibly judgemental-laden issues.

All patients, too, have the right to have their disorders or treatments fully explained to them. Many women lose confidence in the doctor's office; so it is advisable to plan in advance what you want to ask the doctor, and to check how much time he or she has to spare. If the doctor is rushed, and the visit is not an urgent one, it may be better to make another appointment. Many women also find it helpful to make a list of questions, and to work through these.

Finally, but most importantly, any woman patient should remember that it is her body that she is taking to the doctor, not the doctor's body. While not everyone has specific medical knowledge, it is the woman herself who knows how she feels.

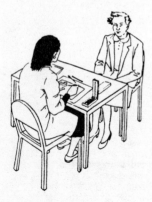

Health care
Health provision can be divided between a doctor and other sources of care. Many women find it most useful to visit the doctor for matters of sickness, and to use Well-Women Clinics for routine examinations or advice on contraception. There is also a wide range of self-help groups covering all aspects of women's health from breast cancer to smoking and sexually transmitted diseases. These groups are rarely medically based but can be a source of considerable information, advice and support.

Sweat does not smell. The unpleasant **body odor** we associate with it only occurs when the sweat has remained so long on the skin that the body's natural bacteria have made it decompose. These bacteria flourish in warm, damp surroundings – in the areas where sweat is trapped by our clothing, for example, or the parts of our bodies where fresh air does not circulate easily, such as under the arms. Removing sweat from the skin before it has a chance to decompose will prevent odor. For most women, this means a daily bath or shower, clean clothes, and an underarm anti-perspirant or deodorant.

Keeping fresh

A mild soap and a clean sponge or washcloth are all that you need to keep fresh. Using anti-bacterial or deodorizing soaps, or adding disinfectant to your bathwater, will only destroy your body's essential natural bacteria that help to fight invading germs. Remember that your hair needs regular washing for freshness, too.

A **bath** is a lovely way to relax and unwind, but make sure it is warm and not hot. Too hot a bath will make you sweat, can damage your skin (making it age more rapidly), and may cause some of the tiny blood vessels in your body to break. Never remain in a bath so long that your body skin takes on a wrinkled, waterlogged look. A **shower** is invigorating, as the pressure of the water helps to speed up your circulation. Like a bath, it should be warm and not hot, or it can have the same damaging effects. Combine the two to get the best of both worlds. Either use a shower to rinse away the soap and scum after your bath, or wash first under the shower and then enjoy a relaxing soak in clean bath water.

Use an **anti-perspirant** or **deodorant** regularly. These products offer extra protection for the underarm area. If used daily, the level of protection gradually builds up. Always apply anti-perspirants and deodorants to clean, cool, dry skin, and allow them to dry thoroughly before dressing. Deodorant sprays for the feet can also be useful in hot weather. Do not use vaginal deodorants: soap and water are all that are needed to keep the external vaginal area clean. The vagina itself is self-cleansing, and deodorant sprays and tissues can upset the delicate balance of its natural secretions and so cause irritations and allergies. The vagina only smells unpleasant if some infection is present. If the odor persists, do not try to mask it with deodorants, but consult your doctor who will advise how to deal with the underlying cause of the problem.

Keeping your body clean will not help you keep fresh, however, unless you change and wash your socks or pantie-hose and underwear daily and clothes regularly. Sweat clings to clothing, especially to synthetic fabrics, and soon becomes stale and smells unpleasant. Loose fitting clothes in natural fibers allow sweat to evaporate away more easily. Remember, too, that poor digestion, heavily spiced food, excessive alcohol, smoking, and poor dental hygiene can all cause bad breath and other unpleasant odors. So taking care of your general health will help you to keep fresh, too.

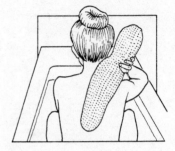

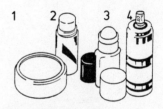

Personal freshness
Anti-perspirants and deodorants are available as creams (**1**), sticks (**2**), roll-ons (**3**), and sprays (**4**).

Spread of disease

Good hygiene is a vitally important requirement in preventing the spread of infectious diseases. Diseases can reach epidemic proportions, for instance, if a water supply is contaminated or if the organisms reach a widespread vector (carrying) population such as flies, rats or mosquitoes. Widespread outbreaks of disease can also occur through contaminated food – when many people have eaten at a restaurant where food has borne germs, perhaps, or when one contaminated animal has been among many prepared in the same batch in a foodstuffs factory.

The illustration shows some of the ways in which disease is commonly spread.

How infections are passed on

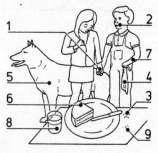

1 Direct contact – such as kissing, sexual intercourse or holding hands – is responsible for spreading many germs.

2 Droplets are frequent carriers of bacteria and viruses. They may be coughed, sneezed or breathed out, and then inhaled by other people.

3 Dust may harbor airborne particles, which are later inhaled by others.

4 Objects such as washcloths, handkerchiefs and tissues that have been used by an infected person are an ideal breeding ground for bacteria.

5 Pets and farm animals may be carriers of diseases or parasites.

6 Insects, especially flies, are frequently carriers of disease, and are particularly drawn to uncovered food, which they then contaminate.

7 Dirt entering a break in the skin often harbors disease.

8 Contaminated food or water, or dirty utensils, can harbor and transmit germs to many people.

9 Parasitic animals such as mosquitoes, ticks and fleas can transmit disease to the host.

FOOD PREPARATION

The following guidelines concerning hygienic food preparation are all-important if contamination is to be avoided.

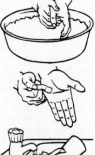

Wash your hands before food preparation: the water should be hot and soapy to be effective. Cover any grazes or cuts on your hands with waterproof adhesive tape. Use clean utensils, and wash them or put them to soak in hot water as soon as possible after use.

Thaw all frozen food slowly and thoroughly, unless the package specifically states it can be cooked when frozen. This inhibits harmful enzyme activity. Wash all raw food thoroughly under running water. Check cans for any unusual color or deposits inside, and do not use any cans with domed ends as this often implies bacterial activity inside.

Cook all pork, poultry and fish very thoroughly and do not eat these meats "rare." Do not keep food warm for long; if it must wait, keep it piping hot; and if it is not needed for an hour or more, cool it as quickly as possible and refrigerate it.

In general, never refreeze food that has been frozen once. But food that has been frozen raw may be cooked and then refrozen in its cooked state. Avoid leaving food where flies or pets can get at it: and, of course, never cough or sneeze over food.

Health in the home

There are many precautions that can be taken to ensure the family home is as safe and healthy as possible.

Children, for instance, need to be taught good hygiene habits as early as possible, since they are not naturally clean beings! Make sure that your child washes his hands after visiting the toilet, and also before every meal; dirt of all sorts accumulates on the hands. Keep children's fingernails short so that they are easy to clean. Encourage your child to clean his or her teeth after every meal. Explain as much as possible the reasons for these measures so that they do not simply seem to be empty instructions. Sanitize a baby's diapers at each wash, and clean your baby's bottom at each diaper change.

Because of forgetfulness and decreased mobility, the hygiene routines of elderly people often suffer. Washing, tooth and gum care and careful food preparation may all be neglected. Those responsible for caring for elderly people should make sure that their food is fresh and that the surfaces and utensils used for preparing food are clean. Food should also be bought in small quantities so that it will not be forgotten. Check for signs of infestation by mice, cockroaches and the like, which may not be noticed by someone with failing eyesight, and which should be dealt with professionally.

Hygiene during illness is a very important concern: good hygiene will help the invalid to recover more quickly, and also prevent (as far as possible) the spread of the illness to others. Keep the sick person isolated if he or she is very infectious; keep dishes and cutlery separate from the rest of the family's; and launder bed linen, washcloths and towels separately too. Give paper tissues instead of cloth handkerchiefs, and discard them after one use. Place a large bag near the bed so that the patient can put tissues and soiled dressings in the bag: in that way, no one else needs to touch them.

Pets can harbor many diseases and parasites that may be transmitted to humans, so good hygiene when there are pets in the house is particularly essential. Don't allow pets to lick your face, or to lick family dishes clean after meals: give them separate dishes, and wash their food bowls separately. Keep your pets clean, and have them given any inoculations your veterinarian advises. Check them regularly for infestations as well. Don't allow pet cats or dogs to sleep on beds: they should have their own sleeping place elsewhere. Keep pets away from babies; and if you have pets in the house, put a net over the crib.

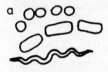 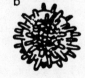

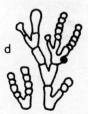 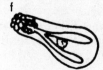

Disease organisms
Most diseases are transmitted by one of the following types of organism.
a Bacteria – microscopic one-celled carriers of infections such as diphtheria and tuberculosis
b Viruses – tiny parasites carrying diseases such as the common cold and influenza
c Rickettsias – germs found in fleas and lice, and causing various uncommon diseases
d Fungi – non-green plants causing ringworm, athlete's foot, thrush and other conditions
e Protozoa – one-celled parasites that cause diseases, including malaria
f Metazoa – many-celled parasites including tapeworms

©DIAGRAM

Health at work

Although women are often barred from occupations which are traditionally perceived as being hazardous (such as mining), there are still many situations in which their health is at risk in the workplace. In developing countries, in particular, there may be little or no legal enforcement of safety standards, combined with lack of union representation and health insurance. Female outworkers also frequently perform low-paid jobs at home where their own and their families' safety are under no supervision.

Women whose work is physically active or who use machinery or chemicals are, of course, subject to the same risks of injury and accident as their male colleagues. On production lines, continuous repetition of the same task – even if each single movement requires relatively little effort – can, for example, often result in pain and disability. Most nurses, whose tasks include the lifting and turning of patients, are women; and back injuries in inadequately trained staff are common. Nurses and other health workers are also at risk of infection if they are not provided with appropriate protection.

Workers in sedentary occupations may also be affected by dust, poor lighting and inadequate ventilation, chemical pollution, unsuitable seating or equipment, and noise. Respiratory, visual, postural, and hearing disorders may all ensue, together with the development of stress-related ailments.

Studies have shown that women actually cope better with stress than do their male colleagues – perhaps because they are more likely to have other compensatory roles outside the workplace, though the demands imposed by these can themselves contribute to stress. Work factors commonly identified with the development of stress-related illness include lack of control over workload and working conditions, unselected job change or relocation (particularly without training or preparation), uncertainty, boring and monotonous work or, conversely, demanding work with unpredictable peaks of intense activity. Problems with other people may cause more stress than the nature of the work itself; and discrimination in selection and promotion, sexual harassment, and aggressive or bullying behavior are additional hazards frequently faced by women.

Employees may often be alarmed by complex new equipment or procedures, and the term "technostress" relates to problems arising from increased office automation. Visual display terminal operators and, especially, those subject to computer monitoring of job performance are known to suffer high levels of headaches, stomach ailments and heart disease.

Common conditions and possible causative factors

Back injury: awkward weights, inappropriate seating.

Respiratory diseases: smoky or otherwise polluted environment.

Eye problems: fine work, VDT operation, chemical pollution.

Infection: dealing with contaminated materials, poor ventilation

Tenosynovitis (repetitive strain injury): production line work, VDT operation.

Hearing difficulties: excessive noise.

Increased risk of fetal abnormality/miscarriage: work with certain chemicals, VDT operation.

Ways to guard your health at work

1 Insist on proper safety measures, and inspection of equipment. If in doubt, see your union or safety representative.
2 Observe existing safety rules and be sure to use protective clothing and devices.
3 Don't carry on working or offer to do overtime when you feel tired.
4 Press management to provide health screening services, child care facilities, relaxation classes, training in first aid and stress management. Such measures could save them money in terms of time lost through illness.
5 If involved in fine work such as computer or VDT operation, look away and focus on a distant object for a few seconds every few minutes.
6 If involved in repetitive work, try to change position occasionally or press for the option of regular, short breaks.
7 Never try to lift heavy weights or cut corners in approved working practices.
8 Report incidents of discrimination or harassment promptly to a personnel supervisor, union representative, etc. Witnesses and documentation will help your case.

Health when traveling

One of the secrets of healthy travel is careful planning. This means consulting your doctor if you are taking medication and for advice on any vaccinations or other preventative measures you may need. (In many parts of Africa, Asia and Central and South America, it is possible to contract malaria through a mosquito bite. When you arrange your journey, check whether you should be taking a course of anti-malarial tablets, and remember to continue taking them for at least a month after your return.) If you are pregnant or suffering from an illness, you should also seek guidance as to whether it is in fact safe to travel: and diabetics should make sure they have an adequate supply of insulin and syringes with them at all times, accompanied by an explanatory letter from their doctor in order to avoid any potentially embarrassing situation. See your dentist, too, before you travel as it may be expensive or difficult to get treatment abroad.

Travel sickness is a common problem, whether traveling by sea or air. If you know from past experience that you are likely to feel queasy, a travel sickness pill should be taken thirty minutes before departure. Make sure you follow the instructions on the pack to avoid side-effects.

If you are taking a long-haul flight, it is sensible to wear loose, comfortable clothing and shoes as the thinner air often causes swelling. Try to avoid alcohol as it acts as a diuretic and can lead to dehydration. Instead, drink plenty of soft drinks. If you are frightened of flying, try a simple relaxation technique by concentrating on your breathing. Inform the cabin crew, too, who will make allowances and reassure you.

Although experimenting with foreign food is part of the fun of traveling, there are certain precautions it is well worthwhile taking. Fruit and vegetables should be peeled whenever possible; and if the local water is not safe to drink, use sterilizing tablets or stick to mineral water, making sure you also avoid ice cubes in drinks.

Check the medical facilities of the country you are visiting and that your insurance cover is adequate. It could be that your country of destination has a reciprocal health care agreement and the cost of treatment may be reduced.

Do not touch animals in countries effected by rabies; but if you are scratched or bitten, get medical help immediately as it can be fatal.

Although nothing beats the sense of well-being that accompanies a tan, sunburn can do terrible damage to your skin. Exposure to the sun should be built up very gradually, starting with as little as fifteen minutes on the first day. Always apply a sun cream, making sure it is the correct factor for your skin. (Note, too, that recent research seems to indicate that very high factor creams may themselves do damage to the skin.) Protection should be increased if you are visiting a very hot country or if you are going skiing. Wear a sunblock on particularly sensitive areas such as the nose, and avoid sunbathing between 11 am and 3 pm even when tanned, as the sun is at its strongest at this time and most likely to do damage. Children and fair-skinned people are particularly vulnerable and should take extra care. Traveling with a small first aid kit is also a wise precaution.

The chart on p.401 shows some of the main diseases you may encounter worldwide and the necessary precautions.

© DIAGRAM

Health checks

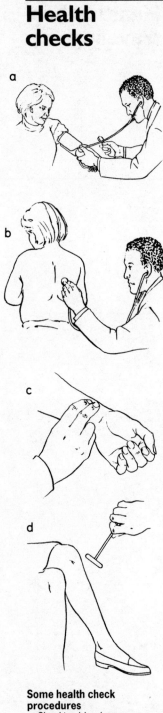

When our grandmothers were young, the doctor was called on only when someone was ill: medical care was expensive and the doctor was a figure of awe-inspiring authority. With the advent of vaccination, nutritional medicine, public health programs, and screening techniques, it became apparent that – in the case of many diseases – prevention was far more cost-effective than trying to treat a condition once it had developed. On the basis of this, most countries now recommend regular health checks to screen for common problems. The availability of certain techniques varies from place to place, and is often based on an economic assessment of the prevalence of a disease in a community and the expenditure likely to be involved in screening part or a whole of the population, compared with the cost of treating those who would develop the full-blown disease.

Many women feel an initial reluctance when they are asked to attend at a family planning, well-woman, or cervical smear clinic for the first time, particularly if they have not previously had a pelvic examination. There are many possible reasons for this anxiety, some of them based on uncertainty about the procedures involved and the way they are performed. Many of us also feel embarrassed about our bodies and their sexual and reproductive functions; medical examination is felt to be a kind of invasion of privacy; we wonder if it will hurt; we are worried about taking up a doctor's time when we are feeling perfectly well; and if anything is wrong, perhaps we would rather not know about it. Older women may feel that, because they have passed the menopause, breast and cervical checks are no longer appropriate (in fact, they are more important than ever).

Many diseases which develop slowly but which have the potential to kill us if left untreated can be detected by a thorough health check; in fact, early treatment can often bring about complete cure. One of the most easily curable conditions is cervical cancer: abnormal cells can be spotted in a smear sample and treatment performed before the

Some health check procedures
a Checking blood pressure
b Listening to your chest
c Taking your pulse
d Testing reflexes
e Mammography

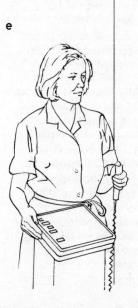
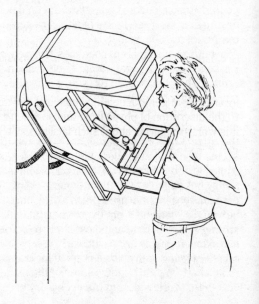

possibility of cancer spread even arises. The risk of developing relatively common conditions like maturity-onset diabetes, osteoarthritis, and hypertension can also be assessed through simple procedures like measuring weight and blood pressure and testing urine. Changes in life style and diet may be all that is then required to forestall or delay the onset of a debilitating disease.

The form that health checks take depends very much on your age and the scope of the screening program. Young women may have their weight and blood pressure measured, be asked about regularity of periods and any contraception used, and be given pelvic (including pap or cervical smear) and breast examinations. This kind of early examination gives a good baseline against which any later changes can be compared. It also provides an opportunity to discuss anxieties and make decisions about which contraceptive method to use. Older women may, in addition to the tests mentioned above, be offered mammography (a low-dose breast X ray) and urine and stool tests. Though the idea of these tests may seem alarming at first, none of them should be painful. Any discomfort will also be lessened if you can relax during the procedures.

Many physicians run well-woman clinics and screening services with the aid of computerized recall systems. Their patients are therefore likely to be sent reminders to come for checks at appropriate intervals. Some women attend family planning, students', or young women's clinics, and these usually offer gynecological screening services. It is often possible to ask to be seen by a woman doctor if you would prefer this; alternatively, a nurse can be present during the examination.

A urine sample may be requested – try to collect early morning urine in a *clean* bottle. Rigorous washing and douching before an examination should be avoided as they can eliminate signs of a discharge. For a mammogram, you will be required to strip to the waist, so it is advisable to wear separates rather than a dress.

Recommendations as to frequency of checks vary widely, but young women are advised to have their first cervical smear test as soon as they become sexually active, with a second test a year later. Subsequent 3-yearly tests may be sufficient, but women at high risk (for example, those with genital warts) should be tested more often. Mammography is usually offered only to women aged 50 or over, though a baseline X ray at age 35 is useful for future comparison. The availability of general health counseling and fitness testing is often left to the discretion of physicians; and so when choosing a family doctor, it is worth enquiring about such facilities as a well-woman clinic.

SELF-EXAMINATION

Monthly breast examination (see p. 102) is a vital part of every woman's health care routine. Some women may also be interested in doing their own regular vulval, vaginal and cervical checks. For the latter, it is necessary to buy a speculum, which should be kept for purely personal use and cleaned thoroughly before and after use. To learn how to use the speculum and establish a baseline, it is best to consult a women's health group or a doctor or nurse.

©DIAGRAM

Stress

Inability to relax is commonly caused by stress, a consequence of the body's physiological reaction to external events. Stressful situations can be pleasant (supporting your team), unpleasant (an accident), physical (running), mental (worrying over past or future events), emotional (a bereavement), prolonged (work or family problems), or instantaneous (cutting a finger). Faced with these or similar situations, the body tenses as part of the "fight or flight" response (see *below*). This response is essential to the survival of animals in the wild. In the modern world, however, man no longer runs after his food, and faced with a dangerous situation cannot always run away. You cannot run in the driving seat of a car or in an overcrowded commuter train, nor can you flee financial trouble, divorce or city noise very easily. Instead, stress is internalized. The unexpressed anger, irresolvable anxiety and frustration become trapped and cause depression, nervousness and irritability. These in turn cause more negative situations until they

Fight or flight response
When your body prepares for action the following changes take place:
1 Forebrain receives stimulus
2a Pituitary gland releases the alarm messenger hormone (ACTH)
2b Lower brain alerts the nervous system
3 ACTH causes the adrenal glands to release the hormones adrenaline (or epinephrine), noradrenaline (or norepinephrine) and cortisone. These cause:
4 Heart rate to increase – blood is diverted to muscles and brain
5 Respiration rate to increase and nostrils and bronchi to dilate
6 Liver to release sugar and fatty acids into the blood
7 Pupils to dilate
8 Sweating to increase
9 Bowels and bladder to empty
10 Muscles to tense

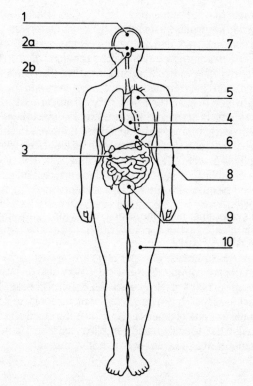

are expressed as physical, "psychosomatic" illnesses such as hypertension, ulcers, muscular pain, aches, neuroses and breakdown. Prolonged stress simply runs the body down, in the same way as a machine wears out. The extra sugars and fatty acids released into the bloodstream, if not burned up with violent exercise, can be converted into cholesterol and give rise to atherosclerosis and other circulatory disorders. Environmental factors, especially noise, uncomfortable living or working conditions and crowding can also cause stress. Misdirected energy (as in constant bad posture), and working in opposition to your natural rhythms are contributory factors to stress, too.

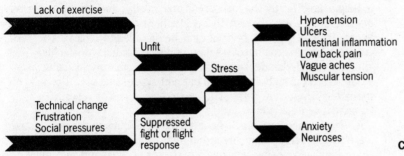

Causes and effects of stress

SIGNS OF STRESS
The following is a list of the most common indications of stress. Check through the list. If you display seven or more of these reactions, you are most probably suffering an undue amount of stress and would do well to follow a relaxation program.

1 Poor sleep
2 Waking up feeling unrested and dispirited
3 Jumping at unexpected noises
4 Impatience and irritability
5 Dissatisfaction with life in general, relationships or your job
6 Any constant, pointless, repetitive action, such as teeth grinding or clenching, nail-biting, chainsmoking, tapping feet, fingers or pencils
7 Habits you know to be bad for you – overeating, smoking, or drinking too much
8 Shallow breathing
9 Hunched, tense posture
10 Obsessions
11 Physical symptoms: migraine, skin complaints, indigestion, stuttering, flatulence, asthma, constipation, or severe menstrual pain
12 Constantly being frustrated in your aims by others
13 Repeatedly being late
14 Use of sedatives
15 Pains in your neck, shoulders, chest or back
16 Sweating for no apparent reason
17 Loneliness
18 Inability to show emotion
19 Inability to enjoy actions
20 A constant desire to change the unchangeable or to be or to do something else

Confidence-building and growth

Some women have a poor image of themselves, and lack of confidence can lead to a variety of problems in dealing with other people. There is a range of techniques for improving self-image and communication skills, however, many of which use elements of psychology and psychotherapy to achieve their aims.

Asking directly for something is seen by some as not being "feminine," and women often feel that they should be compliant to the wishes of others if they want to be lovable. They may consequently experience difficulty in speaking directly about how they really feel and what they want to do. **Assertiveness training** uses techniques derived from transactional analysis, role playing and behavior therapy to help assess firstly the main areas of difficulty; and secondly what is unproductive about the way these situations are currently being handled, as well as how behavior can be modified to achieve a better outcome. It aims to improve self-confidence gradually by tackling situations graded in degree of difficulty, and ultimately to enable women to act in an honest, open but non-aggressive way that will get them what they want without having to back down or resort to manipulative behavior.

Self-confidence can also be boosted by techniques which help women learn to appreciate themselves and their particular skills and abilities. Consciousness-raising sessions, encounter groups, and certain methods of humanistic psychology such as transactional analysis and Gestalt may be very effective in this respect. Creative activities like painting can also act as paths to self-discovery. But a method which works for one woman will not necessarily do the same for another. Women's groups may be able to offer advice on facilities that are available and which is likely to be most appropriate to each individual's aims and needs.

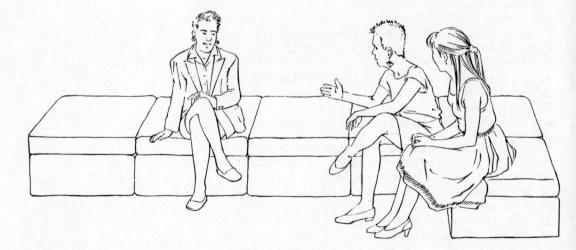

Coping with crises

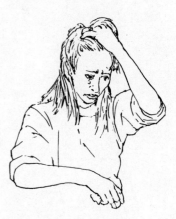

When disaster strikes, it can leave us feeling very alone, even if we have a partner, family or friends to fall back on. Those who are closest to us may not always be the easiest people to talk to, particularly if they are also involved in the situation. In any crisis, it is a good idea to find someone with whom we can openly discuss our feelings. Just talking about what has happened can help put things into perspective and will often help you find an appropriate course of action. Whatever the source of distress, telephone helplines such as the Samaritans offer a listening service; and some are available for a range of special situations. Certain organizations are also able to offer counseling or the fellowship of "befrienders" – people who have suffered from a similar predicament and so can give sympathetic advice.

The list below details some of the crises we may face, the special problems involved, and those who may be able to help us deal with them. You will find many useful addresses on p.408–411.

Death of partner, parent or child (miscarriage, stillbirth, sudden infant death, as well as death in childhood) may bring about feelings of isolation, and possibly depressive illness. Specialist organizations, a family social worker, or a family physician may be able to help.

Serious illness such as cancer, AIDS, disability, stroke or mental disturbance can be devastating. Doctors may only be concerned with clinical aspects; and the general public may be ill-informed. Seek advice from specialist helplines and organizations, a counselor, or a hospital social worker.

Sexual and relationship problems are common, and it can be hard to find someone sufficiently far removed in whom to confide. A partner may also be distrustful of seeking outside aid. A marriage guidance counselor (often able to deal with partnerships outside confines of marriage), a family crisis center, a social worker, or refuge in the case of victims of marital violence or sexual abuse should be consulted.

Family problems range considerably. Seek advice from your family physician, a family therapist or a social worker. If difficult physical circumstances arise, such as homelessness, contact a social worker or an aid agency. Emotional problems can be referred to a family therapist or physician.

In instances of sexual assault, harassment or mugging, unfortunately the police may only be interested in the legal aspects. Rape centers, specialist helplines,or women's, students and racial minority groups may be of help, as may other organizations offering victim support schemes.

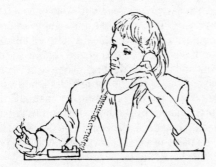

Sleep needs

Sleep is the most important form of relaxation. About one-third of our lives is spent in a state of near unconsciousness. There are two types of sleep. **Non REM sleep** forms about 75% of our sleep. The body is relaxed; and during the deepest periods of sleep, the production of growth hormone and protein is at its highest while the body repairs itself with new cells. **Paradoxical** or **REM sleep** accounts for the remaining 25%. This is the stage in which dreams occur. There is rapid eye movement (REM) behind the closed lids, the heartbeat and breathing become irregular, the brain receives more blood than when awake and its electrical activity is like that of the waking stage.

There are various theories about the nature of sleep. Some say it is due to a reduction in the brain's oxygen supply; others, a reduction in the number of impulses reaching the centers of consciousness, chemical processes or conditioned responses.

Everybody also **dreams**, whether they remember their dreams or not. But the actual function of dreaming, which takes place during REM sleep, is not known. Freud saw them as indications of unconscious fears or desires. They may also serve to help the brain sort out new data from the day's activities.

The amount of sleep we need gradually declines as we get older, but remains fairly constant from age 30. On average, a newborn baby sleeps for 16 hours a day, a 6-year-old for 10 hours, a 12-year-old for 9 hours, and an adult for 7 hours and 20 minutes. Although sleep needs are not dependent upon sex or intelligence, the amount needed is very personal: some adults need as much as 10 hours sleep daily, while others need only 2 or 3 hours. But we are so accustomed to thinking of 8 hours as being the necessary amount that many people use chemical means unnecessarily to prolong their sleep period. **Insomnia** is habitual sleeplessness. It takes various forms: in one, the person cannot get to sleep at all; in another, the person wakes up after a few hours and cannot get to sleep again, or wakes and sleeps continuously and alternately through the night. People sometimes think they have not slept when, in fact, they have just woken at regular intervals and cannot remember sleeping! There are often easily rectifiable physical causes for sleeplessness, such as feeling cold or uncomfortable, or having bad eating habits. Make sure your room is warm but well aired and that the bed gives even and firm support. Avoid eating, and especially refrain from tea or coffee, late at night. Take exercise every day, to tire the body and clear the mind.

But the most common causes of insomnia are psychological factors: tension, depression or emotional upset. The main rule is not to become too concerned over lack of sleep – this only starts a vicious circle of tense worrying. If you really cannot get to sleep, don't lie there and fret about it. Try and reeducate yourself into a positive frame of mind about sleep and have a gentle routine: a relaxing bath, a warm drink and quiet reading or talking to relieve tension. Whatever the psychological reason for insomnia, find a method for taking your mind off it. Try concentrating, for instance, on one part of the body or regularizing your breathing. If you can, get a friend to massage your neck, shoulders, back and legs (see p.122.) Sleeping pills should only be used as a last resort, since they do not give a satisfying sleep and should not be depended upon.

Body rhythms

Day by day, almost hour by hour, rhythms modify the workings of your brain and body.

Asleep, the brain's activity runs in approximately 90-minute cycles, where relative tranquility alternates with a frenzied eruption of electrical discharges to and from the brain's 10 billion cells. While you are awake, daydreaming succeeds periods when you feel mentally alert. In sleep, the rate of brain activity slows down, but even sleep has mental cycles too.

Daily rhythms affect much more than just the brain. Pulse rate, blood pressure, blood sugar level, body temperature, gland secretions, enzyme levels, salt secretion by the kidneys, intestinal contractions, cell growth – altogether more than 40 aspects of bodily activity routinely wax and wane according to established patterns. This helps to explain why we feel lively, hungry, tired or maybe irritable at different times of day.

Biological changes of the kinds just mentioned are called circadian rhythms – rhythms that recur about once daily. Such cycles seem related to the Earth's daily revolution on its yearly path around the Sun. It is as if alarm clocks hidden in the body were set to switch different bodily activities on and off at measured intervals in response to the great celestial cycle of day and night that dominates our lives. Indeed biologists call the mysterious controlling mechanisms "biological clocks."

Many, if not all, circadian rhythms plainly benefit our bodies. For example, reduced urine flow at night helps to ensure a long spell of uninterrupted sleep, and regular sleep itself seems necessary to our health.

However, experiments have shown that within limits our body rhythms change if we are out of touch with regular stimuli of day and night. Cavers, astronauts and others in perpetual light or dark find that their circadian rhythms tend to drift. Two groups of scientists in the unbroken daylight of an Arctic summer set their watches differently. Some adopted a 21-hour day; others a 27-hour day. Both sets found their body rhythms changed to fit the new regimes.

Part of the brain, the hypothalamus, controls a woman's monthly cycle. This works largely as a "feedback" process, triggered by estrogen hormone accumulating in the blood. Interestingly, too, scientists have found that when women work or live closely together, their monthly cycles sometimes begin to coincide.

Upsetting the body's clock
Jet lag is a common example of the effects of altering the body's internal clock. A trans-Atlantic return journey, by air, for instance, means that the clock is desynchronized twice, producing strain on the body and temporarily reducing mental capability. At the start, (**1**), the body is adjusted to US time, but after the outward flight that time zone no longer applies and the traveler finds that she is wakeful at night and sleepy by day. It takes about a week for the rhythm to adjust (**2**) to new local time. On return, the body clock is upset again and does not reset itself properly for another three or four days (**3**).

a US time
b Internal body time
c Continental time

☐ Daytime
■ Night
▨ Duration of flight

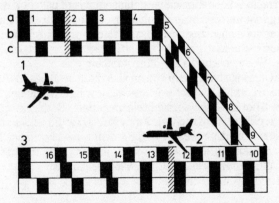

© DIAGRAM

Relaxation

Relaxation should be a concern of everyone who wants to maintain a healthy body. It enables us to escape from the stresses and pressures of everyday life; and the muscles are given an opportunity to rest. Try to spend at least 30 minutes relaxing every day, ideally alone so that you can be as free as possible from interruptions.

Remember, too, that relaxation can be increased by removing stress-creating factors from your environment. Try to organize activities beforehand so you know when you will be doing things. Try to keep tidy so you do not lose things. Maintain good posture, and learn to enjoy physical exertion. Make sure you have complete breaks of attention during the day. Avoid being too hot or too cold, and keep noises to a minimum. Make time to be on your own, and give up any negative habits you know to be bad for you, like smoking or overeating.

AREAS OF TENSION

The illustration shows some of the main areas of muscle tension that frequently affect the body.

1 Tension in the back of the neck is often a result of psychological conditions such as anxiety or stress, and often leads to the so-called nervous headache. Massaging the back of the neck with your fingertips may relieve the tension.

2 Tension in the shoulders may often occur after overwork, or if your desk or workbench is at the wrong height. Stretching and easing the muscles with exercise will often prove effective.

3 Pain and muscle tension in the small of the back may be a result of your posture, wearing high-heeled shoes too frequently, or sagging muscles in the back and abdomen that fail to give proper support to the spine. Menstrual problems, pregnancy or hormonal disorders can also cause low backache.

4 Muscle tension and aches in the arms are usually caused by overworking the muscles concerned – carrying heavy objects, digging, shoveling, pushing, or pulling. Massaging and resting the affected muscles should ease the problem.

5 Tension and stiffness of the thigh and calf muscles are usually caused by strain. Over-enthusiastic exercising such as running or cycling will often produce stiffness the following day, which can be eased by using the muscles gently, for instance in walking or gentle jogging. Pregnancy and its related circulatory problems in the legs will often cause muscle aches. Resting with the legs raised will ease discomfort.

6 Aching foot muscles may result from overwork. Walking, running or even standing for long periods may interfere with efficient circulation in the feet and lead to tenderness and fatigue in the muscles. Warm footbaths are often soothing.

Tension in all parts of the body can also often be relieved by taking a long, warm bath. If the water is too hot, it will be tiring; and if it is too cool, it will not have the desired relaxing effect. Bath salts and other preparations for use in the water may help your muscles to relax: but tension is mainly relieved by the warm water. For muscles that are very painful and stiff, preparations can be bought for massaging into the affected muscles to produce localized heat.

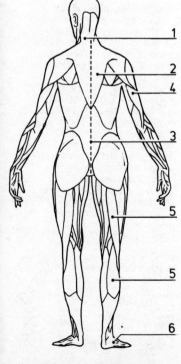

Massage

This is one of the most effective ways of relieving tension in tired, knotted muscles. Techniques of massage vary greatly (see p.122) but the most straightforward ones used for physical relaxation are mainly concerned with manipulating the muscle tissues in order to increase the blood supply to that area and restore suppleness to the muscle. The increased blood flow also speeds the removal of impurities from aching muscles, which helps to relieve the pain. The affected muscles are rubbed with slow, even pressure without losing contact with the skin until the massage is complete.

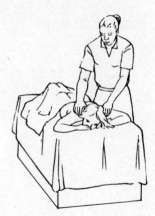

Sitting positions

Relaxation is possible in many positions. One of the best ways to learn to relax is to discover some of the positions that enable your body to rest itself without strain. If you are sitting in a chair, make sure that it gives adequate support. Sit well back on the seat with your back straight and your head supported (**a**). In this position, you can watch television, listen to music, meditate, or just recover from a busy day. The classic lotus position of yoga (**b**) is also a good sitting position to use when relaxing.

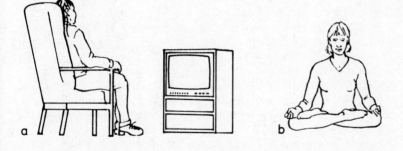

Lying positions

Lying down is one of the most effective ways to relax the entire body completely, and need not be reserved only for sleep. Bend your knee up and cushion your head on a pillow (**c**). Lie flat on your back with your arms by your sides, palms up; allow your arms and legs to go limp so that your feet fall gently apart (**d**). Raise your chin and breathe deeply.

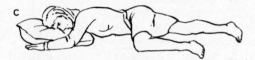

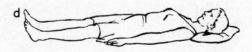

Relaxation exercises

1 Stand upright, as relaxed as possible, and shake each arm in turn. Shake first from your wrist, then from your elbow, then from your shoulder. Repeat with each leg in turn, shaking from the ankle, the knee and then the hip.

2 Stand with your feet apart and your arms by your sides. Take a deep breath as you slowly raise your arms out to shoulder level, then hold your breath as you maintain this position for a few seconds. Breathe out as you lower your arms slowly.

3 Loosen your neck muscles by tilting your head down, to the right, to the back, to the left, then down again.

4 Loosen your shoulder muscles by standing with your arms by your sides and then shrugging your shoulders as high as you can. Hold this position briefly, then relax. Repeat several times.

5 Stand with your arms at your sides. With the backs of the hands leading, move your arms forward, up, back, then down again so that they trace large circles. This will help to relieve tension in the shoulder muscles.

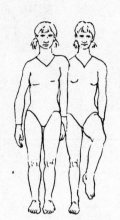

1

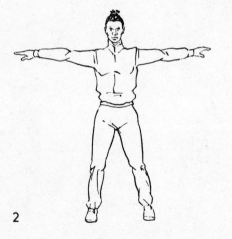

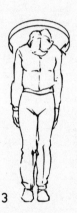

2

3

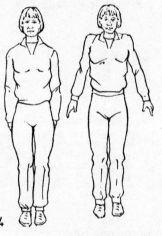

4

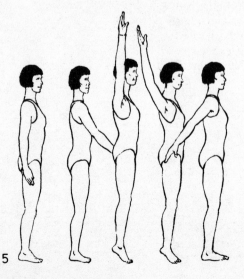

5

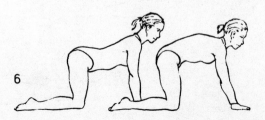

6

6 This is a good exercise for relieving stiff back muscles. Kneel on all fours as shown, and then alternately hollow and hump your back.

7 Sit back to back with a partner and hold hands above your heads. Alternately pull and push forward and back. This will help to stretch and relax your back muscles.

8 First massage your thigh muscles to loosen them slightly, then sit on a chair with your feet slightly apart. Keeping the toes on the ground, move the thigh and knee of one leg from side to side several times until the muscles feel looser. Repeat with the other leg.

9 To relieve tension in your calf muscles, stand upright with your feet flat on the floor. Keeping your heels on the floor, slowly bend your knees and sink down as far as you can: you will feel the muscles of your thighs and calves being stretched.

10 To relieve shoulder tension, do modified push-ups against a wall, as shown.

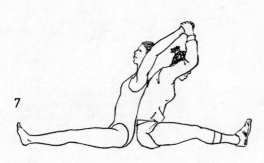

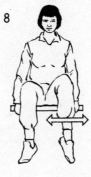

© DIAGRAM

Yoga postures

Many thousands of women are now discovering the physical and mental benefits to be gained from the pursuit of yoga. This ancient discipline, developed in the East over thousands of years, has in recent decades won many enthusiastic followers in North American and European countries. Illustrated on these two pages are representative examples of popular yoga postures. Combined with breathing control, the attainment of such postures produces deep levels of relaxation in both body and mind. Because of the precise nature of yoga, potential students are strongly recommended to attend classes to ensure that all postures are correctly learned. Hard work and dedication are essential for the serious yoga student, and the results will prove well worth the effort.

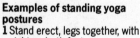

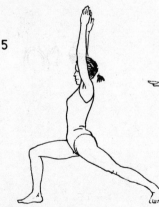

Examples of standing yoga postures
1 Stand erect, legs together, with weight on both feet.

2 With your feet apart, legs straight, and arms stretched, bend to the side and clasp one ankle.
3 Similar to **2** but with one arm above

the head and one knee bent.
4 With your feet apart, legs straight, and hands behind your back, touch your leg with your head.

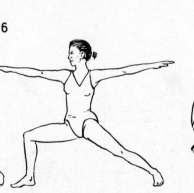

5 Raise your arms above your head, one leg forward, and have the other leg stretched behind.
6 Similar to **5** but with the body turned to the side and arms outstretched.

7 Put your feet together, have your legs straight, then bend your body so that your head touches your legs and your hands are on the floor behind your feet.

8 Stand on one leg, have the other leg bent to the side, and put your hands together.

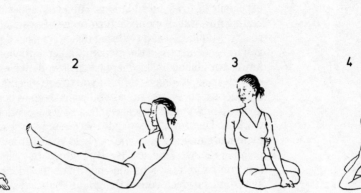

Examples of sitting and resting yoga postures
1 Basic sitting posture.
2 Raise your legs, keeping them straight and together, with your hands at back of your head.
3 Sitting, put your legs to the side, with your back twisted, and one hand behind you.
4 Do a shoulder stand, keeping your back straight.

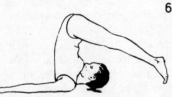
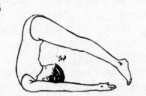
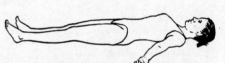

5 Lie down. Then, keeping your arms straight by your sides, hands palms down, lift your legs and feet to touch the floor beyond your head.

6 Lie down. Then, keeping your arms straight behind your head, hands palms up, lift your legs and feet to touch the floor beyond your head.

7 This is the resting posture. It is used with breathing exercises to end each session.

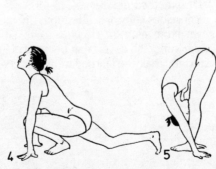
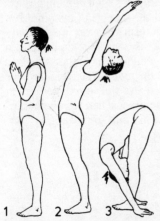
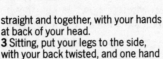

A combination of yoga postures forming a short sequence
1 Stand with your hands and feet together.
2 Inhale, and adopt the posture shown.
3 Exhale, adopting the posture shown.
4 Inhale, adopting the posture shown.
5 Exhale, adopting the posture shown.
6 Inhale, adopting the posture shown.
7 Exhale, returning to the first posture.

©DIAGRAM

Meditation

The mind is, in its usual state, a never-ending series of links. Every impression that enters it sets off a chain of associations which, especially in stressful situations, rebound like a ricocheting bullet, setting up a wall of mental interference between the mind and outer reality. Meditation aims to bring this process under control, allowing you to concentrate on the moment, and not to worry about the past or future possibilities. This increase in attention eventually leads to a new clear-sightedness: it helps you to see objects, people and situations as they are, not as you want them to be. This can in turn lead to a new sense of peace with a new perception of your place in the world and your relation to external circumstances. It gives you a mental breathing space, and can help you to stop wasting energy in pointless anxiety and activity. By bringing the mind under control, you also control your actions and undermine the "donkey and carrot" syndrome in which you do things automatically without knowing why, or even when or how. Meditation helps you to act, and not react automatically in fear, anger or greed.

There are various methods of meditation. Most common is the use of physical or mental objects on which the meditator tries to focus his or her attention. Every time other thoughts or even verbal definitions enter the mind, they must be pushed off, and attention brought back to the object. Natural objects, such as stones or shells, or small personal objects like jewels or plain rings should be used. Alternatively, it is possible to concentrate on the verbal or mental repetition of sounds (transcendental meditation's "mantras," "OM" or prayers); images with uplifting associations (the lotus flower, or pictures of saints and gurus, for instance); or body rhythms, especially breathing. Bhakti, Sufi and transcendental meditations, Raja yoga and Kundalini yoga all use this method.

A second major method is to concentrate on yourself and to cultivate a constant awareness of your actions, thoughts and surroundings. Krishnamurti's "self-knowledge" and Gurdjieff's "self-remembering" typify this method. A third method combines aspects of the other two, the best known examples being Zen Buddhism's "zazen" meditation and use of the "koans" (unsolvable problems), and Tibetan Buddhism.

Despite their differences, all forms of meditation have the same basis – conscious control of attention. Choose the method suitable for your own personality and circumstances, and stress will be relieved. Remember, however, that because of its personal nature, meditation can only really be learned from a teacher on a one-to-one basis.

Conditions for meditation
Try to follow these simple guidelines.
1 Sit in a comfortable position (cross-legged or in a chair) with your back straight.
2 Choose a quiet time and place with no fear of interruption.
3 Let your thoughts and body settle for a few minutes before you begin.
4 Try to meditate for ½-1 hour, if possible at the same times each day.
5 As with all exercises, results are dependent upon the constancy and strength of your effort.

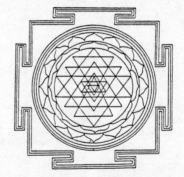

The mandala
Designs such as the example illustrated are often used as aids to meditation and have a spiritual significance as they represent an ordering of the universe and a focus for its forces.

Mind over matter

Some doctors are now convinced that we might help our bodies resist or even overcome disease by mind-control techniques such as **biofeedback**. Subjects cultivate a relaxed mental state by passive concentration, and are wired to electronic devices with lights, tones, or moving meter needles to feed back data concerning their own involuntary bodily activities, notably blood pressure and "brain waves." Properly relaxed patients can often influence these things. Several conditions seem especially well suited to biofeedback treatment. Victims of certain neuromuscular disorders may recover function by learning to reroute nerve signals to affected muscles, for instance. Migraine sufferers can sometimes alter congested blood vessels near the brain by diverting extra blood into the hands. Epileptics may suffer fewer fits and insomniacs sleep better if they can learn to modify the brain's electrical activity. Even some people with allergies may benefit from use of biofeedback.

Similar mind control perhaps explains why certain people condemned to die from cancer literally seem to will their own recovery. Biofeedback has limitations, but its potential may still be largely untapped.

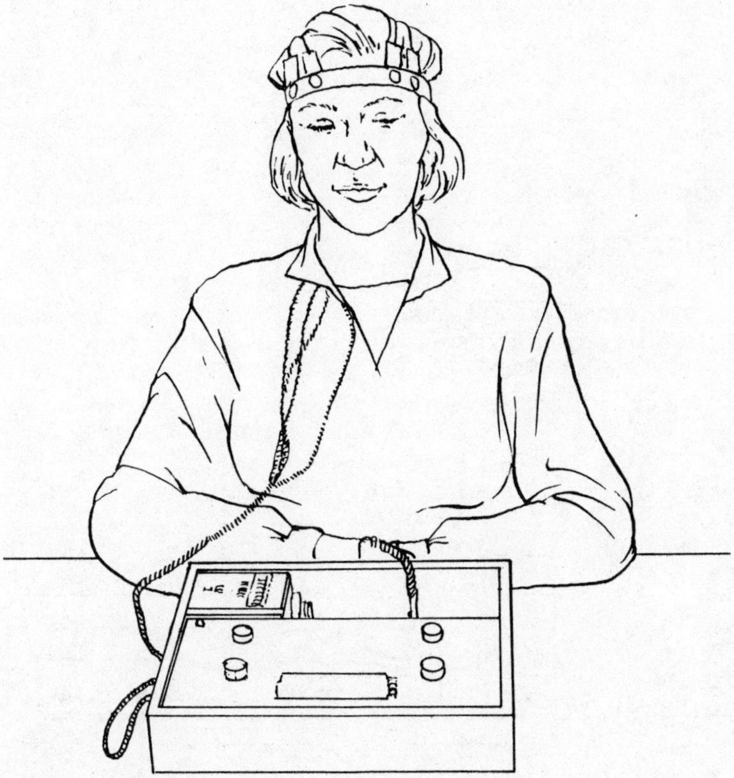

Biofeedback
The woman shown is attempting to alter the way her body normally works by concentrating on the readings given by a biofeedback machine. This kind of relaxation technique, like yoga, has proved that the autonomic nervous system can, to some extent, be brought under conscious control.

© DIAGRAM

145

Hypnosis

Doctors once ridiculed claims that the mind produced effects defying scientific explanation. Hypnosis, psychic healing, extrasensory perception – phenomena like these still largely baffle us, but now scientists at least concede they merit serious attention.

People had unknowingly practiced hypnotism for centuries before Franz Anton Mesmer made his first experiments in 1776. Misconceived by him as "animal magnetism" and later misnamed from the Greek hypnos ("sleep"), hypnotism has been described more fittingly as "a temporary condition of altered attention induced by another person."

Someone being fully hypnotized passes through three main stages: light, medium and deep trance. Only the most suggestible of people – about 1 in 20 – can be deeply hypnotized: unwilling subjects remain quite unaffected. The usual process involves the subject lying or sitting comfortably relaxed while gazing at a shiny object and listening to the hypnotist's voice monotonously repeating suggestions that induce hypnosis. The main point is to shut out all stimuli except those tending to send the subject into hypnotic trance. This can also be accomplished in other ways – for instance, by hearing one's own pre-recorded breathing played back amplified, or by gazing at light shone through revolving prisms. Hypnotized people have a glazed, humorless, withdrawn appearance, yet may behave quite normally unless the hypnotist suggests differently. Then astonishing results may follow.

How hypnotism is induced

Some subjects are hypnotized by the sound of the hypnotist's monotonous voice; others, by a technique that also involves a bright swinging object (**A**).

The subject must be comfortable and relaxed and, above all, open to suggestion. It is impossible to hypnotize an unwilling subject. Self-hypnosis is also possible. The hypnotist's voice may be recorded on tape and played back by the subject. After each suggestion, the subject presses a remote control device to go on to the next stage (**B**). This puts control of the procedure in the hands of the subject and shows that hypnosis is a more simple technique than many of those who use method (**A**) might admit.

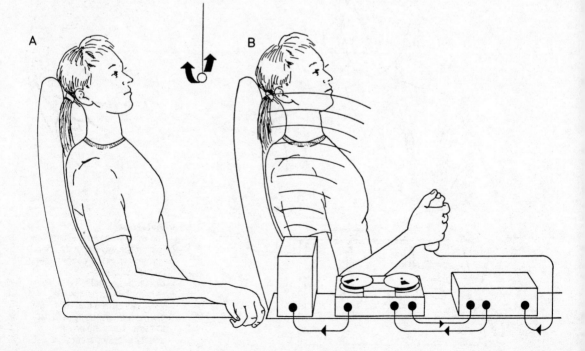

On command, a hypnotized individual may lie rigidly across the backs of chairs while someone stands upon his or her body. Afterward, the subject may not remember anything of what has happened. In fact he or she may go on obeying some instructions received while hypnotized. This is known as post-hypnotic suggestion.

Skeptics claim that unhypnotized people can also remain rigid, withstand pain and mimic other effects supposedly produced by trance conditions. Yet hypnosis does seem to have remarkable effects that cast new light on mind-body interaction. Touching a subject's skin with a pencil may produce blisters if she has been told the pencil is red hot. Touching a hypnotized subject's skin with a Japanese wax-plant, meanwhile, has been shown not to produce an expected skin reaction when the subject has been told it was a harmless chestnut leaf. Yet a chestnut leaf has produced a weal when the subject thought it was a wax-plant leaf. Telling a subject to imagine she has just eaten a large, fatty meal will stimulate her body to secrete lipase (a fat-digestive enzyme). When she thinks the meal was rich in protein, she manufactures pepsin and trypsin (protein-digesting enzymes). Hypnosis can also affect breathing, heart rate, and various kinds of glandular activity. The intriguing aspect of many of these tests is their effects upon body functions that had been long supposed to operate outside the mind's control.

How hypnotism works
There are many theories as to the exact effect hypnotism has on the brain's functioning. One of the most plausible is as follows. When we concentrate our attention on a swinging ball or the hypnotist's voice, messages received through the eyes or ears are relayed to the midbrain. These messages primarily influence and modify the midbrain centers. The effect can be demonstrated by brain wave traces. **A** (shown *left*) is the normal trace of a person who is awake with a characteristic spiky waveform; whereas **B**, taken from a hypnotized subject, shows a different frequency.

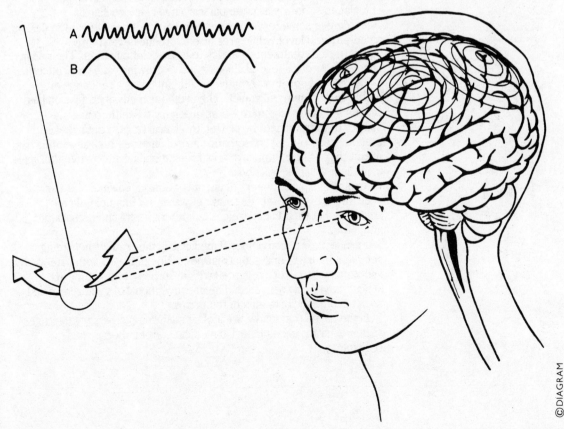

A

B

©DIAGRAM

3.06   Complementary medicine

The alternative approach

Modern orthodox medicine is a development of the last three centuries, based on an increasingly mechanistic view of the universe and the premise that mind and body are separate. The resulting "nuts and bolts" attitude to the physical body, backed by technological advances, of course has a major role to play in the cure of acute disease and infections and the relief of symptoms. But there are other aspects of illness which lie beyond the scope of what is increasingly seen as a rather limited and essentially one-dimensional approach to healing.

Approximately 80 per cent of clients seeking orthodox help are not acute cases, while 40 per cent have been shown by studies to have no apparent physical ailments. Unlike some conventional doctors, the alternative or complementary practitioner takes such invisible complaints seriously as potential warnings of future illness. According to some, orthodox medicine may not be adequate to deal on a non-physical level, while pressure to produce even more sophisticated treatments appears to be no solution either. The rise in iatrogenic or drug-related illness is also a growing cause for concern.

The recent boom in alternative health options is a reflection of increasing consumer disquiet. The orthodox medical profession has responded by tending to reject as quackery those therapies the validity of which cannot be proved by clinical trails. Yet increased acceptance of the psychosomatic basis of illnesses such as asthma has meant that some doctors are now recommending alternative therapies in place of drugs or placebos.

Responsible practitioners of unconventional medicine take a similar line. Alternative therapists treating cancer, for example, do not advocate that their clients reject radiotherapy and chemotherapy altogether.

Alternative or unconventional medicine is thus rapidly becoming complementary to orthodox treatment. Not long ago, both osteopathy and acupuncture were regarded with suspicion. Today, they are almost universally accepted. The unconventional of yesterday could soon become the orthodox of tomorrow.

On the pages that follow, we look at such complementary therapies as homeopathy, shiatsu, herbal medicine, aromatherapy and reflexology.

Holistic medicine

The "holistic" approach (the word is derived from the Greek "holos" meaning "whole"), though apparently a modern concept, has roots about as old as woman herself, and embraces a variety of unique therapies which emphasize the patient or client, not the symptoms.

Oriental therapies in particular regard the organs of the body as being interconnected, and health is seen to be a state of vitalized harmony, each individual being a complex interrelationship of physical, mental, emotional and spiritual energy bodies.

True preventative medicine is the maintenance of this optimum state through a two-way process echoed in the old saying "a healthy mind in a healthy body." Nourishing the mind and spirit is therefore as essential a part of holistic medicine as good nutrition and adequate exercise, as well as immunization and avoidance of such harmful activities as smoking and excessive alcohol intake.

Disease, on the other hand, is regarded by the holistic practitioner as reflecting imbalance or disharmony of the individual as a whole, and problems can be located by a variety of diagnostic techniques, often prior to any symptomatic manifestations. Actual symptoms are usually ascribed by the practitioner to a mental cause which has blocked or misdirected energy on the physical plane. Tension, for example, is said to start in the mind but is soon experienced as a headache.

The function of the holistic practitioner, whose methods may work on many levels simultaneously, is often to stimulate a natural ability for self-healing. Illness can be diagnosed, though in practice this is forbidden by law in many western countries to all but qualified conventional doctors.

There are no instant "miracle cures," so beware of any such claims. Clients of a holistic practitioner will be expected to commit themselves not only to several sessions of treatment but also to change their diet, take exercise, and reduce stress where possible in order to bring about a lasting cure. The emphasis is on re-educating the individual into taking responsibility for personal health, an attitude with far-reaching effects, both personally and globally.

Acupuncture

An ancient skill developed in China at least 3000 years ago as a standard therapy, acupuncture (meaning "to puncture with a needle") forms part of a unique and essentially preventative medical system which also includes diet, herbalism and exercise.

The concept of *chi* or "life energy" is basic to acupuncture. This is said to be inherited at birth and also absorbed daily into the body through food and the breath. Imbalance of *chi* indicates potential or actual disease, and is diagnosed through sensitivity registered by relevant acupuncture points sited on invisible pathways through the body. Location of such imbalance is also identified by direct questions concerning lifestyle and medical history, palpation (touching the body) and pulse diagnosis. The trained acupuncturist can distinguish six different pulses in the radial artery of each wrist, giving clues to hundreds of different conditions.

Chi is stimulated or sedated by needles of varying lengths, usually made of stainless steel and inserted in certain specific acupuncture

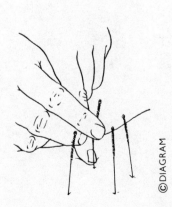

© DIAGRAM

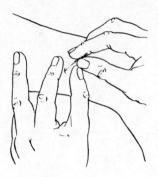

points, which total around 800 and lie along a series of 14 imaginary lines or meridians. The needles are placed at a depth of a few millimeters on the relevant points, perhaps rotated briefly by the acupuncturist and left for approximately 20 minutes. (Sometimes they may be stimulated electrically.) Occasionally, **moxibustion**, the application of burning moxa (mugwort) to the skin, is also employed. Despite appearances, both procedures are almost painless. There is even a whole system based upon points on the ear alone.

Visits can be once or twice a week or more frequently, depending on the condition. Practitioners are both private and increasingly an option in hospital care. Immediate improvements may be noticeable with short-term dysfunctions such as menstrual cramps, bloating and anxiety. It may also be effective for a frozen shoulder, depression, anxiety, lumbago, and digestive problems.

Though often a last resort, acupuncture can boast a very high success rate, but 20 per cent of western clients do not respond to treatment; and despite publicity, acupuncture as an anesthetic is only effective in a few cases. Similarly, acupuncture cannot cure addictions – it can only reduce cravings.

Acupressure and shiatsu

Shiatsu (from the Japanese meaning "finger pressure") and **acupressure** are therapies which depend on thumb pressure applied to acupuncture points or *tsubos*. Both were initially evolved as home preventative remedies; and practitioners of both therapies need a basic knowledge of acupuncture principles. Diagnostic techniques include reading the face, eyes and tongue, pulse readings and palpation. Shiatsu also includes *ampuku*, an additional diagnostic and curative technique based on the *hara* or belly area, which can be helpful with digestive, lower back and sexual disorders.

Shiatsu teachers stress good physical condition as a prerequisite for the practitioner: and concentration, a meditative state of mind and controlled breathing are essential on the part of both the patient and the therapist.

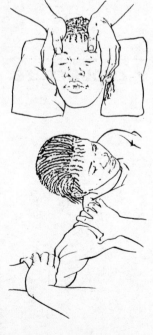

Each treatment lasts about an hour and can involve the use of moxa to increase *chi* energy, and cupping the skin for the reverse effect. Pain is experienced where blockage occurs. Once the *chi* is flowing freshly, the body can exercise its natural healing powers.

Shiatsu, like acupuncture, is a curative and preventative technique. Taking a broader view and applying acupuncture principles, the therapist seeks the underlying cause of the problem: a frozen shoulder, for example, may be caused by liver or gall bladder dysfunction. Shiatsu may be particularly effective for women with menstruation or menopausal problems.

Acupressure takes a more symptomatic view of the client. Set meridians are pressed for specific disorders – heartburn, tinnitus, constipation, hypertension, cramps, carpal tunnel syndrome, toothache or bronchitis, for instance. Acupressure, like shiatsu, is also becoming increasingly popular for sports injuries – everything from tennis elbow to a twisted ankle.

It is worth noting that shiatsu, acupressure and indeed any massage technique should not be used with cancer clients, unless under expert supervision.

Naturopathy

The naturopath views health as a vital state, not merely the absence of disease; and cure is thought to be brought about by the body's own healing power which is undermined by three basic causes. The first is biochemic: inappropriate diet, particularly processed food, may be difficult to metabolize, causing build-up of toxic waste, in turn leading to illnesses such as liver complaints or heart disease. Natural wholefoods are recommended, especially fresh, organic and raw varieties.

The second cause may be structural. Bad alignment of bone and muscle, for example, will ultimately disturb the correct functioning of organic systems as the body attempts to compensate. (Many naturopaths are also osteopaths or will recommend practitioners who can manipulate the body back into alignment.)

Mental and emotional factors may also be involved. Inner conflict inevitably leads to stress which can eventually create illness. Attention to diet and bodily alignment can help to alleviate this.

Diagnosis is carried out by blood tests, X rays, mineral analysis of the hair or iridology (examination of the iris of the eye). A program of natural cures may also be recommended and could include diet, hydrotherapy, exercises and possibly homeopathic or herbal remedies. (Fasting is often prescribed to clear harmful toxins before prescribing specific vitamin or mineral supplements to build up the body).

Naturopathy – particularly effective with recurrent complaints such as allergies, bronchitis and certain digestive and gynecological conditions – is in many respects a self-help therapy that shows the patient that she is ultimately responsible for the correct functioning of her body.

Homeopathy

Samuel Christian Hahnemann's observation that cinchona bark (quinine) produced symptoms similar to those of the malaria that it proposed to alleviate led to the formulation of a new theory of disease. He believed that symptoms were in fact a reflection of the body's natural recuperative powers in action: therefore, rather than being eliminated, they should perhaps be encouraged. Thus homeopathy was born.

Hahnemann (1745–1843) discovered that while large doses of certain plant or mineral extracts were lethal, smaller doses could inhibit disease, and minimal doses were often curative. According to Hahnemann, they operate by replicating on a cellular energy level the correct pattern of response to disease.

Treatment is based on the homeopath first having a detailed case history. Each remedy matches not only a symptom but also temperaments and even physical appearance: sepia, for example, is suitable for short dark-haired people, prone to depression, and also useful for menopausal problems, morning sickness and menstruation difficulties.

Homeopaths use over 2000 remedies suited for most disorders, and prescribe for animals, too. Some remedies are suitable for home treatment of common ailments and can be purchased from pharmacies: but consultation with a homeopathic doctor is preferable.

©DIAGRAM

Herbal medicine

Curing by plants is actually one of the foundations of western medicine. As life has become more complicated, so more complex cures have been sought, but many are still based on ancient plant remedies: atropine, for example, is extracted from deadly nightshade (belladonna), and digitoxin from foxglove (digitalis).

The gathering and preparation of herbs is a complex art and they are difficult to standardize owing to varying climatic conditions, soils, and times of harvest. But a good herbalist will grow his or her own plants, making sure that they are located in an unpolluted environment.

All parts are used, from roots to stem; and in the case of trees, bark and resin, too. These are transformed into the following types of medicine according to set standards.

1 Tisanes or herbal teas. Dried or fresh herbs, brewed briefly in boiling water. Camomile and limeflower are used as stress-relievers, for instance.

2 Infusions. As above, but steeped for a longer period.

3 Decoctions. Hardy roots and bark, simmered in boiling water.

4 Tinctures. Strong alcohol-based preparations adminstered in drop form.

5 Poultices. Macerated herbs in paste form applied to the skin directly or wrapped in gauze.

6 Compresses. Cloth soaked in hot infusions or decoctions and applied to the skin.

7 Creams, lotions and pills.

Tisanes and simple infusions for common ailments such as colds, menstrual cramps or sedatives can be self-prescribed. For more serious problems, it is advisable to consult a trained herbalist.

Plants are powerful drugs which work well for most ailments except the most acute medical and surgical conditions; but if used incorrectly, they can be dangerous. Do not therefore exceed the stated dose or take them over a prolonged period.

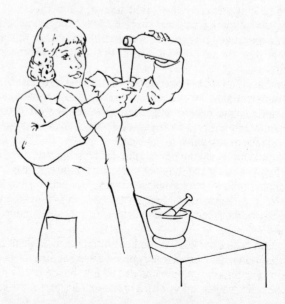

Bach flower remedies

Dr Edward Bach (1880–1936) retired from his London practice in 1930 to dedicate the last six years of his life to perfecting a subtle method of healing by flower essence. The 38 remedies, which bear his name, work on the mental and emotional conflicts which he believed lie at the root of all illness. "There is no true healing unless there is a change in outlook, peace of mind and inner happiness," he wrote.

The remedies are pure plant essences preserved in brandy. As in homeopathy, remedies are sufficiently diluted to cure at a very subtle level. They are classified under seven headings.

1 Fear. (Terror – *rock roses*; specific fear – *mimulus*; fear of loss of control – *plum*; fear of the unknown – *aspen*; fear for others – *red chestnut*).

2 Uncertainty. (Lack of self-confidence – *cerato*; indecision – *scleranthus*; easily discouraged – *gentian*; hopeless despair – *gorse*; lack of physical and mental energy – *hornbeam*; uncertainty as to career or destiny – *wild oat*).

3 Insufficient interest in present circumstances (absent-minded dreamers – *clematis*; living in the past – *honeysuckle*; apathy – *wild roses*; extreme exhaustion – *olive*; continual internal argument – *white chestnut*; black depression – *mustard*; inability to learn through your own mistakes – *chestnut bud*).

4 Loneliness (isolated and self-contained – *water violet*; critical and irritable – *impatiens*; compulsive attention-seekers – *heather*).

5 Oversensitive to influences and ideas (concealed mental torture – *agrimony*; submissive – *centaury*; the "link-breaker," a protection for those during a major life change – *walnut*; strongly negative state of mind – *holly*).

6 Despondency and despair (lack of confidence in abilities – *larch*; guilt and self-condemnation – *pine*; temporarily overwhelmed at magnitude of a task – *elm*; anguish and despair – *sweet chestnut*; sudden shock – *star of Bethlehem*; resentment – *willow*; exhaustion resulting from over-responsibility – *oak*; cleanser for physical and psychological disorders – *crab apple*).

7 Overcare for the welfare of others (overpossessiveness – *chicory*; forceful and argumentative – *vervain*; leadership abilities but misuse of power – *vine*; seekers after perfection – *rock water*).

The appropriate remedy can be selected with the aid of a practitioner, although self-medication is also recommended as an exercise in self-discovery. The stock remedies, also effective for animals, are harmless, inexpensive and can be used in combinations of up to five at a time. Two drops, four times a day, is the usual dose, either neat or in any liquid.

The remedies are said to work almost immediately for temporary states and over a longer period for more entrenched problems. Practitioners also recommend that every home should have a bottle of the Bach "rescue remedy," a combination of five remedies, invaluable for emergencies and sudden shock.

©DIAGRAM

Aromatherapy

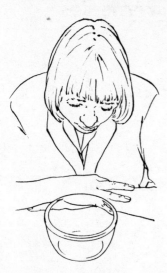

Until the early years of this century, the therapeutic use of essential plant oils was an aspect of herbal lore. The name aromatherapy was then coined by René-Maurice Gattefossé, a French cosmetic chemist, who discovered that such oils also had antibacterial properties which greatly accelerated healing.

Essences, derived from leaves, roots, flowers, bark or resin, can be taken orally (about 3 drops on a sugar lump) for certain complaints – peppermint oil for indigestion and clove oil for toothache, for instance. Investigations have also found three types of eucalyptus oil to have anti-viral properties. Importantly, too, the volatility of aromatherapy oils, which enables them to be readily absorbed into the body, renders them profoundly effective on subtle mental and emotional levels: and in the 1950s, Mme Marguerite Maury established the idea of aromatherapy massage to facilitate penetration via the skin and the breath.

Although essential oils can be used in the home as mood-enhancers to great therapeutic effect, take care with self-dosage as some oils are acutely toxic or can cause allergic reactions.

Drops dissolved in water can also be placed in a bowl and inhaled. Ylang ylang, for instance, is helpful for relaxation; lavender, for headaches; clary sage, for a feeling of euphoric energy as well as uncomfortable menstrual symptoms. Baths can be taken with one or more oils, too: jasmine, will be uplifting; rose, soothing; and peppermint, invigorating.

The Alexander technique

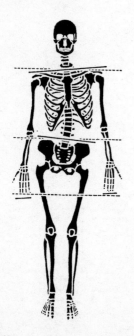

Frederick Matthias Alexander, creator of the postural re-education system which bears his name, was born in Tasmania in 1869. His career as an actor was threatened to be cut short by severe vocal problems which only manifested on stage. When medical help proved useless, he addressed himself to the problem, and finally evolved the technique which is now taught internationally.

Alexander noticed that the natural poise and grace of children gradually disintegrate as they mature into adulthood, sometimes causing physical malfunction. Such bad posture is usually due to laziness and misuse of the body through tension. The Alexander technique aims both to free the muscular-skeletal system from imposed negative habits and to familiarize the body with its own innate natural range of movements.

But Alexander also saw his therapy as having effects beyond the purely physical, declaring that we translate everything – whether physical, mental or spiritual – into muscular tension. Realigning the body is therefore thought also to be effective on a mental/emotional level, imparting a feeling of well-being, exhilaration and greater sense of effectiveness in daily life.

Lessons are generally given by a trained Alexander teacher on a one-to-one basis; and special emphasis is placed on the relationship between the head, neck and trunk, and the pelvic area as the link between the spine and the legs. It is, however, a self-improvement method, not a cure, although very effective in general stress reduction, lower back pain, digestive disorders, speech defects, migraine, asthma, depression and neurosis.

Osteopathy

Dr Andrew Taylor Still (1828–1912), who founded osteopathy, believed that, if we are to be well, the structure of our bodies must be sound – in particular, the spinal column. Many of our illnesses, he believed – headaches, nervous conditions and skin complaints among them – are caused by the spinal vertebrae being out of alignment to a greater or lesser degree; but manipulation could rectify matters.

For many years, osteopathy was not recognized by orthodox medical practitioners. Now, however, in the United States it is generally accepted: in Great Britain, meanwhile, its practice remains controversial and training is given at a specific osteopathic institution rather than a general medical school.

It is a popular form of therapy for back problems especially. Sometimes a simple twist can set things right: in other cases, more long-term manipulation may be necessary. **Cranial osteopathy**, meanwhile, is an off-shoot of more standard osteopathy, and involves treatment via the skull and pelvic area: and **chiropractic**, a similar form of therapy to osteopathy, also involves manipulation but has greater concern with the direction in which this takes place, and also tends to use X rays more often.

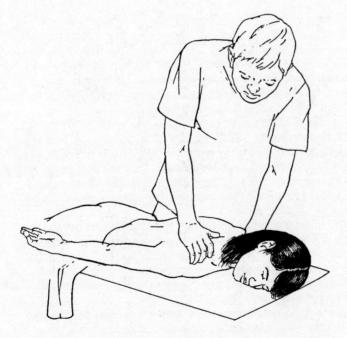

Reflexology

Modern reflexology is based on the zone therapy system, first developed by Dr. W. Fitzgerald in the 1920s, which divides the body longitudinally into ten zones. Organs in the same zone are said to be connected: an untreated kidney malfunction, for instance, could affect sight since they are both located in zone 3, and can be treated by massaging any area in that zone.

Fitzgerald's zone therapy was then extended by his assistant, Eunice Ingham, into reflexology whereby treatment was confined to the feet and to a lesser extent the hands, owing to their extreme sensitivity. She and others subsequently evolved various reflex maps of the feet and schemes of therapeutic massage which are broadly similar.

Diagnosis is made by questioning the patient and examining the condition of the feet both visually and by palpation. As with acupuncture, though the systems are very different, a soreness will register on the skin where there is dysfunction: the ankle area is often tender at particular points in the monthly cycle, for instance. Disorders previously unnoticed by the doctor can often be identified in this way.

Reflex maps of the feet

 1 Side of neck
 2 Sinuses
 3 Ear
 4 Eye
 5 Shoulder
 6 Axilla
 7 Gall bladder
 8 Spleen
 9 Transverse colon
10 Small intestine
11 Ascending colon
12 Descending colon
13 Ileocecal valve/appendix
14 Sigmoid colon
15 Brain
16 Hypothalamus
17 Pituitary
18 Nose
19 Throat
20 Neck/thyroid
21 7th cervical
22 Lungs
23 Thymus
24 Heart
25 Diaphragm
26 Solar plexus
27 Liver
28 Adrenal glands
29 Stomach
30 Kidneys
31 Pancreas
32 Spine
33 Ureter tubes
34 Bladder/rectum
35 Sciatic nerve
36 Pelvis

Bottom of feet

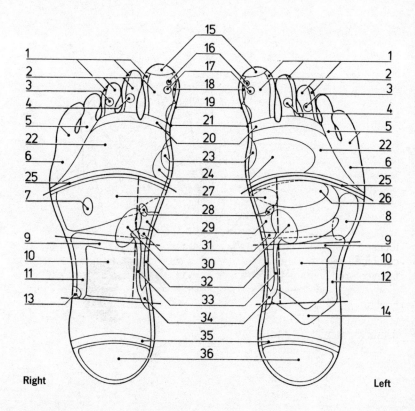

Right   Left

With kind permission of The British School of Reflexology

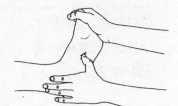

Both feet are treated as a microcosm of the human body: the big toe is the reflex for the head, and the inside edge of the foot represents the spine. Thumb massage and manipulation are employed over the total area of the foot, thereby treating the whole body system. In the case of foot injury, however, treatment can be applied to reflexes on the hand where necessary.

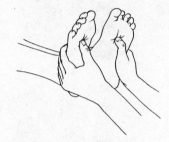

The experience should be relatively painless since the main object is to promote relaxation, thus enabling the body to heal itself. Eunice Ingham also believed that the massage was effective in breaking up crystalline deposits of uric acid, helping to eliminate toxic build-up, though this remains unproven.

A client will be expected to have a number of treatments lasting about 45 minutes until the condition has cleared. Often symptoms will worsen initially, but this is considered indicative that the healing process is under way.

Metamorphic technique, also known as **prenatal therapy**, takes a more metaphysical approach. Focusing on the spinal reflex, practitioners aim to clear psychological blocks which may have rooted themselves in the spine during the gestation period.

Color therapy

The psychological effect of color has played a therapeutic role since ancient times because of its ability to produce direct emotional responses. According to Rudolph Steiner, the founder of modern color therapy, "color is the soul of nature."

Color therapy is based on the concept of the aura, an invisible field which is linked to seven energy centers or *chakras* which interpenetrate the physical body. White light is absorbed from the atmosphere by the aura and split into component color energies to revitalize different parts of the body. This is one explanation of SAD (Seasonal Affective Depression) where winter "blues" have been linked to lack of ultra-violet light.

Color therapy is regarded by some as a subtle art, and employs several different techniques. The auric colors can be seen directly if the therapist views through a Kilner screen which penetrates the UV spectrum. (Some also claim to be able to do this psychically.) Illness manifests as a dark or discolored patch over the affected area.

Therapy may involve use of a color lamp or cabinet, so that the client is either totally bathed in colored light or a particular area of the body focused upon; and color filters (a maximum of three at one time) are combined with rhythm and pattern for greater effect. Drinking water from colored containers that have been exposed to sunlight; eating food of the requisite color; and suitable colors for clothes and the home or work environment may also be suggested. (Blue, for instance, is calming and may reduce blood pressure, while red is energizing and useful for menstrual cramps.)

Color therapy should not be tried without expert advice since wrong combinations can be disturbing both mentally and physically.

© DIAGRAM

Music, art and dance therapy

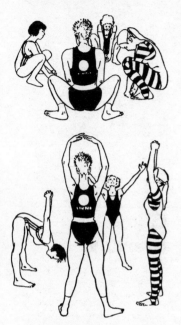

All forms of art are essentially creative and as therapy, they can free the individual from past conditioning. **Art therapy** is carried out by specially trained therapists and psychotherapists of various schools. Clients are encouraged to create spontaneously in a variety of media ranging from wax crayons to modeling clay, and the therapist is on hand to interpret results.

Dance therapy was pioneered by Rudolph Laban (1879–1959). His freer dance forms were designed to promote harmony between body and mind, and to inspire creative interaction between members of a group. Although the nature of dance therapy is as varied as its teachers, great emphasis is generally placed on helping the student to strengthen personal identity through increased awareness of physical body-image. Creative eurythmy, established by Rudolph Steiner, blends movement and vocal sound, and specific exercises are designed to benefit various parts of the body such as the digestive tract, respiratory system and the skin, as well as many psychiatric conditions.

The way in which sound can stir emotions makes **music therapy** an ideal tool for those, particularly the autistic and physically handicapped, whose feelings are blocked by a deep sense of isolation. It is based on improvisation, encouraging the individual to externalize feelings by playing an instrument or using the voice. Participation in a group also inspires a meaningful sense of community.

All three therapies are group-orientated and primarily used to encourage self-expression in the handicapped or psychologically disturbed. But dance, and art therapies in particular, are also popular with those wishing to externalize a problem or to renew contact with their own creative vitality.

Psychic and spiritual healing

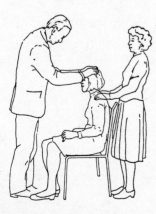

The healing of one person by another has been practiced from earliest times. Despite disapproval from certain elements in both orthodox medicine and many religious bodies, the laying on of hands and absent healing continues.

While in practice there is little to distinguish the psychic from the spiritual healer, they differ philosophically. Spiritual healers believe that healing power comes from God. The psychic healer, however, accepts responsibility for personal powers but claims that these serve to activate the body's own healing processes. But whatever their stance, healers always require the cooperation of the patient to bring about cure. Diagnosis tends to be either clairvoyant or by use of the hands, often an inch or so from the body, to sense areas of heat and cold which in turn may indicate areas of energy imbalance. Treatment can often be sensed as heat, tingling, and surges of energy along the limbs or up the spine.

Many healers are a "last resort" for the apparently incurable: but though there is claimed to be a high rate of cure, depending on the caliber of the healer, do not expect miracles. Failure, it is said, can be due to incompatibility. Often several visits may be required and prescriptions, perhaps involving diet or imaging techniques, must be followed.

But healing can apparently also be practiced at a distance. This is done either by a group or on an individual basis. Some claim to be able to tune into a patient thousands of miles away, and will proceed to describe symptoms and prescribe precise remedies.

Medical **radiesthesia** and **radionics** can also operate at a distance, often relying on a pendulum to diagnose from a blood or hair sample. Practitioners of radiesthesia may prescribe homeopathic or Bach flower remedies; while radionics practitioners claim to be able to cure by transmitting the energy of the selected prescription to the patient simply through the power of thought.

T'ai chi

Often described as meditation in motion, t'ai chi is a complex physical discipline derived from a richly inspirational combination of Taoist, Buddhist and Confucian esoteric teachings. It continues to be studied in the West today for its incalculable benefits as a total physical, spiritual, and mental training.

At the root of t'ai chi is the *chi* or life energy with its subtle divisions of *yin* and *yang*. Practice increases the student's awareness of self-constructed blocks. The result is a dynamic and harmonious combination which blends breathing, circular rhythmic movement, and meditative concentration into an energized and total experience.

The "forms" or series of flowing movements through which the inner being of the student is expressed are modeled on the graceful rhythms of the natural world and have names such as "Grasp the Sparrow's Tail" and "Snake goes down into the Water." The correct traditional long form takes around 25 minutes, though many schools prefer shortened versions of five to ten minutes.

Relaxed and fluid, the forms gently stir the circulation, breath and *chi*, enabling their flow to nourish and balance the body, mind and spirit. Regular practice increases mental clarity, endurance and flexibility; and physical benefits include improved body tone and elasticity (particularly useful in pregnancy), flexible and open joints, and reduction of stress-related symptoms such as high blood pressure. T'ai chi, as with Chinese medicine generally, is most effective as a preventative health measure, and is open to everyone, unless severely disabled.

Commitment to at least 1½ hours each week of group training is essential, as well as daily practice. Like yoga, t'ai chi cannot be taught from a book: a good teacher is all-important.

Yin and yang
According to ancient Chinese belief, the life-force or *chi* moves through our bodies along a number of meridians or paths that connect different organs of the body. Two elements known as *yin* and *yang* (which correspond roughly to female and male or negative and positive forces) are thought to activate the *chi*. While you are in good health, *yin* and *yang* are in perfect harmony; but when you are ill, imbalance occurs. Therapies such as acupuncture and shiatsu aim to correct this, so that *chi* can once again flow freely.

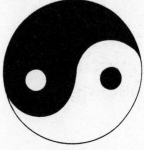

The yin/yang symbol

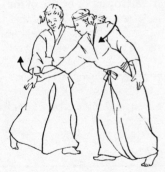
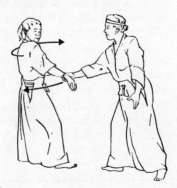

WHAT CAN GO WRONG?

Sometimes, however vigilant you are over health care, illness strikes. What are the symptoms and danger signs? And what can you do to stem the course of such serious conditions as heart disease and cancer, as well as many specifically female complaints and sexually transmitted diseases? All-importantly, too, who should you turn to for advice?

In an age of tremendous stereotype pressures, many disorders also have social roots. What is the true nature of psychosomatic illnesses? How can you allay depression? And what form of therapy might be right in particular circumstances? This is your guide to modern methods of diagnosis and successful treatment.

Chapter four

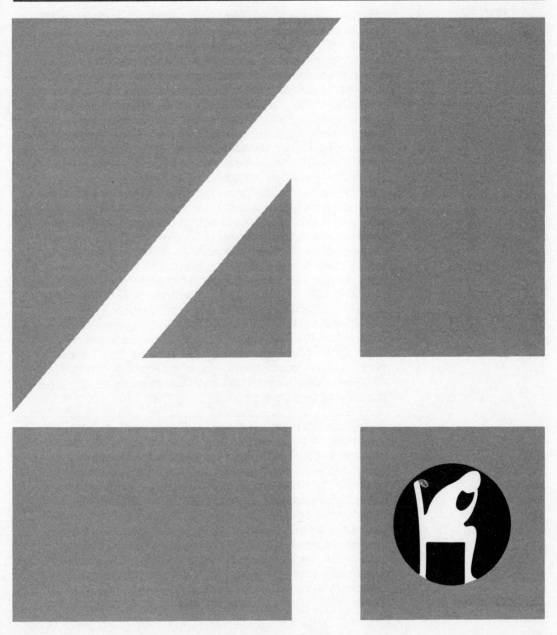

4.01 Physical disorders

Defining illness

When we speak of illness, it is usually the more obvious forms of physical illness that spring to mind – rashes, infections, a damaged organ, and the like. But stress and mental illness are also very common disorders and can have severely disabling effects on those who suffer from them, often for long periods. The physically exhausting results of high levels of stress also demonstrate that mental health has a direct relationship with physical well-being. The way we feel about ourselves, our lives, and our dealings with other people all have a bearing on how we view our bodies. An anorexic whose image of her body is distorted, for example, will try to starve it to make it thinner, and severe depression is often accompanied by self-neglect and loss of sex drive.

A reverse situation may also occur, in which physical conditions influence mental processes. Many women are aware of the emotional effects of changes in hormone levels, manifesting themselves when severe as premenstrual tension or depression following childbirth. Similarly, lack of thyroid hormone is accompanied by feelings of lethargy and depression as well as physical symptoms.

So the boundaries between physical and mental disorder are frequently blurred. This means that doctors can be misled, either by factitious physical "signs" or the apparent lack of them, and it is not easy if we are feeling unwell to sort out what is likely to be the root of the problem. No health guide can hope to describe all the ailments that afflict us: the following pages outline some of the more common physical disorders (including diagnosis and established forms of treatment), dependencies, factors which commonly result in stress, and psychological disorders.

INFECTIONS

Infections can be caused by a wide variety of organisms. Sometimes the organism is already present in the body but normally causes no symptoms and only gives trouble if it gets into the wrong place, or if immunity is lowered or the body's chemistry changes, allowing it to flourish. For example, the yeast **candida** often proliferates during pregnancy and after antibiotic treatment, causing the condition of **thrush** or **moniliasis**. Many acute diseases are also caused by invading organisms; and infection may be limited to the site of entry and surrounding tissues, as in a boil, or it may spread widely as a "systemic" illness. The body's response to infection depends on the immune system (see pp. 58–59).

VIRUSES

These tiny organisms rely for survival on an ability to penetrate the cells of a host, where they then utilize the host cells' own systems for their multiplication. Replicated viruses leave the damaged cell and invade further cells, thus spreading the infection. Illnesses caused by viruses include the **common cold**, **influenza**, **measles**, **rubella**, **herpes**, **chickenpox**, **mumps** and **AIDS**. Some viruses, such as herpes, are capable of lying dormant after initial infection only for symptoms to reappear after some triggering incident. The chickenpox virus is responsible for the painful condition of **shingles**, experienced often decades after the original infection. Viral infections can also pass through the placenta, and an illness which is mild to the mother (such as **German measles** or **rubella**) may be very serious to her unborn baby. Research has even implicated certain viral infections in specific types of cancer, but it is often unclear whether the virus is a cause or a "co-factor" (only one of several combined causes).

Vaccines have been created to prevent infection by the more common, most dangerous viruses, though vaccine development is a time-consuming and costly process. The numerous strains of virus causing the common cold and the illness' relative mildness make vaccination impracticable, but vaccination against the most prevalent influenza strains can be offered each year to groups at risk of severe infection, such as the elderly.

Antibiotic drugs are useless against viral infections, though they may combat any opportunistic bacteria causing secondary infections. Antiviral drugs are few, the problem being the close relationship between the virus and the host's cells. If powerful enough to kill viruses, the drug is liable to damage the body's cells as well. However some available drugs work principally by slowing down the virus' rate of replication. Interferon is a substance having this effect and is actually produced by the body's own cells to combat the virus.

COURSE OF INFECTION

All infections involve the same basic process – invasion by a foreign organism, and the body's response – so all tend to show a common pattern (though the stages are more obvious in an acute illness). The process is as follows.

1. Incubation, beginning with the movement of infection. The organisms multiply inside the body.

2. Prodrome, a short interval of generalized symptoms (such as headache, fever, nasal discharge, irritability, and other feelings of illness). The infection at this stage is usually very communicable to others – but diagnosis is difficult.

3. Peak, when illness is at its height. Each infection shows its own characteristic symptoms. Temperature is at its highest, and the rash appears where relevant.

4. Termination, the end of the illness, marked either by a period of 12 to 48 hours in which the symptoms rapidly disappear or by a more gradual termination.

5. Convalescence, after the illness, the patient regains health and strength.

BACTERIA

Bacteria are larger than viruses and can survive and reproduce without invading a host's cells. They are present in soil and water, on and in food, and live on our skin and in our bodies. Some of them are beneficial – for example, Vitamin K is manufactured by bacteria living in the intestines. However, certain kinds of bacteria in the wrong parts of the body, can cause severe illness. Symptoms of illnesses caused by these microorganisms are frequently consistent with their mode of entry into the body. **Cholera** and **salmonella** germs are swallowed in water and food, respectively, causing diarrhea; **typhoid**, though it enters the body by the same route, results in a more general illness with fever. Many germs get into the body via the respiratory system – **tuberculosis**, **whooping cough**, **Legionnaires' disease**, **diphtheria**, **bacterial meningitis** and **tonsillitis** are caused by a variety of bacteria invading by this route. Sometimes the organism itself is not harmful but produces a toxin or poison which can be lethal, as in **diphtheria** and **tetanus.**

Antibiotic drugs are effective against most of these germs, but because of often indiscriminate and incorrect use, many microorganisms have developed resistance to certain antibiotics. If you are prescribed an antibiotic drug, it is most important that you finish all the medication, unless you feel that it is not working or you suffer side-effects, in which case you should consult your physician.

Vaccination is available against diseases such as **tuberculosis**. The injection contains weakened organisms which do no harm but are capable of stimulating the body to produce antibodies. If a germ causes illness through its toxin, an altered non-harmful toxoid can be given to program the body's defences.

INFECTIOUS MONONUCLEOSIS (GLANDULAR FEVER)

Also known as the "kissing disease" because it is sometimes thought to be spread in that way (although this is not certain), mononucleosis can have a variety of symptoms, including swollen glands and a fever. It is often mistaken for flu, but sometimes a rash also develops, as may jaundice. It is not in itself a cause for concern but it may run a protracted course, or occasionally recur in the immediate convalescent phase. Antibiotics will not help because, like flu, it is a viral infection.

YEASTS AND FUNGI

Several kinds of yeasts and fungi can live on the human body, and many people carry the **candida** yeast in their digestive system. Common infections caused by yeasts and fungi include **thrush**, **athlete's foot** (**tinea pedis**) and **ringworm**. There are effective antifungal drugs.

PROTOZOA

These are tiny one-celled animals, often living a parasitic existence in an animal host. They may be passed on in food and water, as in **amoebic dysentery**; by contact with animal feces; by insect bite (**malaria**) or by sexual contact (**trichomoniasis**). Drugs are available to treat these infections.

FOOD POISONING

The diagram shows the course of a gastrointestinal infection as a result of food poisoning. Salmonella and other germs may well be present in uncooked foods such as chicken; and refrigerated storage at a suitable temperature (below 5°C or 41°F) and thorough defrosting prior to thorough cooking are therefore vital. Different foods (that is, raw meat, fish, dairy products and cooked foods) should also be stored separately to avoid contamination from one to another.

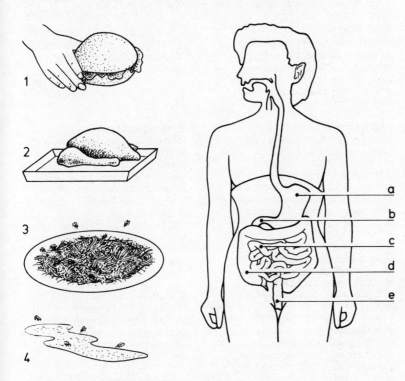

Gastrointestinal infections
1 Infected food handled
2 Undercooked food contaminated
3 Flies
4 Polluted water

a Stomach
b Certain germs may enter bloodstream
c Multiplication of bacteria in small intestine causing diarrhea
d Large intestine
e Germs can be passed on to others through infected feces in unhygienic conditions

WORMS

Humans can be infected by worms and flukes of all sizes, from the large tapeworm to the tiny flukes which cause **bilharzia**. Part of the parasite's life cycle may be spent in another animal host, such as the pig, and the infection acquired by eating uncooked or undercooked infested meat. **Toxocariasis** affects children who take in the worm eggs found in cat and dog feces. Small worms, like threadworms which remain in the intestines, do little harm, but those which invade the bloodstream and tissues can cause serious illness. There are effective drugs to treat worm infestations.

MITES AND INSECTS

Insects in the environment are important carriers of diseases such as **malaria** and **plague**, but actual infestations are few. The most common in developed countries are **scabies**, **nits**, **fleas** and **pubic lice**, all of which can be treated satisfactorily.

©DIAGRAM

Symptoms guide

Periodic changes brought about by female sex hormones and the extensive body area taken up in women by the breasts and reproductive tract help to give rise to many (mostly minor) symptoms suffered only after puberty. The hormonal changes that usher in the menopause can cause further problems. For various reasons, women also suffer more than men from migraine, gall bladder troubles and some other conditions such as fainting and varicose veins. This chart stresses symptoms related to female problems, but includes some symptoms caused by ailments also found in men or children.

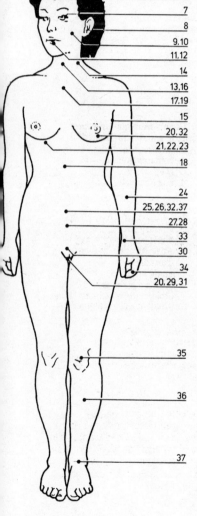

1, 2, 3
4, 5, 6
7
8
9, 10
11, 12
14
13, 16
17, 19
15
20, 32
21, 22, 23
18
24
25, 26, 32, 37
27, 28
33
30
34
20, 29, 31
35
36
37

1 Headaches
Women may suffer premenstrual, menstrual, or tension headaches, or migraine. Most headaches have minor significance, but new or severe types should be investigated.

2 Dizziness
Migraine, the contraceptive pill, toxemia of pregnancy, the menopause and anemia may produce dizzy spells. Rising after kneeling can also make you dizzy. Dizziness can mean ear, heart or circulation problems, brain injury or heat exhaustion.

3 Fainting
Women faint more easily than men, for instance in stuffy rooms, in early pregnancy, or when suffering from emotional stress or anemia.

4 Fatigue
Premenstrual tension, emotional disturbances, the menopause, infections, diabetes, anemia and hypo-thyroidism all produce fatigue.

5 Depression
Childbirth, job loss, bereavement or organic disease, marriage problems or the menopause may all be to blame.

6 High temperature
Many infectious diseases and chest and kidney infections produce high temperatures, but the height of a temperature during illness is not necessarily an indication of the severity of the illness, since a high fever often implies good bodily resistance to the disease. However, a doctor should be called if the fever is prolonged. Appendicitis, blood-poisoning, bronchitis, chickenpox, croup, gastroenteritis, German measles (rubella), influenza, measles, mumps, roseola, sinusitis, tonsillitis and whooping cough may all be accompanied by a fever.

7 Blurred vision
Nearsightedness, farsightedness, migraine, and toxemia of pregnancy can all blur vision, as may various disorders of the eye, kidney or pancreas.

8 Earache
Ear, nose or throat infection or injury to the eardrum (perhaps the result of an explosion, deep diving, or a sudden blow) can all cause earache.

9 Pallor
Blood loss due to piles or menstrual flow can cause pallor, as may shock and heart attack, anemia, motion (travel) sickness and blood loss.

10 Discoloration
Liver and gall bladder diseases produce jaundice; and bruising produces skin discoloration. Addison's disease browns skin on the knees, elbows and knuckles; and heart or lung disease may tinge the lips and face blue.

11 Thirst
Anemia, dehydration, diabetes and certain poisons are among factors that produce excessive thirst.

12 Toothache
Impacted wisdom teeth and tooth decay (a risk in pregnancy), and severe throat and nose infections may all produce pain that seems to be located in the jaw.

13 Sore throat
This may be due to the common cold, pharyngitis, laryngitis, tonsillitis and also (more rarely) quinsy, syphilis and cancer.

14 Stiff neck
This may be due to arthritis, neck injury or slipped disk. Other common causes are sleeping awkwardly, exposure to cold, and tonsillitis.

15 Swollen glands
Swollen glands in the neck, armpits, or groin indicate infection; mononucleosis (glandular fever) causes swollen glands in many parts of the body; and some cancers may cause swollen glands nearby.

16 Hoarseness
Laryngitis, upper respiratory tract infections, benign tumors and cancer of the larynx or esophagus can all make someone hoarse. Hoarseness persisting for two weeks should be investigated.

17 Coughing
Colds, smoking, asthma, bronchitis, pneumonia and other respiratory conditions or irritants make people cough. A persistent cough should definitely be investigated.

18 Backache
This is sometimes linked with menstruation, pregnancy, the menopause or a prolapsed uterus. Other causes may be strained muscles, a slipped disk, fatigue, depression, stress and other emotional problems.

19 Breathlessness
Obesity, heart trouble, asthma, lung disease, anxiety, chronic bronchitis, pneumonia, a perforated ulcer and high altitudes may all cause breathlessness.

20 Discharge
Benign cysts and breast cancer may produce nipple discharge. Unusual vaginal discharge suggests infection or possibly a cervical or uterine tumor. Ear discharge often indicates a perforated eardrum. The common cold, hay fever and sinusitis yield nasal discharge.

21 Indigestion
Gall bladder trouble, pregnancy, the menopause, emotional stress, overindulgence in food or alcohol, hasty eating, bad teeth, hiatus hernia, constipation and appendicitis can all cause indigestion.

22 Nausea and vomiting
Migraine, early pregnancy and some infections cause these symptoms. Food poisoning, dyspepsia, infections and alcohol abuse are also likely to produce nausea and vomiting.

23 Loss of appetite
Anorexia nervosa, depressive illness, menopause or intestinal infection may be to blame.

24 Rashes
Rashes of special significance to women include those produced by rosacea and German measles (rubella).

25 Stomach ache
This may accompany menstruation or be due to food poisoning or disease inside the genital tract. Agonizing cramps radiating to back and shoulder may mean gallstone trouble. Gastrointestinal inflammation and salt deficiency are also possible causes.

26 Painful periods
Hormonal changes in the uterus and sometimes diseased reproductive organs cause these.

27 Constipation
This often coincides with painful periods, pregnancy and childbirth. Lack of exercise and insufficent roughage in the diet are common causes of constipation; only rarely the problem may be a bowel obstruction.

28 Diarrhea
This may be caused by infection, certain drugs, eating foods that disagree with you, or gastrointestinal disease.

29 Flatulence
Belching or passing wind may indicate air-swallowing or disease of the digestive tract.

30 Itching
Itchy genitals may mean infection or pelvic infestation. Other skin irritations may be due to allergy.

31 Painful urination
This may mean urinary tract infection, bladder stones, or inflammation of the vagina or vulva.

32 Aches and pains
These range from minor muscle problems to arthritis. Women are liable to pains in the breast, lower back and abdomen.

33 Pulse changes
Normal heartbeat for women is 70-80, slower in old age. Rapid heartbeat (tachycardia) often occurs in menstruation, pregnancy and menopause. High blood pressure and fever may raise the rate. Extra beats, missed beats and a slow pulse seldom indicate disease.

34 Trembling
Anxiety, cold, fear, drugs and old age may all produce trembling.

35 Stiff joints
Stiff knees and hips may signal osteoarthritis. Rheumatoid arthritis also affects many joints.

36 Aching legs
Obesity makes legs ache. Cramping leg pains may be caused by painful periods or varicose veins.

37 Swelling
Premenstrual tension, the contraceptive pill, toxemia of pregnancy and kidney trouble can cause general edema. Pregnancy and ovarian cysts may also cause swelling of the abdomen.

©DIAGRAM

Diagnosis

On first seeing a patient who is ill, the physician has to make an informed guess about the nature of the illness in order to select an appropriate technique which will provide quick and accurate confirmation of the diagnosis. The techniques below are described in connection with their role in diagnosing female complaints but are also used for a wide range of illnesses.

Blood tests

A small sample of blood tested in the pathology laboratory can provide extensive information. Blood cell counts and smears indicate the presence of anemia or other bleeding disorders; microorganisms can be identified; immunity to certain infections assessed; and levels of sugars, hormones and other chemicals measured.

Urine tests

Urine can be analyzed to detect the presence and nature of any infection in the kidneys and urinary tract. The presence of a protein called "albumin" indicates that the kidneys are damaged and failing to carry out their role of filtering the blood. Untreated or uncontrolled diabetics have large amounts of sugar in their urine, and pregnant women are given urine tests to screen for diabetes.

Body fluids

Sputum and other discharges, cerebrospinal fluid, stomach contents and sweat can all provide useful information in certain illnesses. Microorganisms contained in the fluid can be made to grow (cultured) under laboratory conditions and their susceptibility to antibiotic drugs assessed.

Smears

Microscopic examination of smears containing cells from a suspect lesion (injury), growth or ulcer gives valuable data on the cause. Cervical smears from the cervix are easily obtained and are valuable screening for cancerous and precancerous conditions.

Biopsy

In this procedure, a piece of tissue is taken so that the cells can be examined under a microscope for signs of abnormality. Some organs such as the liver, lung and breast can be biopsied using an instrument like a large hypodermic needle, without the need for surgery. Biopsies of the respiratory and digestive tracts can be taken during endoscopy with tiny cutting devices incorporated in the endoscope. When the surgeon has obtained a sample of tissue, smears or sections are examined for signs of abnormality while the patient is still in theater. When the biopsy results are known, the surgeon can decide on treatment.

X rays

Radiography has been a valuable medical tool for nearly a century and its uses have been continually refined and enhanced. Mammography (see p.131) is increasingly being used as a screening technique for breast cancer. Apart from the slight discomfort of having the breasts squeezed between two plastic plates, the procedure is painless and harmless and uses a low dose of X rays. Contrast X rays, in which an opaque fluid is injected into the appropriate area to give a clear outline, are sometimes used for the investigation of infertility to detect blockage of the Fallopian tubes or malformations of the uterus. If you need to have an X ray, you should always be asked whether or not you are pregnant, as exposure to radiation can harm the fetus.

Cat scans

The CAT (computerized axial tomography) scanner creates detailed pictures of "slices" of the head or body by sending out beams of X rays and measuring the amount absorbed in the tissues. The clear images obtained aid the specialist or surgeon: for example, a tumor looks very different from a fluid-filled cyst.

Radioisotope imaging

Certain body organs take up particular elements: the thyroid gland, for instance, absorbs iodine to synthesize one of its hormones. Radioactive isotopes of iodine and other elements can be injected into the bloodstream and, after a few hours, a special scanner measures their emissions. Useful information is thus obtained about the organ's functioning.

Ultrasound

This diagnostic technique is widely used in gynecology. As it employs high-frequency sound waves, it is considered to be a much safer imaging method than radiography, particularly during pregnancy. Sound waves emitted by a hand-held transducer placed against the skin pass into the tissues and are reflected back by the internal structures to be received by the transducer. A computer builds up a picture from the data and can display it on a screen or print it. (See p.324.)

Magnetic resonance imaging

Like the CAT scan, this technique provides detailed pictures of "slices" through the body but it utilizes a powerful electromagnetic field rather than X rays.

Thermography

A heat-sensitive camera builds up a picture showing hot and cold spots in the body. Areas which should normally be cool but show up as hot may indicate problems such as inflammation or a tumor.

Endoscopy

This literally means "looking inside." **Colposcopy**, a routine gynecological procedure in which a colposcope is inserted into the vagina to enable examination of the cervix, is a simple form of endoscopy. Most people, however, think of endoscopy in terms of more complex procedures such as **gastroscopy** (looking inside the stomach); **cystoscopy** (the bladder); **sigmoidoscopy** (the lower intestine); or **hysteroscopy** (the uterus). These techniques involve passing an endoscope (a usually flexible tube containing fiber-optic light filaments, suction devices and tiny cutting tools) through one of the body orifices. Endoscopy is usually carried out with the patient under mild sedation or with the use of anesthetics.

Gynecological and obstetric examinations

Examinations likely to be performed at a well-woman clinic are described on p.130, and standard tests at an antenatal clinic on p.315.

Urinary disorders

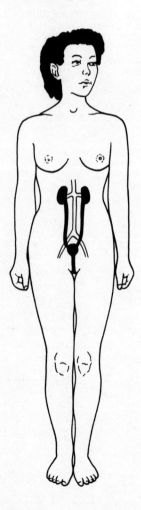

SYMPTOMS

For a doctor, the urine and urination are among the most useful signs of disorder, relating sometimes not just to the urinary system, but to the general health of the body.

Characteristics of urination that may interest a doctor include changes in quantity and frequency (including rising at night; slow and weak, or unusually forceful flow; stopping and starting, and dribbling; difficulty in beginning or continuing; inability to restrain (incontinence); sudden stopping; and, of course, pain or other unusual sensations on urinating, or inability to urinate at all.

Characteristics of the urine that may be of interest include unusual color, odor, cloudiness, frothiness, and content. Abnormal chemical content can include albumin (which may indicate kidney disorder) or sugar (indicative of diabetes). Chemical testing can be carried out very easily, using a treated paper that changes color when moistened with urine. Other abnormal contents can include bacteria, parasites, kidney tube casts, bile pigment, and especially blood or pus. However, many unusual characteristics of the urine or urination will more usually be due to insignificant causes than to disorder. For example, having to get up from bed to urinate is often due to drinking tea or coffee last thing at night. Strikingly unusual colors can also be produced just by certain medicines and foods.

Other symptoms of disorder include itching, redness, or stickiness at the urethral opening; discharge or fluid from the urethra; pain or swelling in the area of the kidneys, and shivering, temperature, or fever.

TYPES OF DISORDER

Infection can reach the urinary system in two ways: "downward," via the bloodstream and then the kidneys; or "upward," via the urethral opening in the genitals. An example of the first can be tuberculosis. But the second is much more common, and especially in women because the closeness of anus and urethral opening helps bacteria pass between them and because the shortness of the female urethra allows bacteria to reach the higher parts of the tract more easily.

Most bacteria entering the tract from outside are killed by the urine; but 5% of women (both adults and children) do have active bacteria in the bladder. Often there are no symptoms. If there are, frequency of urination and pain on urinating are typical. Diagnosis is by bacteriological examination of a urine sample. Treatment is with an antibiotic.

Inflammation of the tract is mostly caused by infection, but also by dietary irritation due to alcohol, and perhaps food allergy; use of chemicals (vaginal deodorants, contraceptive foams, etc); and tissue damage during sexual activity, childbirth, or surgery. Inflammation of the urethra is called "urethritis," and that of the bladder "cystitis" (see p.172). Symptoms again include pain on urinating. Treatment depends on the cause, but drinking large quantities of fluid usually helps.

Flow abnormality includes obstruction of flow, complete or incomplete and apparently normal flow that nevertheless leaves stagnant pools of urine in the tract. Causes include blockage by extraneous objects such as stones or blood clots; malfunction of the tract itself through congenital malformation, tumors and other growths or tissue changes, or temporary spasm; and outside pressure on the tract (perhaps from fibroids, a displaced uterus, or pregnancy).

Stagnant urine is always a likely site for infection. Where there is flow blockage as well, pressure builds up behind the obstruction, and that section of the tract may be stretched and dilated. Eventually, the pressure and dilation may reach back up the ureter toward the kidneys. Kidney infection may result, and rapid surgical treatment is needed before the kidneys suffer permanent damage.

Urinary problems
1 Normal tract
2 Obstructions
3 Sites of infection

Obstructions include
a Stones
b Strictures
c Tumors
d Blood clots
e Foreign bodies, and
f TB fibrosis or external pressure from
g Pregnancy
h Tumors and
i Congenitally displaced arteries
Infections include
j TB
k Kidney infection
Bacteria may be
l In the bladder
m In stagnant or obstructed urine
n In stones
o In foreign bodies
p In structural inflammations

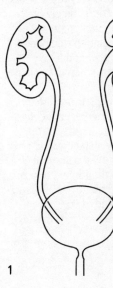
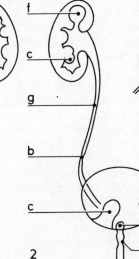
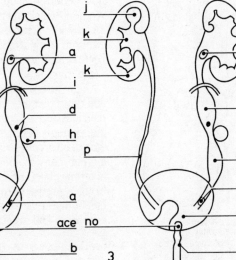

Incontinence

This is inability to control urination. For incontinence in the old, see p.390; but it also occurs in younger women. Causes include psychological stress; disorders of the bladder; congenital defects; tissue damage occurring as a result of childbirth or surgery; and impairment of the nerves due to injury or disease. Two types are fairly common: urge incontinence occurs where there is a shortened time gap between the desire to urinate and uncontrollable urination. (this is experienced quite often by women over 40); and stress incontinence, typified by small amounts of urine escaping when the person strains, coughs, or laughs – whether the bladder is full or virtually empty. This is usually only seen in post-menopausal women; and special exercises, or sometimes surgery, are needed.

KIDNEY DISORDERS

These include congenital defects; tumors, or stones; damage through injury; inflammation without infection; and infection.

Infection is especially common in women. It can arrive via the bloodstream or the urinary system. In acute attacks, bacterial infection via the urinary tract is typical. Symptoms are shivering and fever, acute pain in the loins or under the ribs at the back, and frequent urination. Qualified medical attention is vital, as are prescribed antibiotics, bed rest, and plenty of fluids. Long-term infection may follow acute infection, or arise from urinary obstruction or blood-borne infection. (Stones are frequent sites.) Treatment depends on causes. In neglected cases, kidney damage may result, with possible high blood pressure and blood poisoning.

CYSTITIS

Strictly, this means inflammation of the bladder. However, the term is now generally used for a certain collection of symptoms, usually in women, which can arise in a variety of ways. The main symptoms of an attack of acute cystitis are great frequency of urination (perhaps every few minutes); pain on urination – often extreme; and a recurrent or even continuous desire to urinate, even when there is no urine to pass.

As the attack continues, there may also be increasing incontinence, and often blood in the urine. Other associated symptoms can include pain just above the pubic bone, or in the loins; and a foul smell from, and perhaps debris in, the urine. Extreme pain may also be felt if sexual intercourse is attempted. This syndrome is very common; a great many women suffer from it at some time in their lives, and it is often recurrent and hard to eradicate. In its extreme forms, it can bring depression, disrupted career and home life, and even (since it can both derive from sexual intercourse and interfere with it) broken emotional and marital relationships.

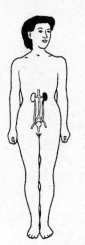
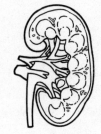
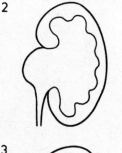
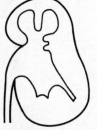

Kidney problems
1 Normal kidney
2 Kidney damaged by back pressure
3 Kidney damaged by infection

CAUSES OF CYSTITIS

There are two main alternative causes: infection or inflammation without infection (which may also set in later).

Infection is usually by Escherichia coli (E. coli), bacteria from the rectum, finding their way into the urethral opening. E. coli are often found on the perineum (the skin between anus and genitals.) Their progress toward the vulva is often helped by careless use of toilet paper or by sexual activity (petting, or just the movement of the penis.) Other sources of infection are cross-infection from the vagina (as in candidiasis, trichomoniasis, or gonorrhea); lack of male hygiene or infections from the kidneys that pass downward.

Infections may be aided by stones; stagnant pools of urine due to retention; lowered resistance, as in anemia; and (for bacteria preferring non-acidic urine) diabetes.

Inflammation
In cystitis, the normal cause (apart from infection) is bruising or skin cracking through sexual activity. Relevant here are frequency of intercourse (hence "honeymoon cystitis"); insufficient lubrication; use of certain positions (depending on the individuals); and over-forceful petting. Other relevant causes are tissue irritation through use of vaginal deodorants, foam contraceptives, or unsuitable lubricants; strain on the bladder due to prolapse of the uterus; damage through childbirth or surgery; and possibly allergic reaction of the urinary tract to certain foods.

Inflammation can, in turn, provide a breeding ground for infection (and an entry for infection into the bloodstream).

Chronic cystitis
Repeated attacks of acute cystitis may involve long-term tissue changes, including changes in the urethra due to the menopause, and changes in the bladder lining from bacterial or other infection. Occasionally, there may be psychological factors involved too.

INVESTIGATIONS

The sufferer should always see a doctor and always try to get proper tests made to pinpoint the cause. The first step should be laboratory testing of a urine sample for infection and (if present) during treatment. The patient should drink before going to the doctor, so as to be ready to pass urine for this test. A clean sample is important: the vulva should be swabbed, and only a small midstream sample (that is, from halfway through urination) taken into a sterile container. During menstruation, a tube (catheter) inserted by the doctor into the urethra should be used. The patient may also be able to give useful information, such as the amount of time between the attack and the last previous intercourse. (Cystitis due to inflammation alone will follow intercourse sooner than that due to infection, since bacteria need time to multiply.)

Unfortunately, estimates vary from "very soon after" for inflammation and "12-24 hours after" for infection, to "24 hours after" for inflammation and "36 hours after" for infection. If no infection is found, or if it fails to clear after a course of drugs, hospital investigation may be needed, and may include physical examination by a specialist; taking of bacteria samples from vagina and perineum; early morning urine samples; blood samples; X rays of the urinary tract, often using injections of dye into the bloodstream to show up obstructions, or introducing dye into the bladder to show its action; and cystoscopy, which is the surgical inspection of the inside of the urethra and bladder, using a "periscope tube" inserted into the urethra under general anesthetic.

Urinary tract X rays
The diagrams show "intravenous pyelograms" (IVPs). These X rays of the urinary tract are taken after iodine dye has been injected into the bloodstream. The iodine passes out through the urinary system.
1 IVP showing normal functioning of the kidneys and urinary tract.
2 IVP showing blockage in one ureter, distention above the blockage, and a growth in the bladder.

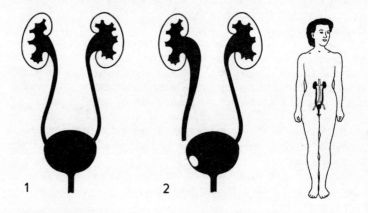

1   2

TREATMENT
Depending on the cause of the trouble, treatment may include antibiotics and similar drugs to combat urinary and/or kidney infection; increase of the patient's fluid intake; drugs to relax the muscles of the bladder; drugs to combat vaginal infection; hormone therapy to restore mucus and tissue characteristics; surgery for urinary blockages; or surgery to deal with other causes of inflammation (such as repair for a prolapsed uterus).

When on a course of drugs, the symptoms may vanish soon after starting the course or there may be side-effects (such as nausea or depression). But it is very important to finish the whole course or to consult a doctor if serious side-effects occur.

Drinking a Vitamin C source may be requested to bring urinal acidity into a range where the drug works best.

SELF-HELP
At the first hint of trouble, pass a urine specimen into a sterile container for the doctor; drink 1pt (½liter) of cold water; take a mild painkiller; lie or sit down with two hot water bottles, one against the back, one (wrapped in a towel) high between the legs; drink ½pt (¼liter) of water, diluted fruit juice, or barley water, every 20 minutes; use diuretic pills if prescribed; and after urination, wash the skin between anus and vulva, and dab dry. After half an hour, the attack should begin to ease.

Menstrual disorders

PREMENSTRUAL SYNDROME (PMS)

For many women, the imminent arrival of a period is heralded by a variety of unpleasant symptoms. These comprise headaches, bloating, irritability, depression, breast tenderness and nausea. Hormone treatment in the form of progesterone may be prescribed in severe cases, particularly when tension and depression cause disruption of normal life; and effective self-help measures include alterations in diet and supplements of pyridoxine (Vitamin B_6) or evening primrose oil. Diuretic (water-reducing) drugs should be used with caution for, while they help to reduce bloating, they can have side-effects.

PAINFUL PERIODS (DYSMENORRHEA)

Cramp-like abdominal pains sometimes occur during menstruation, especially in young women. There may also be diarrhea and nausea. The cause is thought to be excessive contraction of the muscular wall of the uterus. Anti-prostaglandin and pain-killing drugs may be prescribed in severe cases. Self-help treatments include herbal remedies (such as raspberry leaf and peppermint teas), heat applications, massage, relaxation techniques, and over-the-counter drugs such as aspirin. Cramping dysmenorrhea often disappears after pregnancy; but if it starts for the first time in older women, pelvic inflammatory disease or endometriosis may be the underlying cause.

IRREGULARITY

Menstruation is often irregular during adolescence. But in a mature woman, disturbance of a previously regular cycle may be caused by some of the factors which also cause amenorrhea (see *below*). The menopause is also frequently heralded by irregular periods.

ABSENCE OF PERIODS (AMENORRHEA)

There are two types of amenorrhea – primary and secondary. Primary amenorrhea (not having had a period by age 18) may be an aspect of delayed puberty, chromosomal abnormality, or a congenital defect of the reproductive tract. Secondary amenorrhea is the term used to describe absence of periods in a woman who has already begun to menstruate. This is, of course, normal in pregnancy. However, secondary amenorrhea can also be caused by emotional stress, endocrine disorders, weight loss, the Pill or injectable progestogens, drug-taking, or poor general health.

UNUSUAL BLEEDING

Spotting between periods sometimes occurs at the time of ovulation. If it happens at other times, it should be investigated. **Heavy periods** have many possible causes – IUDs, hormonal imbalance, fibroids, polyps, pelvic inflammatory disease, endometriosis, hormonal methods of contraception, or cancer. Occasionally there is no detectable cause. Self-help measures include a diet rich in vitamins, fiber and iron to prevent anemia. A D&C may be performed.
Breakthrough bleeding describes bleeding which takes place during use of hormonal contraceptives (but not the withdrawal bleeding experienced by users of the combined Pill). It may be a sign that the method is not fully effective and should be reported.

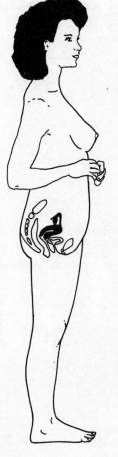

©DIAGRAM

Uterine disorders

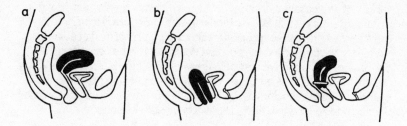

Prolapse (right)
a Normal uterus
b Prolapsed uterus
c With pessary

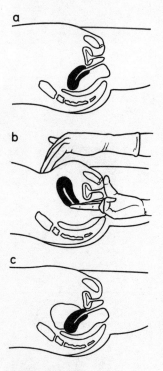

Prolapse of the uterus is a not uncommon condition in which the uterus sags down into the vagina, and may even protrude out between the legs. The symptoms include frequent and difficult urination; incontinence; vaginal discharge; low backache; a feeling that something is coming out of the vagina; and, especially, that all the above symptoms immediately disappear on lying down. The condition is produced by weakening of muscles that support the uterus. The cause is usually damage in childbirth: 99% of women with prolapsed wombs have given birth. But aging and heavy physical activity also contribute, and the symptoms often appear only after the menopause, when the affected muscles may lose tone and ligaments atrophy. Mild cases require no treatment, but more serious or troublesome ones need a pessary inserted by a doctor, or sometimes surgery.

RETROVERSION

In most women, from puberty on, the upper end of the uterus is tilted forward in the body, and moves backward only as the bladder fills or when the woman lies on her back. But in about 10% of women, the uterus is always retroverted (tilted backward). Once blamed for many ailments, in fact this may be troublesome only in pregnancy, when the enlarging uterus may fail to rise into the abdomen. Urine retention in the bladder results. A doctor can usually correct the situation by hand. Untreated, it could cause cystitis, and even miscarriage. Retroversion can also start after childbirth. Doctors disagree whether this can cause backache. If it seems very troublesome, surgery is needed. Other causes can include pelvic tumors (such as ovarian cysts) and connective tissue joining to other structures. Surgery can deal with these if necessary.

Retroversion
a Retroverted uterus
b Manual correction
c Retroversion due to a fibroid

ENDOMETRIOSIS

Endometrial cells can grow in the wrong place, forming cysts in the uterus muscle, the ovaries, or other parts of the pelvis. This is most common in unmarried or infertile women in their thirties. On menstruation, these cells bleed a little, so the cyst swells, causing pain in the lower abdomen, especially before or at the end of menstruation, and sometimes pain on intercourse. Where ovaries or Fallopian tubes are blocked, infertility results. Treatment may be with hormones or surgery.

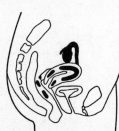

Endometriosis
Typical endometriosis sites

FIBROIDS

These are lumps of fibrous tissue, growing in the muscle wall of the uterus, sometimes singly, sometimes in large groups, usually pea-sized, but occasionally as large as grapefruits. They occur in about 20% of women over 30, especially the infertile, the sexually inactive, and those who only bear children late in life (also, for some unknown reason, in black women more than white). Their cause is unknown, but it may be hormonal. Most give no trouble and need no treatment. Large ones can cause pain, heavy and irregular menstrual bleeding, womb enlargement that interferes with urination and bowel action, and infertility through spontaneous abortion. They can usually be removed by surgery, but in extreme cases hysterectomy is necessary. Long-term emotional stress can also enlarge the uterus and give heavy periods. This has occasionally resulted in unnecessary surgery. **Polyps** are another type of lump, developing from mucus tissue and forming dangling shapes: they are usually harmless.

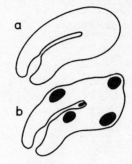

Fibroids
a Normal uterus
b Uterus with fibroids

DILATATION AND CURETTAGE

Also known as "D&C," this involves enlargement of the cervical opening, using dilators; and gentle scraping of the uterine wall with a metal curette. It is used to diagnose cancer, or causes of abnormal bleeding or discharge; to clear waste from incomplete delivery or abortion; to help fertility; to cause abortion and, sometimes, as routine preparation for gynecological surgery.

Anesthesia is needed. Recovery takes 6 hours – 2 days.

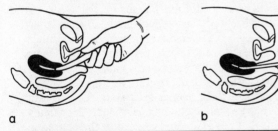

a   b

D&C
a Enlargement of the cervical opening
b Scraping of the uterine wall

HYSTERECTOMY

This is surgical removal of the uterus (womb). It can be **subtotal** (removal of the uterus except for the cervix); **total** (removal of uterus and cervix); or **radical** (removal of uterus, surrounding tissue, and part of the vagina). With any of these, the ovaries and Fallopian tubes may also be removed.

If the uterus is not enlarged by disease, removal can be via the vagina. Otherwise, an incision is necessary: a vertical one below the navel or a horizontal one just above the pubic region. The operation takes less than an hour.

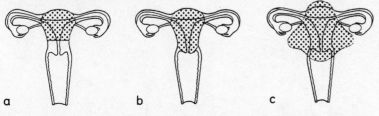

a   b   c

Hysterectomy

░░░ Area removed

a Subtotal
b Total
c Radical

© DIAGRAM

Possible reasons for hysterectomy
a Fibrosis
b Endometriosis
c Cancer or pre-cancer
d Heavy periods

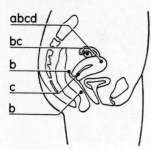

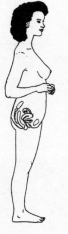

WHY A HYSTERECTOMY?

In the USA, 25% of all women aged 50 and over have had hysterectomies. The diagram shows some valid reasons for the operations; but very often it occurs for no good reason (as for removal of small fibroids). Some doctors even favor routine hysterectomy once childbearing is over, to forestall any risk of cancer; but many others view this as a surgical racket or unnecessary. Some American doctors have also urged hysterectomy as combined abortion and sterilization for poor women with large families. But again, most doctors are against this, because hysterectomy within 13 weeks of conception can endanger the mother's life and the patient may not be able to have the hormone therapy necessary to combat the resulting severe menopausal depression if the ovaries also are removed.

PHYSICAL AFTER-EFFECTS

Following a hysterectomy, menstruation ends immediately, and with it fertility and the need for contraception. Subtotal hysterectomy usually has no effect on the libido. With other forms, some women claim loss of sexual pleasure. Some also complain of shortened vaginas. If the ovaries remain, female hormone production continues. If they have been removed, severe menopausal symptoms may result. Hormone therapy may be given to combat these. Obesity does not follow hysterectomy unless the patient eats too much and exercises too little (but psychological factors may encourage this).

PSYCHOLOGICAL AFTER-EFFECTS

A hysterectomy affects women differently. Some enjoy the relief given from heavy bleeding or threat of disease, feel more active and healthy, and are happy that they can no longer conceive accidentally. But younger women often resent the loss of fertility, and many become depressed. Research shows that hysterectomy patients in the USA tend to grow more dissatisfied with the operation as time passes; are more likely to be dissatisfied if the ovaries are also removed (blaming the operation for hot flashes, lethargy, and obesity); are four times more likely to become depressed in the 3 years after the operation than other women; are likely to remain depressed for twice as long (2 years on average); are especially liable to depression if under 40 when operated on; and are five times more likely to make a subsequent first visit to a psychiatrist than older women, with the peak period 2 years after surgery.

In fact, all such statistics probably reflect a situation in which many hysterectomies have been performed unnecessarily. Even so, 41% of a typical sample were still satisfied with the operation 4 years afterward. Where the operation is genuinely necessary, serious or long-term psychological disturbance is much less likely.

CERVICAL EROSION

The cells lining the cervical canal sometimes extend down till they show as a reddened area at the head of the vagina. This happens naturally in puberty and a first pregnancy, and needs no treatment unless it persists over 6 months after childbirth and causes much vaginal discharge. It then needs electric cauterization, which produces a heavy, discolored vaginal discharge for 4–6 weeks until healing is complete. It may also occur in women on the pill or using IUDs. Again, it usually disappears without symptoms or treatment, but needs regular Pap or smear tests to check for signs of cancer.

AN INCOMPETENT CERVIX

Often a cause of repeated miscarriages, a weak cervix may be due to problems during a previous birth, or to previous termination of pregnancy. Treatment is by means of a "cervical stitch" which is made to keep the cervix closed throughout the pregnancy but then removed prior to the birth.

OVARIAN CYSTS

Swelling of the abdomen, pain during intercourse and irregular periods can all be symptomatic. A doctor may also be able to feel an enlarged ovarian cyst during a pelvic examination. Large cysts will need to be removed surgically to prevent further problems such as bursting and leakage of infected matter into the pelvic cavity. Sometimes this will be possible without affecting the ovary itself.

REMOVAL OF OVARIES

This is usually to deal with or prevent cancer of the ovaries, which eventually affects 1% of US women over 40. It often accompanies hysterectomy, especially if this is peformed for cancer of the uterus (about 10% of US women with the uterus only removed do later get ovarian cancer.) Removal of large cysts can be another reason.

Where one ovary needs removal, the other may also be taken out to prevent it being a future site of disease. Post-menopausal women who lose both ovaries experience no special effects. Younger women have a menopause, but with symptoms treatable by hormone therapy.

PELVIC INFLAMMATORY DISEASE

If harmful microorganisms enter the uterus and Fallopian tubes, they may set up a site of infection and cause any of the following symptoms: fever, abdominal pain or swelling, discharge, bleeding or spotting, nausea, menstrual pain, malaise, and backache. Symptoms tend to be persistent; and inflammation and scarring of pelvic tissues can lead to infertility and general abdominal pain. Gonorrhea and the organism commonly linked with NSU (chlamydia) are frequent causes of PID. IUDs, childbirth, and gynecological treatments may also allow bacteria to pass through the cervix. PID is hard to diagnose and treat; antibiotics are not always effective, and surgery may be necessary to remove infected tissue, particularly if there is a risk of ectopic pregnancy.

Cervical disorders

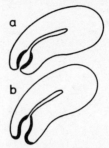

Cervical erosions
a Uterus with normal cervix
b Uterus with eroded cervix

Ovarian disorders

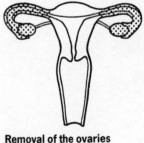

Removal of the ovaries
▓ Area removed

Pelvic cavity disorders

© DIAGRAM

Vaginal infections

VAGINAL DISCHARGE

Apart from the contribution of the uterus at menstruation, normal vaginal discharge consists of clear watery mucus from the cervix (especially midway between periods): clear fluid that has "sweated" through the walls of the vagina (usually only a small amount, but more in pregnancy or emotional upset, and a great deal during sexual excitement): dead cells from the vaginal wall; and a small contribution from the Bartholin's glands at the vaginal entrance during sexual excitement.

The resulting discharge is transparent or slightly milky, with little or no odor, slippery in feel, and perhaps yellowish when dry. It keeps the vagina moist and clean, and may be more noticeable at certain points in the menstrual cycle than at others.

Signs of disorder

What is significant is not increased amount, but irritation, unpleasant odor, or unusual color. Irritation includes itching, chafing, soreness, or burning of the vagina, vulva, or upper thighs.

Causes

There are several possible causes of abnormal discharge such as forgotten foreign bodies, tampons, or contraceptive caps. These can cause a very thick odorous discharge, which clears up when the cause is removed and the vagina washed out. Disinfectants in bathing water can also cause soreness, as can vaginal deodorants, contraceptive foams, and even some soaps. Symptoms may take time to clear after the cause is eliminated. Post-menopausal atrophy, cervical erosions and infection (including candidiasis, trichomoniasis, gonorrhea and NSU) are other causes.

Infection

Many bacteria live harmlessly in a normal healthy vagina. Some help keep its surface a little acidic, and this restricts the development of other harmful organisms.

Factors favoring infection include generally lowered resistance (due to lack of sleep, bad diet, or illness); cuts or abrasions perhaps from childbirth or intercourse without sufficient lubrication); and potentially, all factors which affect the quantity and acidity of the vaginal mucus, including menstruation and pregnancy; taking birth control pills, other hormones, or antibiotics; excessive douching; diabetes or pre-diabetes; and the menopause.

TOXIC SHOCK SYNDROME (TSS)

This occurs very rarely but is a medical emergency. It happens when microorganisms present in the vagina multiply and cause a sudden, severe illness with fever, shock, vomiting, diarrhea, or rash. TSS usually arises during menstruation; and factors linked with its development include the use of highly absorbent tampons and other materials, such as the diaphragm or sponges, which retain menstrual flow in the vagina and may thus provide the conditions under which certain bacteria can thrive. Rapid onset of high temperature and other symptoms during menstruation require urgent medical advice; and hospitalization is likely to be necessary.

TRICHOMONIASIS ("TRICH")

Trichomoniasis vaginalis is a one-celled animal parasite, and one of the most common infectious causes of vaginal discharge. A great many women carry it at some time; and about 15% develop symptoms at least once. The discharge is often greenish-yellow or grayish, thin and foamy, but may be thicker and whiter if other infection is also present. Other symptoms include itching and soreness of vagina and vulva; clusters of raised red spots on the cervix and vaginal walls; and an unpleasant odor. If it spreads to the urinary tract, it can cause cystitis.

Transmission can occur sexually (men carrying it generally have no symptoms) and also very occasionally via moist objects such as towels, washcloths, and toilet seats. (The parasite can live briefly outside the body but it cannot be passed on to a baby in childbirth. Qualified medical treatment is vital, especially as it often occurs in conjunction with gonorrhea or chlamydia which should be checked for once the symptoms of trichomoniasis clear up. Both partners should be treated. The usual treatment is with oral drugs. Prescribed vaginal suppositories or gels may be adequate alternatives, though infection may recur.) However, do avoid oral metronidazole if you are pregnant, and do not take alcohol with it. Avoid intercourse until tests show clear.

CANDIDIASIS (THRUSH)

This is caused by a yeast organism (a type of fungus). It can be passed on sexually, men usually having no symptoms. But it often occurs in the vagina anyway, kept at bay by the acidic conditions, and only thriving if these get milder. Itching and soreness of the vagina and vulva then result, especially when the body is warm. There may also be a thick creamy discharge that smells of yeast and looks like cottage cheese. Self-treatment may help (one or two plain, unsweetened yoghurt applications, for instance, or vinegar douches twice a day for 3 days). But these will not usually clear up an established infection. Normal treatment is with nystatin suppositories, inserted to the top of the vagina – one each night for 1 or 2 weeks. (These have fewer side effects than oral doses, and can be used during pregnancy.) Tampons cannot be worn, as they will soak up the medication; but a pad and old pants are needed, as nystatin gives a yellow stain. Other suppositories have also begun to be used recently, and creams are still sometimes prescribed for direct application to the vagina, cervix, and vulva; but these destroy all vaginal bacteria, so when treatment ends it is important to encourage normal bacterial growth. Very recurrent infection suggests lack of hygiene by the partner (thrush can live under the male foreskin); developing sugar diabetes; or the effects on the vaginal mucus of taking oral contraceptives and/or antibiotics.

If a woman with thrush gives birth, the baby may have the infection in its digestive tract, and should be treated with nystatin drops.

OTHER INFECTIONS

Non-specific vaginitis (also known as "anaerobic vaginosis") presents with cystitis-like symptoms followed by a discharge that is often white or yellow and may be streaked with blood. The vaginal walls may be puffy and coated with pus, and there may also be lower back pains, cramps, and swollen glands in abdomen and thighs. The usual treatment is with sulfa creams or suppositories (such as Vagitrol, Sultrin, or AVC cream).

The Gardnerella vaginalis bacterium has now been identified, and in some areas is found to be more common than trichomoniasis or candidiasis. Symptoms are similar to trichomoniasis, and it is often misdiagnosed; but the discharge is usually white or grayish, creamy in consistency, and smells especially unpleasant after intercourse. It is often transmitted sexually, and treatment of both partners is necessary.

Hepatitis B can be spread through blood or semen and is a contagious disease that can go on for several months. An infected individual may have no symptoms but still pass on the infection, even through saliva.

Venereal disease

The term venereal disease (VD) is used for certain infections which are passed on by sexual contact. The microorganisms that cause a sexually transmitted disease (STD) usually live in the infected person's genitals or in some other place (such as mouth or anus) where they have been put by sexual activity. To infect another person, they usually have to enter his or her body through an orifice (such as the genital opening, anus, or mouth), and sexual activity gives them this chance. The first symptoms of disorder appear on the part of the body that has been in contact with the infected part of the infected person.

Otherwise these disorders have little in common. Some are caused by bacteria, some by viruses, some by other microorganisms. Some are rare in our society; others are virtual epidemics. Some may only be painful or troublesome; others, if untreated, crippling or fatal. At the same time, there are also a number of other infections, not officially classified as VD, but typically passed on by, or associated with, sexual activity.

Although new and very powerful antibacterial treatments have been developed during recent years, certain venereal or sexually transmitted diseases are still on the increase, among them gonorrhea and genital herpes – and, of course, AIDS.

Prevention is of great importance, since no one is immune; and so, too, is prompt treatment if any symptoms are recognized by yourself or your partner (see p.184). If in any doubt, see your doctor or visit an STD clinic, where complete confidentiality is assured.

PREVENTION

There is no immunity to sexually transmitted diseases nor a vaccine against them. But various measures can greatly reduce the chances of infection: use of a condom by the male partner can help enormously; and so may use of some contraceptive foams, some contraceptive creams and some contraceptive jellies. Other useful preventative means (though none is guaranteed) include use of some non-contraceptive vaginal products; inspection of the male penis, for an ulcer or sore, or for infectious discharge from the penis tip; use of a "morning after" antibiotic, under prescription from a doctor or clinic (but this may be very difficult to obtain in an adequate dose); urinating immediately after intercourse, and possibly washing the genitals before and after intercourse. As an anti-VD measure, a condom needs to be put on before any sex play begins. It then guards fairly effectively against **gonorrhea** (see p.186) and **AIDS** (see pp.189-191) but not against **syphilis** (see p.185). To wash out the vagina after intercourse, a low-pressure douche can be used. But no vaginal washing should be carried out if the contraceptive method used involves a foam, jelly, or cream, whether alone or with a diaphragm or condom.

To check a penis for discharge, roll back the foreskin, if necessary, and squeeze the penis firmly – preferably before it becomes erect. One or two drops of thick white, gray, or colored fluid, appearing at the tip, may indicate infection. Clear liquid is usually just urine or semen.

It is important to stop infection spreading if you do develop a sexual infection. You therefore need to:

a Get cured properly, and follow qualified medical instructions, returning for prescribed checks and tests even if they seem unneccessary. In fact, ask for repeat tests if these are not offered.
b Avoid sexual contact with anyone until you are sure you are cured; and
c Make sure that all your recent sexual contacts know what has happened, and that they all get themselves thoroughly tested and, if necessary, treated.

SAFER SEX

The following will not only help you guard against AIDS (see pp.189-191), but also other sexual infections.
1 Always ensure your partner wears a condom. (This is important for oral and anal sex, too.)
2 Cut down on the number of partners with whom you have a sexual relationship.
3 If everyone ensured he or she was free from infection (by means of checks at a Special Clinic – see p.184) before embarking on a sexual relationship, sexually transmitted diseases would virtually disappear.

SYMPTOMS

The diagrams below show possible signs of venereal disease in a woman. All these symptoms usually have some other cause other than venereal disease. But do not delay in getting proper medical advice. If symptoms disappear, it may just mean that the infection has progressed naturally to its next stage. You may still have a venereal disease; and you may still be able to infect others.

Signs of venereal disease

a Sore, rash, or ulcer on, in, or around the genitals
b A sore, rash or ulcer on, in, or around the anus
c Unusual vaginal discharge
d Pain or a burning feeling on urinating
e Increased frequency of urination
f Itching or soreness of vagina or vulva
g Swollen glands in the groin

Possible symptoms on the head and body include
h Sore, ulcer, or rash on, or in the mouth (or sometimes the nose)
i Eye infection
j Loss of patches of hair
k Persistant sore throat after fellatio
l A rash on the body
m Sores in soft folds of skin
n Swollen glands in the armpits
o A sore, ulcer, or rash on the fingers or hand.

Possible symptoms if infection spreads up the reproductive tract include
p Nausea
q Backache
r Abdominal pain
s Pain during intercourse
t Painful or excessive periods and fever

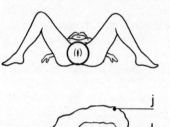

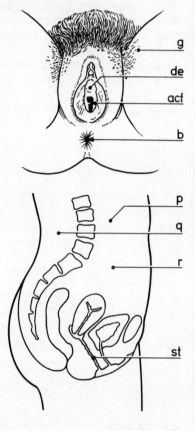

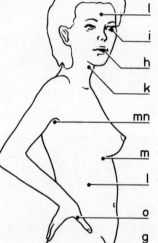

WHERE TO FIND HELP

If, for some reason, you do not wish to see your doctor about a suspected venereal infection, your hospital may have a Special Clinic (also known as a Genito-Urinary or VD Clinic). They have particularly good facilities for diagnosis and will provide both treatment and advice. You will be assured of absolute confidentiality; but, of course, you should be ready to give information about recent relationships since, to prevent spread of infection, partners may have to be traced, again with every respect for confidentiality.

SYPHILIS

Syphilis is sometimes nicknamed "the pox" or "scab." Its prevalence varies, and it is caused by tiny bacteria shaped like corkscrews and known as "spirochetes." These thrive in the warm, moist linings of the genital passages, rectum, and mouth, and can live in concentrated sites as sores on the skin surface, but die almost immediately outside the human body. So the infection is always spread by direct physical contact, and in practice almost always by sexual contact. Very occasionally syphilis does occur from close non-sexual contact but it cannot be spread by objects such as lavatory seats, towels, or cups.

Incubation

There is an "incubation period" between catching syphilis and showing the first signs – always between 9 days and 3 months, and usually 3 weeks or more. About 1000 germs are typically picked up on infection. After 3 weeks these may have multiplied to 100–200 million.

Primary stage

The first symptom is in the part that has been in contact with the infected person: genitals, rectum, or mouth. A spot appears and grows into a sore that oozes a colorless fluid (but no blood). The sore feels like a button; round or oval, firm, and just under ½in (1.27cm) across. A week or so later, the glands in the groin may swell but they do not usually become tender, so it may not be noticed. There is no feeling of illness, and the sore heals.

Secondary stage

This occurs when the bacteria have spread through the body. It can follow the primary stage straight away, but usually there is a gap of several weeks. The person feels generally unwell. There are breaks in the skin, and sometimes a dark red rash, lasting for weeks or even months. The rash appears on the back of the legs and the front of the arms, and often too on the body, face, hands, and feet. Other symptoms can include hair falling out in patches; sores in the mouth, nose, throat, or genitals, or in soft folds of skin; and swollen glands throughout the body. The sores – like the original primary stage sore – are very infectious. All these symptoms eventually disappear

Latent stage

This may last for anything from a few months to years. There are no symptoms. After about 2 years, the person ceases to be infectious (though a woman can still sometimes give the disease to a baby she bears). But presence of syphilis can still be shown by blood tests.

Tertiary stage

This occurs in about one third of those who have not been treated earlier. The disease now shows itself in concentrated and often permanent damage in one part of the body, but tertiary syphilis is more serious if it attacks the heart, blood vessels, or nervous system. It can then kill, blind, paralyze, cripple, or render insane.

Tests and treatment

Testing sores for bacteria, or blood for antibodies, is necessary. Repeat tests are important too. Treatment involves antibiotics – usually penicillin. Given in primary or secondary stages, it completely cures most cases. Tests and examination often continue for more than 2 years. In the latent and even tertiary stages, syphilis can still be eradicated and further damage halted.

Stages of syphilis
1 Incubation
2 Primary
3 Secondary
4 Latent
5 Tertiary
The primary sore may develop in or on the
a Genitals
b Anus
c Mouth or sometimes the
d Hand
Secondary stage symptoms include
e Skin rash
f Patches of loose hair
g Swollen lymph nodes, and
h Secondary sores in the mouth, nose, throat, genitals, or skin
Tertiary syphilis can attack almost any part of the body.

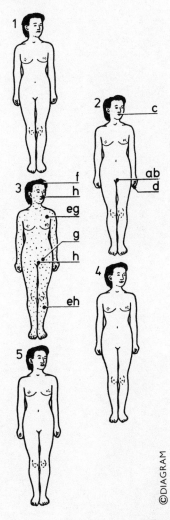

©DIAGRAM

GONORRHEA

Sometimes nicknamed "the clap," gonorrhea has become epidemic in recent years – partly because it is so easy for a woman to have it without knowing it. Several infections in a person in a single year is not too uncommon. Worldwide, there are probably about 150 million cases.

Causation

Like syphilis, gonorrhea is caused by a bacterium that thrives in the warm moist lining of utethra, cervix, rectum, or mouth. It is normally only passed on by sexual contact, but sometimes by close body contact or by inheritance from an infected mother. It cannot be picked up from objects (though perhaps it can be carried by pubic lice, which can sometimes be picked up from objects such as lavatory seats).

Unlike syphilis, the form of sexual contact involved is normally only genital or anal intercourse. Oral contact does not often pass on gonorrhea. (If it does, it is usually fellatio rather than cunnilingus that is responsible: but some scientists even allow possibility of infection through kissing).

Symptoms in men

These are more noticeable. Incubation usually takes under a week, but can extend to a month. It is followed by discomfort inside the penis; thick discharge, usually yellow-green, from the penis tip; and a burning feeling on urinating. Later, there may be swollen glands, a urethral abscess, and swollen infected testes (with danger of sterility).

Symptoms in women

In women incubation is longer, and the eventual symptoms, if any, are much less severe or identifiable. There may be discomfort on urinating, more frequent urination, and vaginal discharge. The discharge is distinctively yellow, and unpleasant to smell – but this may be unnoticed due to the typically small quantities involved. Often there are no other symptoms. So up to 90% of cases in women occur without the woman being aware of the disease. But she is still just as infectious – and just as much at risk. For if untreated, the infection may spread to glands around the vaginal entrance, making them swell; the rectum (because of the closeness of the two openings), causing inflammation and perhaps a discharge; and/or the cervix, uterus, Fallopian tubes, and pelvic interior. Fallopian infection can result in fever, abdominal pain, backaches, sickness, painful or excessive periods, and pain during intercourse. If not treated quickly, sterility can result. It can also possibly kill the fetus by causing any pregnancy to be ectopic. Even where gonorrhea does not affect the Fallopian tubes, it can result in premature birth, umbilical cord inflammation, maternal fever and blindness in the child. It can also spread to the bloodstream and infect bone joints, causing arthritis. If oral contact results in infection, it is mainly as a throat disorder that is often not recognized as gonorrhea. This form is unlikely to infect others, because the lymph tissues are deep in the tonsil area.

Tests and treatment

Gonorrhea is diagnosed by laboratory analysis of any discharge or of a smear from an affected part. Treatment is with antibiotics – usually penicillin, though many forms of gonorrhea are becoming more resistant to it. Qualified medical surveillance is vital. Alcohol can interfere with a cure.

OTHER VENEREAL DISEASES

Soft chancre (chancroid) is caused by a bacillus (a rod-shaped bacterium) and is contracted sexually (usually by intercourse). After 3–5 days' incubation, it generally produces an ulcer on the genitals and painful swollen glands (but either sex can carry it without symptoms). Treatment is with antibiotics and other drugs.

Lymphogranuloma venereum is caused by a very small bacterium, and can be contracted from infected bedding and clothing as well as (more usually) from sexual intercourse. After 5–21 days' incubation, it produces a small genital blister or ulcer. Later there can be internal complications. Treatment is with antibiotics.

Granuloma inguinale is caused by a bacillus, and is contracted sexually (usually by intercourse.) After 1–3 weeks, it produces bright red painless genital sores. Treatment is with antibiotics.

OTHER SEXUAL INFECTIONS

Genital warts are fairly common and very contagious. They are spread by sexual contact (perhaps caused by a virus), and appear, after 1–6 months' incubation, on or around genitals or anus. They are usually cured by repeated use of resin application. Importantly there is now thought to be a link with carcinoma of the cervix.

Infestations are passed on by sexual or sometimes other close bodily contact, and are not especially common. **Scabies** or "the itch" is caused by a tiny mite, which mainly lives on or around the genitals. The female mite burrows beneath the skin to lay her eggs. The symptoms – itchy lumps and tracks – become noticeable after 4–6 weeks. They can occur between the fingers, on buttocks and wrists, and in the armpits, as well as on the genitals. The itching is worse in warm conditions. **Pubic lice**, or "crabs," are genital versions of lice that can also occur in other hairy parts of the body. Treatment of these parasites involves painting the hair-bearing parts with appropriate chemicals.

Non-specific urethritis (NSU)

NSU is the most common of all sexual disorders in men, but in women the symptoms are often insignificant or hard to diagnose but it may cause vaginal discharge. It may be present alongside other infections. In some people it is caused by a small organism called chlamydia trachomatis. This infects the cervix and/or the urethra. In other people there may be other organisms, or sometimes no organism at all is found.

The infection can spread up into the pelvis to cause pelvic inflammatory disease, and it is an important cause of tubal blockage with resulting infertility. NSU can also occasionally spread to Bartholin's gland at the opening of the vagina, where it may cause an abscess that requires medical treatment.

Symptoms in men resemble gonorrhea; principally discharge and discomfort when urinating. It can be recurrent. Occasionally in men and rarely in women, NSU may be associated with certain types of arthritis and inflammation of the eyes. If a woman's partner has NSU, she should also be treated with an antibiotic such as tetracycline.

©DIAGRAM

GENITAL HERPES

One type of herpes simplex virus can affect the genital/anal area and is sexually transmitted. Genital herpes is highly dangerous if the ulcers are present at the end of pregnancy, as they can cause a life-threatening infection in a newborn baby. Mothers are therefore usually advised to have a Cesarian section to prevent the baby coming into contacts with the ulcers. It can be very uncomfortable for the sufferer; and it is thought, too, that there may be some link with cervical cancer since women who have had this infection seem more likely to develop it.

Symptoms

These include a stinging sensation or intense irritation, a feeling of being generally unwell, a high temperature and perhaps backache. There may also be signs of the typical highly contagious blisters and small ulcers; but if these are inside the vagina or on the cervix, they will not, of course, be visible. In both sexes, they can also occur in the rectum. It may be painful to pass urine because of the sores.

Treatment

If you experience any of the above symptoms, you will be wise to see your doctor or to visit a Special Clinic (also known as an STD, VD or GU Clinic), perhaps attached to your local hospital. Swab tests and possibly an internal examination will confirm the diagnosis. You will be given one of the many forms of medication available. This will shorten an attack but cannot cure the condition completely, and it may recur from time to time. Bathing the infected area with a salt solution (one teaspoonful of salt, to one pint or ½ liter of water) may also help, as may adding salt to your bath. Cold packs can also relieve pain, and a cold shower may help. Leave the sores exposed, if you can, which may mean that you leave off underwear as much as possible. Keeping the sores dry (perhaps by dabbing them with witch hazel) may also be effective. Avoid use of a sunbed which may exacerbate pain. Other frequent recommendations include checking that your diet contains good quantities of Vitamin C, all the B vitamins, zinc and calcium as well as a daily kelp tablet.

Other frequent recommendations include checking that your diet contains good quantities of Vitamin C, all the B vitamins, zinc and calcium, as well as a daily kelp tablet.

Prevention

To prevent spread of infection to your partner, avoid sexual intercourse, oral sex or any genital contact while you are infected. A condom will not provide complete protection. Be sure to try to avoid getting run-down as some women find this brings on the infection. This is important because once you have the infection, the virus remains and may flare up. It is highly contagious, and over recent years has increased considerably, particularly among women. If you (or your partner) have a herpes blister, the chances of passing on the infection are very high: but you can also pass it on (or be infected by someone else) even if there are no obvious signs of the virus.

The disease AIDS first came to public attention as a "plague" afflicting San Francisco homosexual men during the late 1970s. But the virus which causes AIDS, though only identified and named in 1983, was around perhaps as long ago as 1959 and is capable of infecting anyone, no matter what their sexual orientation.

The virus is present in the body fluids (blood, saliva, semen or vaginal secretions) of an infected person and can be transmitted either through sexual activity, or from a mother to her baby or through blood transfusion or injection with infected needles. It is not the sort of virus that can be caught by ordinary social contact.

The HIV virus attacks the body's immune system, but the syndrome of full-blown AIDS does not develop immediately after the initial infection. Some individuals who are HIV-positive do not show any symptoms for years, and indeed may never show any, though still capable of infecting others. There are several recognized stages through which the disease may evolve, and other factors such as stress or new infections may be involved in precipitating progression from one stage to the next.

There is no vaccine or cure for AIDS as yet. But drugs which slow down the growth rate of the virus are effective in dealing with some of the symptoms and may delay further progression toward full-blown AIDS.

AIDS (Acquired immune deficiency syndrome)

RISK GROUPS

There are well-defined high-risk groups for infection with the HIV virus. These include male homosexuals, drug users, prostitutes and hemophiliacs who may have received transfusions of infected blood. Once established, the virus can be passed on by heterosexual relationships to those who do not necessarily consider themselves in a high-risk group. In Africa, AIDS has spread extensively through heterosexual contact.

Sexual habits, such as promiscuity, encourage spread of the virus, as does anal intercourse, and the virus in semen passes more easily through inflamed or torn membranes. Drug users may pick up and spread the virus through shared needles. Some drug users finance their habit with prostitution, another means by which infection can be widely spread. Hemophiliacs have become infected because of contaminated Factor VIII (a blood derivative) used in their treatment. But most countries now test donated blood for HIV virus and discourage members of high-risk groups from becoming donors.

AIDS is still a relatively rare disease in most countries outside central Africa, but its growth is hard to measure, partly because those already infected may not feel ill and unwittingly go on passing the virus. In the absence of certainty, it makes sense to assume that everyone who participates in sexual activity and has more than one partner takes some level of risk. The only absolute protection against infection with HIV is celibacy, but condoms are capable, if manufactured to sufficiently high standards and used correctly, of containing the virus.

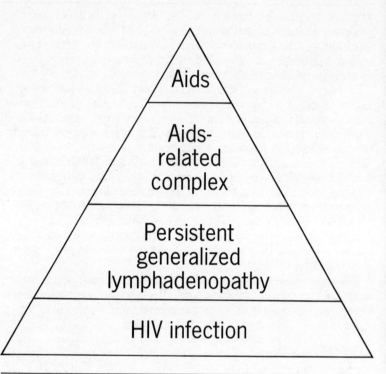

HIV infection
Full-blown AIDS does not develop immediately after infection with the HIV virus. There are several stages through which the disease may evolve. But even if symptoms never show themselves, someone who is HIV positive may still infect others.

HIV-POSITIVE

Blood tests to detect infection with HIV are available; and about 12 weeks after contact it is usually possible to say whether or not someone has contracted the virus. There may be flu-like symptoms lasting for up to 14 days, but frequently there are no symptoms at all. Being diagnosed as HIV-positive can be a frightening experience; apart from worries about getting full-blown AIDS, patients are unfortunately likely to suffer discrimination in employment, life insurance and possible loss of social and economic status. It is therefore very important for patients to seek counseling and for their families and friends to offer love and support. To be diagnosed as HIV-positive is not in itself an immediate "death sentence" – in one survey 75% of HIV-positive men were well and symptom-free two years after diagnosis.

PERSISTENT GENERALIZED LYMPHADENOPATHY (PGL)

About 30% of people with the HIV virus develop persistent swelling of the lymph glands. This is often accompanied by tiredness and malaise. Patients with PGL may be advised to avoid stress as much as possible and keep to a healthy diet in order to avoid worsening of the condition.

AIDS-RELATED COMPLEX (ARC)

A proportion of patients infected with HIV go on to develop definite symptoms of immune system damage. These include infections like thrush and skin disorders, fever, diarrhea, weight loss and constant tiredness.

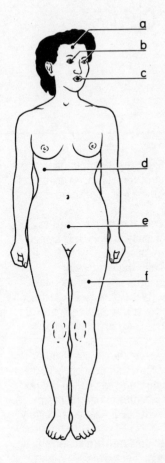

When AIDS may strike
a The brain
Problems include "AIDS encephalopathy," a progressive shrinking of the brain resulting in dementia; and infections causing symptoms ranging from headaches to convulsions and partial paralysis
b The eyes
Infection may lead to blindness
c The mouth
Oral thrush, pain on swallowing
d The lungs
Pneumonia caused by parasitic bacterial or fungal infection.
e The digestive system
Chest pain and difficulty in swallowing due to severe oral thrush. Also colicky pains. Persistent diarrhea
f The skin
Kaposi's sarcoma, usually noticed first on the skin, is the second most common condition by which AIDS is diagnosed. Skin rashes may also occur.

AIDS

Full-blown AIDS is the last stage of HIV infection. The immune system is destroyed, making sufferers vulnerable to a variety of infections which would normally be trivial but are now potentially fatal. In about a third of patients there are symptoms caused by infection of the brain. An otherwise rare tumor, **Kaposi's sarcoma**, is common in AIDS – sometimes it is the first symptom. While certain symptoms and infections can be successfully treated, the underlying immune damage cannot be repaired and full-blown AIDS is a terminal illness.

PREGNANCY AND AIDS

Pregnancy in a woman who carries the HIV virus can be a two-fold tragedy: not only may the baby be born already infected, but the mother also runs an increased risk of developing ARC or full-blown AIDS. A great many of the babies born to HIV-positive mothers are infected at birth. The virus can also be transmitted in breast milk. Babies progress to the late stages of AIDS more rapidly than adults because their immune systems are relatively undeveloped.

©DIAGRAM

4.03   General disorders

Cancer

WHAT IS CANCER?

Cancer is one of several disorders which can result when the process of cell division in a person's body gets out of control. Such disorders can produce tissue growths called "tumors." Cancer in some form or other attacks one in every five people.

The body is constantly producing new cells for the purposes of growth and repair – about 500,000 million daily. It does this by cell division: that is, one parent cell divides to form two new cells. When this process is going correctly, the new cells show the same characteristics as the tissue in which they originated and they are capable of carrying out the functions that the body requires that tissue to perform. They do not migrate to parts of the body where they do not belong; and if they were placed in such a part artificially, they might not survive.

When the process of cell division goes wrong, however, a tumor can result. Cells multiply in an uncoordinated way, independently of the normal control mechanisms. They produce a new growth in the body that does not fulfill a useful function; this is a tumor, or "neoplasm." A tumor is often felt as a hard lump, because its cells are more closely packed than normal.

Tumors may be "benign" or "malignant." In a **benign tumor**, cells reproduce in a way that is still fairly orderly. They are only slightly different from the cells of the surrounding tissue; their growth is slow and may stop spontaneously; the tumor is surrounded by a capsule of fibrous tissue, and does not invade the normal tissue; and its cells do not spread through the body. (A wart is a benign tumor.)

Benign tumors are not fatal unless the space they take up exerts harmful pressure on nearby organs. This usually only happens with some benign tumors in the skull.

In a **malignant tumor**, the cells reproduce in a completely disorderly fashion and differ considerably from those of the surrounding tissue. (Generally, they show less specialization.) The tumor's growth is rapid compared with the surrounding tissue. There is no surrounding capsule, and the tumor can therefore invade and destroy adjacent tissue. The original tumor is also able to spread to other parts of the body by a process known as "metastasis" and produce secondary growths there. A malignant tumor is usually fatal if untreated, because of its destructive action on normal tissue.

A **biopsy** is the most certain way of distinguishing between benign and malignant tumors. A piece of the tumor is surgically removed, and then studied under a microscope.

CAUSES OF CANCER

In cancerous cells, the characteristics of malignant growth are passed on from one generation to another. This means that the genetic code must have been damaged. This is seen if the chromosomes of cancerous cells are examined.

Normal cells have 46 chromosomes arranged in 23 pairs. Almost all cancer cells are abnormal in the number and/or structure of these chromosomes. Cells with genetic defects appear in the body every day: so many millions of cells are being made that some mistakes are inevitable. But most die almost immediately, because they are too faulty to survive, or because they are recognized as abnormal and swallowed up by white blood corpuscles. Others are only slightly defective, and not malignant. Only very rarely do malignant cells survive and reproduce successfully.

Appearance of cancer may simply be due to this unlucky chance. Alternatively, it may be that the body's immunity to such malignant cells sometimes breaks down. This would explain why cancer can sometimes remain dormant for many years.

A few factors have been recognized that make genetic damage in cells more likely. But they only explain a tiny proportion of cancers. Certain chemicals can cause cancer to form if they are repeatedly in contact with the body over a period of time, for example. Such chemicals are called **carcinogens**; but apart from tobacco smoke, they usually only affect workers whose jobs necessitate regular contact with them.

Certain **viruses** are also known to pass malignant tumors from one animal to another, and the same may occur in humans. Viruses have, for example, been implicated in the development of **cervical** and **liver cancer, Burkitt's lymphoma** and **Kaposi's sarcoma**.

Without correct protection, X rays can cause **skin cancer**, and radiation may cause **leukemia**. Ultraviolet rays (as in prolonged exposure to intense sunlight) may also cause skin cancer in some circumstances. Some experts also believe that continued physical disturbance of the skin or mucous membranes can cause cancer (not just accelerate it). Some individuals also seem more likely to develop certain forms of cancer than others. Actual cancerous growths are not inherited; but it seems that a predisposition for cancer can be passed on.

Most cancers occur in the 50 to 60 age group. However, children and adolescents are susceptible to leukemia, brain tumors, and sarcomas of the bone. In almost all countries, cancer occurs more frequently in men than in women. Diet is often implicated, and the range of foodstuffs locally available, their preparation and preservation are all likely to have an effect. It has also been found that cancer of the cervix is much less common in societies where male circumcision is usual.

As always, prevention is better than cure. A high fiber diet, minimum stress, and cutting out smoking are therefore strongly recommended, as are regular cervical smear (Pap) tests, and other precautions listed on p. 195.

For information on **leukemia**, see p.204.

CANCER GROWTH

Generally, cancerous cells cannot divide faster than normal cells. But normal cell division reaches its maximum rate only in times of injury and repair. Cancerous growths are continually producing cells at this maximum rate without check. They are, however, less successful than normal tissue could be. This is because many of the faulty cancerous cells die. Nevertheless, the result is that cancerous growths develop much faster than normal tissue.

Metastasis is the process by which cancerous cells travel from the original (primary) cancer site to other parts of the body. It occurs when cancerous cells get caught up in the flow of blood or lymph. The cells are carried along in the vessels until they lodge in another part of the body. If they succeed in establishing themselves, this becomes a new (secondary) cancer site; and if a secondary site gets large enough, it can also metastasize in turn.

Cancer that has metastasized along the lymph vessels normally sets up its secondary sites in the glands. Cancer that has metastazied in the bloodstream sets up secondary sites in the bones, lungs, and liver. Cancers in the brain do not normally metastasize outside the skull or spinal column, but cancers elsewhere can metastasize to the brain. Some sites are more receptive than others.

The most common locations for secondary growths are the bones, brain, lungs, kidneys, and adrenal glands. Others are much rarer. A cancer can also spread through the body simply by the process of growth.

Normal and abnormal cell replacement
a Normal body tissue
b Damaged body tissue
c Normal cell replacement
d Abnormal malignant growth

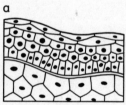
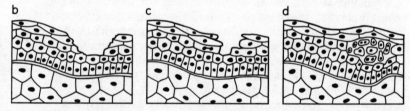

a   b   c   d

SYMPTOMS

Any unusual bleeding or discharge from mouth, genitals, or anus (including, in women, bleeding from the nipple and menstrual bleeding between periods) should be reported to a doctor, as should any lump or thickening or swelling on the body surface, any swelling of one limb, and increase in size or change in color or appearance of a mole or wart. Other symptoms may include a sore that will not heal normally; persistent constipation, diarrhea, or indigestion that is unusual for the person; hoarseness or a dry cough that lasts more than three weeks; difficulty in swallowing or urinating; or sudden unexplained loss in weight or persistent pain.

If you develop any of these symptoms, you should visit your doctor. Nearly always, the cause will be something else, not cancer. But do not delay. If it is cancer, quick diagnosis is essential.

SITES OF CANCER

Cancers can grow almost anywhere in the body, but the most common sites are listed *right*. Cancers are classified by the kind of tissue in which the primary growth occurred. Tumors originating in the "epithelial" cells (for example, skin, mucous membrane, and glands) are called **carcinomas**; those in connective tissue (such as muscle and bone), **sarcomas**. Secondary tumors are classified by the kind of primary tumor from which they came. Cancer in general has become vastly more prevalent in the present century. In the UK, for instance, almost 1 in 4 of all deaths are caused by it, and it has been estimated that about 250,000 new cases occur every year. This seems to indicate that as many as 1 in 3 will develop some form of cancer during their lifetime. (Some experts believe this is simply because people are living longer, for the likelihood of cancerous growths increases with age. Diagnostic and autopsy skills have also, of course, improved.)

Nevertheless, some types of cancer have shown a dramatic fall in recent years – stomach cancer for instance. This particular example may be linked with changes in techniques of food preservation and also with the diet. (For information on **leukemia**, see p.204.)

REDUCING RISK OF CANCER

There are many preventative measures that can be taken – none of them absolute guarantees but all thought to cut down considerably the risk of several forms of cancer.

1 Give up smoking. Lung cancer (the second most common form of cancer in women) causes hundreds of thousands of deaths worldwide each year. If you smoke regularly, your chances of getting lung cancer are 10 times more than that of a non-smoker. Chewing tobacco also increases risk of cancer of the mouth. It has been estimated, too, that non-smokers continually exposed to other people's smoking have 10–30 percent higher risk than other non-smokers of developing lung cancer.

2 Avoid having too many X rays. Try to limit dental X rays to not more than once every 2 years, and wear a protective apron. If you work with radiation, always ensure that you follow safety regulations.

3 Do not expose your skin to excessive sunshine, and always use a sunscreen cream or lotion with a factor suited to your skin type to help filter out harmful rays.

4 Restrict your alcohol intake. Cancers of the mouth, throat and liver are found more frequently in those who drink heavily. Up to 14 units per week for a woman is considered sensible. (One unit equals half-pint beer, one glass of wine, or a single measure of spirits.)

5 Avoid being overweight, cut down on fats, and include fiber or roughage in your diet.

6 If you are or have been sexually active, be sure to have a cervical smear test at least every 5 years.

7 Examine your breasts regularly.

8 Avoid contact with asbestos dust and other substances which you might meet in the course of work: some wood dusts, raw material for PVC, some types of soot and tar, for instance. This means observing occupational health and safety regulations very carefully.

The ten most common forms of cancer in women and approximate percentages of incidence
a Lung 9%
b Breast 24%
c Stomach 4%
d Pancreas 3%
e Colon and rectum 12%
f Ovary 5%
g Cervix 4%
h Uterus 3%
i Skin (excluding melanoma) 10%

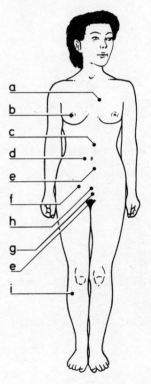

©DIAGRAM

TREATMENT

Treatments for cancer have a good chance of success only if the tumor is still localized. Early diagnosis is therefore vital. Once a tumor has metastasized, successful treatment is far more difficult.

Surgical removal of localized malignant tumors at an early stage is the only completely successful form of treatment known at present. But **lasers** allow very accurate destruction of abnormal tissue. In later stages, surgery may be attempted in conjunction with other techniques. Cancer cells are killed by radiation more easily than normal cells, and **radiotherapy** seeks to destroy cancerous tissue by focusing beams of radiation on it. This can be done only if the cancer is still localized, and can be destroyed without causing excessive damage to the rest of the body. New techniques (**implanted radioisotopes** and **monoclonal antibodies**) enable radiation to be delivered more precisely to the site of the tumor.

Chemotherapy treatment includes administration of chemicals. Again, the major difficulty is finding drugs that will destroy cancer cells without harming normal cells. Three main types of chemical are used: those that interfere with the cancer cells' reproductive processes; those that interfere with the cells' metabolic processes; and those that increase the natural resistance of the body to the tumor cells.

These chemicals can affect the whole of the body, specific regions, or the tumors themselves, depending on how they are applied.

The development of monoclonal antibodies, which preferentially attach to malignant tissue, has enabled chemicals to be delivered directly to tumor sites.

Hormone therapy is used mainly for tumors of the endocrine glands and related organs. It is also useful in the treatment of metastases originating from these areas (in women, against disseminated breast cancer, for example). Success depends on whether the cancerous cells still have the specialized relationship with the hormone that the original tissue had. In women, hormone therapy may also include removal of the ovaries.

Other more recently introduced forms of treatment include complementary therapies such as **massage, visualization, relaxation, art and drama therapy,** and regimes such as the **Bristol and Gerson diets.** The Gerson diet, still somewhat controversial, includes detoxification, supplements and natural remedies over a period of 18 months. The Bristol diet, developed at the Bristol Cancer Help Center, England, is based on similar principles but takes a less rigid approach. Both stress the importance of organically-grown foods, however.

CANCER OF THE REPRODUCTIVE TRACT

Statistics show that, as far as **cervical cancer** is concerned, 2 women in 100 get it, and one of these dies from it. It can occur at any age, but 45–50 is most common. A possible symptom is unusual vaginal bleeding between periods, after intercourse, or more than 6 months after the menopause. But analysis of the cervical tissue is the only sure evidence. The well-known "Pap" or smear test involves the painless gathering of a few sample cells on the end of a wooden spatula. (The physician may well do a pelvic examination to check the uterus and ovaries at the same time.) It takes only a few minutes, and can be done at the doctor's office, a family planning clinic or a well-woman clinic. The sample is sent to a specialist laboratory, fixed in alcohol, stained in solution, and examined for abnormal cells. In 1000 smears, 20 might show some abnormality; and perhaps 3, the early signs of cancer. (The other abnormalities may include signs of vaginal infection.)

A woman should have had such a test within 6 months of first having sexual intercourse. Thereafter, the smear test should regularly be repeated at least every 3 years. (Occasionally cancer can appear after a recent negative smear; but this is rare.) There is, incidentally, a link between cancer of the cervix and a wart virus called HPV, which can be transmitted sexually. A condom will reduce risk of infection.

If possible signs of cancer are found, a repeat smear may be taken, followed by a larger specimen using curettage or a tiny punch. If cancer is then confirmed, alternatives include **conization**, in which cervical tissue is cut away (the cervix is stitched, and rapidly heals with little pain and usually no after-effects:) or **hysterectomy**. Which is used depends on the state of the tumor. Hysterectomy is necessary once malignant growth has begun to spread. It gives almost total success, but a few very advanced cases may need radiation therapy or further surgery. Other possibilities include laser treatment, diathermy (heat treatment), or cryosurgery (cold treatment) which may mean extensive surgery can be avoided.

Cancer of the body of the uterus usually only occurs in older women (typically 50–60.) The diabetic and obese seem susceptible, and it can run in a family. Tumor growth is slow; and bleeding symptoms are significant. Diagnosis is by curettage of the uterus under anesthethic; treatment, by hysterectomy and X ray therapy. If treated early enough, 80 percent of patients survive more than 5 years.

Cancer of the ovaries accounts for 5 percent of cancers in women. It is more frequent after 40, and especially after the menopause. Its slow growth is hard to detect. The first sign is enlargement of the ovaries, showing up on pelvic examination – but only 4 percent of ovary enlargements are cancerous. Pelvic examinations at least every 5 years should catch them in time.

Cancer of the vulva is rare, and usually only found in older women. It is typically preceded by long-standing vulval itching, and sometimes an ulcer (but in 99 percent of cases these symptoms do not signify cancer). Diagnosis is by examination of tissue samples taken under anesthetic.

Cancer of the vagina is also rare, except in girls and women whose mothers were prescribed the drug diethylstilbestrol (DES) in pregnancy.

©DIAGRAM

Breast cancer

Almost a quarter of all cancers in women take the form of breast cancer and about 5 per cent of women develop it. If it is caught at an early stage, 9 out of 10 survive. But metastasis can occur within a month of the tumor appearing.

The disease is most common in women aged 40–60. Heredity, diet, and estrogen levels in the body are all under investigation as possible significant factors. Research suggests, too, that early first childbirth, and breastfeeding for several months, may both make breast cancer less likely in the mother. It is vital to check the breasts once every month for any changes. (See p.102 for the procedure and what to look for. Anything you find – lumps or other changes – will usually be due to some other cause, not cancer; but do check with a doctor immediately. Early detection can save your life.)

If a lump is confirmed, it is not necessarily cancerous. The doctor may insert a needle into the lump to see if it collapses (indicating a cyst). If not, a biopsy will be taken to distinguish between cancer and a benign tumor. Again, sometimes a needle may be used for this, but usually a surgical examination is necessary.

For speed, it is usual for some surgeons to obtain and then examine the suspicious tissue while the patient remains under anesthetic and then to go on to operate at once if the tissue is judged cancerous. You should therefore see about this likelihood before any biopsy.

Benign and malignant tumors
1 Growth of malignant tumor
2 Growth of benign tumor

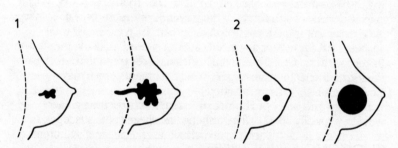

NON-CANCEROUS DISORDERS

Other disorders have symptoms similar to breast cancer. These include **fibroadenosis (chronic mastitis)** which features a permanent increase in the breast's glandular content, due to hormonal effects. The breast may feel lumpy or rubbery, all over or in patches, and there may be tenderness, particularly before menstruation or after heavy lifting. Most common between the ages of 30 and 50, fibroadenosis is a normal condition for many women. Treatment may not be needed but always check with a doctor.

Perhaps 75 per cent of lumps are non-malignant. **Breast cysts** are small sacs in the breast tissue, filled with liquid, and usually harmless. Most common in women aged 35 to 45, they may be drained or have their linings surgically removed. Benign tumors may swell until pressure on nerves or neighboring tissues requires their removal; but they cannot invade or destroy other tissue, as cancer can.

SCREENING TECHNIQUES

Mammography is often used as an aid in the diagnosis of breast cancer, and in some countries has been introduced as a routine check for women over 50. It involves placing the breasts in direct contact with the X ray plate. Usually two views of each breast are taken. Malignancy shows up as an irregular opaque patch in the breast. One run of 2000 mammograms detected 92 percent of cancers present. Mammography alone is not usually thought sufficient for certain diagnosis, but in combination with clinical examination and biopsy, around 97 percent of lumps examined can be correctly diagnosed. The whole procedure takes only half-an-hour. (See p.131)

Thermography is another method used in the detection of breast cancer. In a normal person, 45 percent of the heat given off by the skin is infrared radiation. Thermography records in a photograph the way in which this heat is given off. A malignant growth emits more heat than the surrounding tissue, and so shows up as a different shade on the photograph. Thermography, however, is less successful than mammography and clinical examination.

TREATMENT

Breast cancer usually spreads in the lymph system, beginning with the armpit nodes and those of the chest and spine. Surgical possibilities include removal of the lump alone (**lumpectomy**); removal of the breast (**simple mastectomy**); removal of breast and some armpit nodes (**modified radical mastectomy**); removal of breast, some armpit nodes, and some chest wall muscles (**radical mastectomy**); and, occasionally, removal of breast, all armpit nodes, some chest wall muscles, and some chest nodes (**superradical mastectomy**).

   Which type of treatment is chosen depends on the tumor's size, type, position, and spread. Surgery may also be accompanied by drug and/or radiotherapy. More extensive operations will be followed by **physiotherapy**, to minimize the effects of muscle loss on arm movement and breathing abilities, and also the fitting of a **prosthesis** or artificial breast. Support groups can also help enormously in providing advice and guidance, both practically and emotionally.

CHOOSING A PROSTHESIS

There are several types available, and some are so successfully fitted that it is possible to wear a swimming costume without the operation being noticed. The art is in matching the other breast so that there is no obvious difference. Breast reconstruction by various other methods is also a possibility; and a surgeon will always discuss with the patient the sort of cosmetic success that can be expected.

Mastectomy
1 Simple mastectomy: area removed and stitching
2 Radical mastectomy: area removed and stitching.

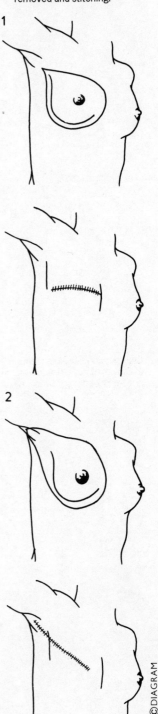

1

2

©DIAGRAM

Skeletal disorders

BONES

Apart from the likelihood of their being fractured by extreme force, bones are prone to only a few disorders. Apart from obvious crookedness in a limb, signs that a bone has been fractured include pain, redness, and swelling. A fracture to part of the skull, meanwhile, may be indicated by bleeding or loss of clear cerebrospinal fluid from the nose or ear. Fractures of the neck or back should always be suspected in the case of a fall or automobile accident: symptoms include numbness and inability to move. *The victim should not be moved until medical help arrives.* Treatment of a fracture consists of replacing the bone ends so that they will knit satisfactorily; and a plaster cast or metal pins and plates may be used to keep the bones together. Healing takes much longer in older people and it may be several months before full use of a fractured limb is regained.
Osteoporosis is a gradual thinning of the bones which affects older people, especially women.
Osteomyelitis is infection of bone by bacteria which may be carried there in the bloodstream or enter through a wound. Prolonged antibiotic treatment is necessary to prevent bone from being eroded, and surgery may also be needed to remove infected material.

JOINTS

Dislocation occurs when the two bone ends forming a joint are forcibly pushed away from each other, tearing the ligaments which normally hold the joint together. Joints most commonly dislocated include fingers, shoulder, jaw, hip, and knee. Symptoms of dislocation are obvious deformity, pain, and swelling. Larger joints must be repaired in hospital, often with the use of a general anesthetic, and then rested for several weeks. However, once dislocation has taken place it is liable to recur, particularly if the joint has not been properly repaired or given insufficient time to heal. Repeated dislocations are sometimes treated with surgery to restrict the potential range of movement.

   A **sprain** is damage to one or more ligaments holding a joint together. Blood from the torn tissues causes bruising, and leakage of fluid results in joint swelling. Pain and swelling can be reduced by resting the joint and applying an elastic bandage. Surgery may be required if a ligament has been completely torn away from its attachment to the bone.

   Bursae, ligaments, and tendons become inflamed if there is excessive unaccustomed movement of a joint. **Bursitis** is inflammation of one of the protective fluid-filled sacs in a joint.
Tendinitis and **tenosynovitis** refer to inflammation of a tendon and its surrounding sheath, respectively. **Fibrositis** (not a specific term) denotes general swelling and irritation of tissues around a joint. Treatment of all the above conditions is likely to include resting the affected joint (perhaps with splints), injection of steroid drugs and physiotherapy. **Osteoarthritis (osteoarthrosis)** and **rheumatoid arthritis** usually occur in older people.
Gout is caused by crystals of uric acid being laid down in joints and other tissues due to excessively high levels of this substance in the blood. Affected joints become inflamed and very painful. Avoidance of

alcohol and certain foods may prevent recurrence, otherwise drugs which lower blood levels of uric acid may be used.

Backache and **back pain** have a multitude of possible causes, the most dramatic of them being **slipped disk** and also degeneration or displacement of vertebrae. Most often backache is due to bad posture or unaccustomed bending and lifting movements straining the back muscles. This backache responds to rest, special exercises to strengthen the muscles and avoidance of activities likely to produce pain. Slipped disk, in which pain is largely produced by the disk pressing on a nerve (**sciatica**), is treated with bed rest, painkillers and application of heat. The spine is particularly prone to inflammatory and degenerative joint disorders which may result in loss of flexibility of the back or neck.

Cardio-vascular disorders

CIRCULATORY PROBLEMS

Arteriosclerosis is thickening and loss of elasticity in artery walls. It is a normal part of the aging process but appears to start earlier and proceed faster in some people. **Atheroma** is a cholesterol deposit in the artery linings which impedes and alters blood flow, making clots more likely to occur. Arteriosclerosis and atheroma are often found together and the condition is then called **atherosclerosis**. Atherosclerosis is the cause of coronary heart disease.

An **aneurysm** is bulging of an artery where there is a weak point in the muscular lining. If an aneurysm ruptures, a severe hemorrhage will occur. Small aneurysms within the skull may cause a "**stroke**" when they burst.

Thrombosis is the blockage of a vein or artery by a blood clot (thrombus). Clotting results from a clotting disorder or impaired blood flow caused by dilated vessels, inactivity, inflammation or atheroma. Thrombosis in a superficial vein causes **phlebitis** – the vein looks hard and reddened, and feels very tender. Action must be taken to prevent the clot from spreading and the clotting's cause dealt with to prevent recurrence. **Deep vein thrombosis** may occur, particularly in the lower leg. Symptoms include pain and swelling. Both phlebitis and deep vein thrombosis carry the risk of **embolism**: part of the clot may break off and be carried to small vessels of another organ such as the brain or lung where blockage results in loss of blood flow to vulnerable tissues leading to their death (infarction). Treatments for thrombosis include anticoagulant drugs, vascular surgery and supportive bandaging.

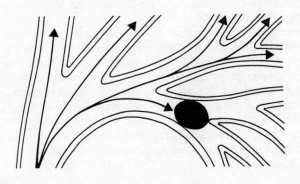

Embolism
If a clot lodges in an artery, the area depending on that blocked artery for blood supply will be severely affected without treatment.

©DIAGRAM

High blood pressure (hypertension) is a complex condition with a multitude of possible causes including genetic and environmental factors, obesity, excessive alcohol intake, and kidney and endocrine disorders. Taking the contraceptive pill may raise blood pressure, and women in the last stage of pregnancy are at risk of **eclampsia** (see p.328) if pressure gets too high. Blood pressure normally rises gradually with advancing age; but sudden sustained increases are most likely to cause harm. Several drugs can be prescribed to reduce high blood pressure.

Varicose veins are swollen superficial veins in the lower leg. Incompetent valves in deep veins allow blood to pool in these superficial veins, stretching them and increasing the likelihood of phlebitis because of slow blood flow. Around 10 percent of people have a congenital abnormality of one or more valves; and pregnancy and obesity are likely to exacerbate the condition. Thrombosis, eczema and skin ulceration are common complications; and treatments include support hose (to relieve aching), exercising the legs, injections to narrow the veins, and surgery.

Varicose veins
Support hose or elastic bandages will help if you have varicose veins, as will sitting with your feet up.

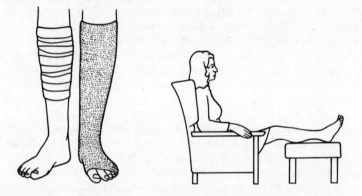

Hemorrhoids or **piles** are varicose veins inside and around the outside of the anus. They are subject to the same complications as those in the leg and may bleed if irritated by straining at hard stools. Creams and drugs help soothe pain and itching (which can be severe), and extra fiber should be included in the diet to avoid constipation. Injections or surgery may be needed. (See also p.205.)

Raynaud's syndrome arises in the fingers when cold, cigarette smoking or other factors cause painful narrowing of the arteries, making them blue or white. Sufferers should avoid situations which aggravate the condition.

Peripheral vascular disease is a complication of atherosclerosis. The development of a blood clot in an affected artery prevents sufficient blood flowing to the area it supplies. Other blood vessels may provide enough oxygen to prevent the tissues dying but not enough for muscles which demand high levels during exercise. The main symptom is therefore pain on exercise. The feet and legs are principally affected: sufferers should avoid getting cold or causing any injury to the feet and legs. Arterial insufficiency can also affect the brain, heart and kidneys, causing serious loss of function.

Stroke, see p.209.

HEART DISORDERS

Congenital heart defects arise while the heart of the fetus is developing in the early weeks of pregnancy. Several types of defect may occur, many of which can be corrected surgically in infancy.

Rheumatic heart disease is caused by streptococcal infection (including scarlet fever). Unless treated with antibiotics, the infection results in inflammation of the heart and damages the heart valves. In some cases, the valves can be surgically repaired or replaced.

Coronary heart disease is a major cause of death, particularly in developed countries. Many risk factors have been proposed: those with firmest scientific evidence to back them up include lack of exercise and obesity, hypertension, bad diet (excess alcohol and high saturated fat levels) and smoking. Stress and personality type have also been thought to have some effect but evidence for these is less conclusive. The condition is caused by narrowing (**atherosclerosis**) of the coronary arteries which supply the heart muscle with oxygen and nutrients. If the muscle's blood supply is impaired, it is no longer capable of efficiently maintaining its pumping operation. The principal symptom of coronary artery insufficiency is **angina pectoris**, a pain in the chest whenever the heart is called on to exert itself. Drugs are available to relieve angina and control disorders such as hypertension and clotting tendency, but the only remedies for the underlying condition are surgical procedures such as coronary bypass in which a piece of vein is used to bypass the narrowed section or balloon angioplasty in which a balloon catheter is introduced into the narrowed artery and then inflated to widen the vessel.

A **heart attack** (myocardial infarction) may be the first sign of coronary heart disease. Blood clot or sudden artery spasm reduces the blood supply to an area of the heart muscle so drastically that tissue begins to die, causing severe chest pain. The outlook for the patient depends upon the size of the area supplied by the blocked artery, the ability of other arteries to make up the deficiency, and the speed with which treatment is available. Equipment to restart and regularize the heartbeat and drugs to dissolve the clot may be used in the early stages. Long-term treatment may include a variety of drugs, change in diet and life style and, possibly, coronary bypass surgery.

Congestive heart failure is a sign that the heart has been affected in some way – possibly by myocardial infarction, damaged valves or chronic lung disease – and is no longer capable of pumping blood efficiently. The left or right side of the heart may fail separately but "knock-on" effects of raised pressure may result in both sides failing. The main symptoms are breathlessness with wheezing and fluid accumulation in the tissues (edema), particularly in the legs. Drugs such as digitalis and water-reducing diuretics, and treatment of any aggravating illness are often effective.

Arrhythmias (irregularities of the heartbeat) may be caused by heart disease or stem from disorders elsewhere in the body, such as hyperthyroidism. If the heart's own nerve pacemaker is failing to give the correct sequence of signals, an artificial electric pacemaker can be used to impose a normal heart rhythm. **Ventricular fibrillation** is a potentially fatal complication of a heart attack. The muscle, instead of pumping regularly, flutters in an uncoordinated way and normal rhythm must be reestablished with a defibrillator.

Use of a pacemaker
This device provides a regular electrical impulse to replace that in the heart. It is inserted under the skin on the chest wall, but can be worn on a belt if only needed for a short period.
a Heart
b Pacemaker
c Electrode connecting pacemaker with heart

©DIAGRAM

203

Blood disorders

ANEMIAS

Anemias are disorders of the blood's red cells. Only the most frequent are described *below*.

Iron deficiency anemia is a common cause of feelings of tiredness and weakness among women, particularly those who are pregnant, who suffer from heavy menstrual periods or who have a diet poor in iron. If regular blood loss is suspected, it should be investigated to rule out serious disease. Iron deficiency anemia can readily be diagnosed by a physician and remedied with iron supplements.

Folic acid deficiency causes a form of anemia if not enough folic acid-containing foods (such as leafy green vegetables, liver, and yeast) are included in the diet or if intestinal absorption is impaired. Supplements may be needed in pregnancy.

Pernicious anemia occurs in older people and is associated with changes in the stomach and nervous symptoms such as numbness of hands and feet. The condition used to be fatal, as its name indicates, but it can now be controlled with Vitamin B_{12} injections.

Sickle-cell anemia is an hereditary disease. The sufferer inherits the sickle-cell trait from both parents and is prone to painful crises in which abnormal hemoglobin distorts the red blood cells, causing them to disintegrate. Hospital treatment is usually needed to deal with the effects and, while oxygen and transfusions may help alleviate symptoms, there is no cure. Carriers of the trait may be offered genetic counseling.

Thalassemia is also hereditary and can cause severe symptoms in affected children. The red blood cells are very small and easily broken down. Blood transfusions may be helpful.

LEUKEMIA

Leukemia is characterized by presence of too many white blood cells of a particular type. White cells protect against infection, but in leukemia the cells are often immature and other blood cells are correspondingly reduced in number, leading to symptoms such as increased infection, tiredness and bleeding disorders. The most common leukemia in older people has a chronic form which often does not require treatment for some time, and life expectancy may be many years. Acute forms usually arise in children or young adults; some types respond better to treatment than others, and continuing improvements in techniques such as **bone marrow transplant** and **cytotoxic drug therapy** hold out real hope of long remission or even cure.

BLEEDING AND CLOTTING DISORDERS

Deficiencies of certain vitamins or clotting factors (as in **hemophilia**) lead to excessive bleeding from small bumps or cuts.

Treatment consists of remedying the underlying deficiency or giving transfusions of whole blood, platelets or the missing factor. Just as hemophilia is an inherited lack of clotting factor (found only in men but passed on by female carriers), so some people have a tendency for blood to clot too readily. This can be treated to some extent with anticoagulant drugs.

Hiatus hernia is common in women, particularly in those who are overweight and those who have had children. The upper stomach protrudes upward through the diaphragm, making the valve between the esophagus and the stomach less effective. The most characteristic symptom is heartburn, which tends to come on when bending or lying down. Pain is caused by the stomach's acid contents spilling back into the esophagus and irritating its lining membrane. Simple measures like losing weight, using extra pillows and not bending over are usually helpful. An operation to repair the diaphragm may be performed if the condition is very troublesome.

Indigestion is a very common complaint. Possible causes include smoking and alcohol; taking of aspirin and similar substances; eating spicy foods; eating too fast and not chewing food properly. Discomfort, belching and heartburn are common symptoms and can be relieved in the short term by taking antacids. In the long term, avoidance of the causative factors (particularly alcohol and smoking, which irritate the stomach) is the best medicine. **Peptic ulcers** are not uncommon in women; and the warning sign is persistent indigestion that is worse when the stomach is empty and improves when food is taken.

Abdominal pain is not always linked with a digestive disorder. Problems in the ovaries, Fallopian tubes and uterus can cause sudden severe pain; and an ectopic pregnancy or twisted ovary may give rise to very similar symptoms to **appendicitis** (inflammation and possible rupture of the appendix). Persistent pains and **diarrhea** are indicative of **irritable bowel syndrome, ulcerative colitis,** or **Crohn's disease.** Bleeding may also occur in the last two.

Diarrhea and vomiting associated with **gastroenteritis** are best treated by drinking small amounts of water or rehydrating solution at first, gradually reintroducing bland foods as the condition improves. Kaolin is a simple but effective remedy.

Constipation can be reduced by eating extra dietary fiber. Wholemeal bread and high-fiber cereals are good sources, as are fresh fruit and vegetables. Regular use of laxatives is likely to worsen constipation by disrupting the normal working of the bowel. Medical advice should be sought if constipation lasts for more than a few days or alternates with diarrhea.

Hemorrhoids (piles) come about through the enlargement of veins in the wall of the rectum or in the anus. This may be due to acute constipation or overstraining during excretion. It can also result from tumors. The swellings cause the mucous membrane to press against passing feces, leading to discomfort, pain, and sometimes bleeding.

Internal hemorrhoids occur at or before the rectum's junction with the anus. If they protude beyond the anal opening, the pressure of the anal muscle (the "sphincter") often causes great and constant pain: this is known as "strangulation."

External hemorrhoids occur under the skin just outside the anus. In addition to the usual causes, they can also result from a ruptured vein under the skin. Sometimes they burst, discharging blood.

Digestive disorders

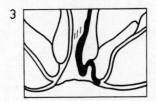

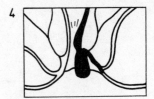

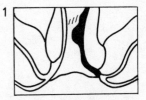

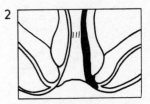

Hemorrhoids (piles)
1 Internal hemorrhoid
2 External hemorrhoid
3 Enlarged hemorrhoid
4 Strangulated hemorrhoid
Small hemorrhoids do not usually need treatment besides removing their likely cause which may mean, for instance, following a high-fiber diet to avoid constipation. More troublesome piles may require injections to shrink them, or surgical removal.

© DIAGRAM

Respiratory disorders

THE NOSE

Injury

The nose is very vulnerable to injury and the cartilage plate which separates the nostrils may be left crooked, resulting in possible congestion and increased risk of **sinus infection**. The nose can be straightened immediately or later on by an operation carried out inside the nose so that the scar is not visible.

Infections

Colds are the commonest infections to afflict the nose, causing sneezing and vast outpourings of clear mucus because the virus causes inflammation of the nasal membranes. Decongestant sprays can help but should only be used for a limited period. Bacteria may also rarely invade the membranes if they become too dry or have previously been damaged by viral infection. The result may be persistent **postnasal drip** or an unpleasant smell or discharge needing treatment with antibiotics.

Allergies

Hay fever and other allergies may cause sneezing, as well as congestion and swelling of the membranes and a runny nose which can be alleviated by antihistamines or other anti-allergy drugs.

Nasal polyps

These are small fleshy growths hanging from the lining membrane of the nose which often occur in people with allergies. The usual symptom is a feeling that the nose is blocked on one or both sides. Polyps can be removed by a simple operation in which they are cut off at the base by a wire snare. Nasal polyps are almost always benign.

Sinusitis

The entrances to the sinuses are tiny openings in the nasal cavity which can be blocked by thick mucus or inflammation caused by an infection. Mucus produced in the sinuses can no longer drain out into the nose and infection may result. Areas of the face overlying the sinus swell and redden and are often very painful (**acute sinusitis**). Sometimes decongestant treatments can unblock the sinus opening and allow it to drain; while antibiotics might be prescribed to deal with the infection. **Chronic sinusitis**, in which the nose is permanently stuffy, is usually dealt with by decongestants, antibiotics or, as a last resort, sinus irrigation where the sinuses are flushed out with saline.

THE THROAT

Infections

A sore throat is often the first sign of an infection entering the respiratory system. The tonsils and adenoids swell as they try to combat the infection, and the surrounding membranes may also be red and sore causing pain on swallowing. If a **cold** or **influenza** is the cause, gargling with aspirin or sucking throat lozenges will usually help, but a painful sore throat accompanied by fever or lasting for more than a few days should be seen by a physician. Tonsils or adenoids are not removed unless they repeatedly become infected or swollen, causing swallowing or hearing problems.

The larynx is the throat's lower part where the vocal cords and epiglottis are situated. **Laryngitis** is inflammation of the larynx resulting in hoarseness or complete loss of voice. The cause may be infection, irritants like dust or smoke, or strain from unaccustomed or untrained use of the voice. Treatment depends on the cause, but complete rest of the voice is important. Small nodules, usually benign, sometimes grow on the vocal cords and can be surgically removed. Severe infection can result in dangerous narrowing of the airway, particularly in children, so that any throat inflammation that makes breathing noisy or difficult should be treated as an emergency.

THE LUNGS

Coughing is one of the lungs' defense mechanisms. Infections or foreign bodies such as inhaled objects or dust cause swelling of the respiratory tube linings and an outpouring of mucus. This mucus, containing dead cells or dust, is then coughed out or swallowed.

As air passes in and out of the lungs, it makes sounds that can be heard through a doctor's stethoscope. In a healthy individual, these have a sighing or rustling character. But in an unhealthy person, unusual sounds and their location can indicate lung disorders. Tubes that are constricted cause wheezes or whistling noises; those filled with fluid, bubbling noises.

Influenza and some other viruses invade the lungs producing a hard, dry cough along with other symptoms such as headache, feverishness and runny nose. The most effective treatment is to rest in bed and antiviral drugs may be prescribed for the elderly or infirm. If a cough does not clear up after a few days or causes pain, then a bacterial infection may be cleared up with antibiotics.

Bronchitis literally means inflammation of the bronchi; and acute bronchitis with coughing up of thick mucus is a common sequel to colds and influenza. Chronic bronchitis is a condition that is created by damage to the normal mucus-clearing mechanisms resulting from prolonged exposure to cigarette smoke or other irritant substances. Patients suffer from repeated chest infections, breathlessness and bouts of coughing, especially in the mornings. The most helpful part of treatment is avoidance of the underlying cause, which means stopping smoking or avoiding a polluted environment. Antibiotics, inhalations and expectorants may be prescribed.

Treating bronchitis
In an acute attack, stay in bed in a room with warm, but not dry, air until your temperature is normal. Antibiotics and a soothing inhalant help; use a cough suppressant only if you have an irritating unproductive cough. Treat aches with analgesics that do not irritate the stomach. Chronic bronchitics should practice breathing out, sitting relaxed with fingernails on the lower rib cage. As you gently breath out, you feel your rib cage sink below your fingertips. As you gently breathe in, you feel the rib cage rise. Practice controlled breathing for several minutes twice daily.

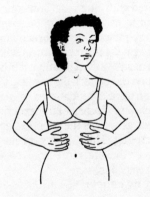

© DIAGRAM

Emphysema mainly affects older people, especially those who have suffered from other illnesses such as chronic bronchitis and asthma. The normal aging process of loss of elasticity is accelerated and the linings of the smallest air chambers break down to form larger air sacs, thereby reducing the potential surface area for exchange of gases to take place. Breathlessness may be severe, requiring oxygen inhalation, and patients are prone to pneumonia and heart problems.

Pneumonia may be caused by viruses, bacteria or other factors such as immobility after surgery or in elderly patients. The tiny chambers of the lung which should be full of air become fluid-filled, making breathing difficult, and the patient becomes feverish. Bacterial infections can be successfully countered with antibiotics so that pneumonia is normally only fatal in elderly people or those with low resistance. Pneumonia caused by one particular microorganism, *Pneumocystis carinii*, is a life-threatening disease in those with AIDS.

Treating pneumonia
Severe pneumonia needs hospital care and treatment with antibiotics. The patient sits up in bed in a well-ventilated warm room, at first taking only milk, orange juice or similar fluids, with some solid food after a day or two. Postural drainage (lying tilted with the affected part of the lung uppermost) may assist coughing up sputum, as may placing a hand on the part of the patient's chest and punching the hand with a clenched fist. Similar treatment aids lung abscesses, bronchoectasis and cystic fibrosis.

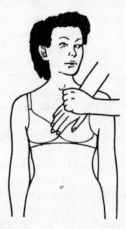

Legionnaires' disease and **psittacosis** are illnesses which cause pneumonia-like symptoms; but both respond to antibiotics.

Tuberculosis can affect many parts of the body but the primary site of infection is usually the lungs. Active disease is characterized by coughing (blood only appears in sputum at a late stage), weight loss, night sweats and tiredness. People in good health living in sanitary conditions are at relatively little risk from TB but it is a serious disease in developing countries and for those with compromised immune systems. Vaccination is available to prevent preliminary infection and the disease can be cured with long-term antibiotic treatment.

Pleurisy is a condition in which the membranes surrounding the lung become inflamed. There may be pain on breathing or painless accumulation of fluid between the membranes which interferes with breathing. Pleurisy is usually a complication of other lung diseases and treatment depends upon the underlying cause.

For information on **asthma**, see Allergies (p.215).

Cystic fibrosis is a chronic disease of the exocrine glands and affects the respiratory system, as well as the pancreas and sweat glands, causing excessive secreting. Thick, sticky mucus is typical of the disease. In order to keep the lungs free from mucus, daily respiratory or physiotherapy is usually necessary.

For information on **lung cancer**, see p.195.

Nervous disorders

INJURIES

Accidents such as a blow or penetrating wounds to the head, neck and back may result in serious damage to the central nervous system. The spinal cord is likely to be bruised or even ruptured unless fractures of the neck and back are immobilized. Tissue in the central nervous system rarely regenerates, though the brain is sometimes able to create new "pathways" through remaining nerve cells. The degree of disability caused by injury depends largely upon the injury site and tissue damage sustained: for example, damage to the spinal cord in the back results in loss of feeling and paralysis in the legs and lower body, whereas a neck level injury can affect the whole body except the head. Peripheral nerves may also be damaged by blows and cuts; but surgical repair cannot always restore full function.

Concussion means brief unconsciousness following a head injury. Confusion and headache are typical symptoms, and there is rarely any permanent loss of function. More severe blows may cause prolonged unconsciousness and brain swelling or bleeding.

Stroke is a term describing interruption of the blood supply to part of the brain, resulting in death of tissue. Strokes usually occur in older people. The underlying cause may be a clot in a narrowed artery or a ruptured aneurysm. If only a tiny amount of tissue is affected, symptoms may be slight and fleeting, but if a large artery is put out of action the tissue damage will be extensive. Signs that a major stroke has occurred include dizziness or unsteadiness, sudden paralysis of an area of the body, and inability to speak, see or hear. Immediate treatment consists of drugs to prevent further clotting or an operation to stop bleeding or remove a clot. Subsequent physical therapy and rehabilitation training enable many stroke patients to regain their confidence and independence.

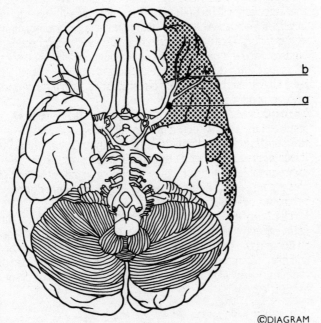

Stroke symptoms
Sometimes there may be loss of consciousness. Other possible symptoms include numbness, headache, blurred vision, dizziness, and inability to move or speak. Medical assistance should be sought immediately.
a Clot causing blockage
b Blocked artery
▨ Area of brain deprived of blood

©DIAGRAM

HEADACHES AND MIGRAINE

Headache causes include stress, tiredness, muscle tension in shoulders and neck, anxiety, alcohol hangover, food allergy, hormone changes, sinus infection, hypertension (rarely), eye disorders and diseases of the brain and meninges. The last category is a very rare cause – viral or bacterial infection of the meninges (**meningitis**) results in severe headache and neck stiffness. **Migraine** is a headache occasionally preceded by disturbances of vision, frequently confined to one side of the head and accompanied by nausea and vomiting. Painkillers and rest, together with avoidance of aggravating factors, are usually effective treatment, and drugs to prevent migraine attacks are available.

OTHER NERVOUS DISORDERS

Neuralgia is pain in a nerve, most commonly the face's trigeminal nerve. Any stimulus, such as touching a part supplied by the nerve, may result in severe pain. Drug treatment or surgery may be needed.

Neuritis is inflammation of a nerve, leading to weakness or paralysis. Treatment is directed at removing the cause, if it can be determined.

Shingles (herpes zoster) is caused by the chickenpox virus attacking sensory nerves. Blisters, which burst and then dry up, appear on the area of skin supplied by the nerves. Pain may linger for several months. Antiviral drugs can help if the condition is diagnosed sufficiently early.

Epilepsy is the tendency to suffer from seizures or "fits." A group of cells in the brain suddenly becomes overactive and disturbs the normal electrical pattern of part (**focal seizure**) or all of the brain (**generalized seizure**). Epilepsy can first occur at any age; and injuries, infections or strokes are sometimes responsible. A young child may have a seizure (**febrile convulsion**) when infection causes a high temperature – but these convulsions seldom recur and do not mean that the child will be epileptic. Focal seizures are characterized by localized symptoms such as uncontrollable jerking of a limb or visual disturbance. **Grand mal seizure** is sometimes preceded by warning signs before the person loses consciousness and falls. Victims should be turned onto their side once muscle spasm has subsided and reassured when they regain consciousness. Drug treatment to prevent seizures is highly effective.

Multiple sclerosis is patchy destruction of the fatty sheath which insulates nerves. Affected nerves are no longer capable of transmitting nervous impulses efficiently and symptoms depend on which nerves have been attacked. Progress of the disease is unpredictable: symptoms may disappear temporarily but gradual worsening of the condition usually results in some degree of permanent disability.

Parkinson's disease results from gradual deterioration of nerve centers, and the symptoms include tremors and involuntary shaking of the hands or head, or both, rubbing together of the thumb and first finger, excessive salivation, and sometimes loss of memory. It affects men slightly more often than women. Drug treatment can be quite effective.

Glandular disorders

There is a wide range of glandular disorders, many quite rare. A gland's failure to produce sufficient hormone will cause such symptoms as stunted growth caused by lack of growth hormone from the pituitary. Overproduction of a particular hormone can also cause problems: too much prolactin released from the pituitary, for instance, results in infertility because it suppresses the hormones responsible for ovulation. Loss of production often results from the gland's inactivity or destruction; and overproduction can be caused by cysts or tumors. Only the most common endocrine disorders are described *below.*

Thyroid disorders are relatively common: **hyperthyroidism**, for example, or excessive thyroxine production (also called **Graves' disease** and **thyrotoxicosis**) produces symptoms of increased metabolic rate with loss of weight, anxiety, palpitations and, sometimes, protruding eyeballs. The cause may be a tumor but is usually an "autoimmune" process in which immune system elements attack the body's own tissues. Treatment consists of drug therapy to control hormone levels; surgery to remove part of the gland; or injection with a radioactive isotope of iodine (which accumulates in the thyroid), to destroy the overactive tissue.

Hypothyroidism (myxedema) is also usually an autoimmune disease. As thyroxine-producing tissue is attacked, symptoms of lowered metabolic rate appear. The sufferer puts on weight and feels cold, lethargic, and tired. Treatment with thyroxine reverses the condition but has to be continued for life in many cases.

Goiter is a general term for swellings of the thyroid. Common causes include lack of iodine; tumors (usually benign and causing few symptoms); and autoimmune disease, resulting in hypothyroidism.

Diabetes mellitus results when insulin-producing cells in the pancreas no longer make enough insulin to enable body cells to make proper use of sugar. Levels of blood sugar build up and the person feels thirsty and has to urinate frequently. A simple urine test shows high levels of sugar, confirming the diagnosis. Diabetes is thought to have an hereditary component in that some families have more sufferers than others, but there must be additional factors at work – perhaps viral infections or dietary habits. By no means every member of an affected family will develop it. Physicians tend to divide diabetes patients into "juvenile-onset" and "maturity-onset" categories. In children, the insulin-producing cells' destruction is often total, causing rapid onset of symptoms and, usually, the need for insulin injections to control blood sugar. Diabetes arising in older people (particularly in overweight women) tends to develop more slowly: some insulin is still produced and the condition may be treatable by weight and dietary controls and, if necessary, tablets which stimulate the pancreas to make more insulin. Occasionally diabetes symptoms occur during pregnancy (see p.328). Diabetics may also suffer from slowly-developing complications such as eye changes (which can lead to blindness unless treated), increased arteriosclerosis (requiring special care of feet and legs) and kidney problems. Good control of blood sugar levels helps prevent these complications arising or progressing: this means avoiding the

©DIAGRAM

dangerous and distressing state of **hyperglycemia** (too much sugar in the blood) and **hypoglycemia** (too little sugar in the blood). Hyperglycemia tends to develop when a diabetic does not take enough insulin; and unless it is treated, the patient may lapse into a coma. Hypoglycemia can come on very suddenly due to too much insulin, causing symptoms that include aggression, unsteadiness and even unconsciousness. It can quickly be remedied with glucose.

Restricted growth in childhood may be the result of long-term illness, achondroplasia (a form of hereditary dwarfism), thyroid disorder or failure of the pituitary to produce adequate growth hormone. Genetically engineered human growth hormone can restore a normal rate of growth in certain cases.

Adrenal disorders are rare: the most common are **Addison's disease** and **Cushing's syndrome**. Addison's disease is caused by lack of cortisol and aldosterone, making the body unable to deal with any kind of stress such as infections. Treatment is with corticosteroid drugs. Cushing's syndrome is caused by too much cortisol, produced either by pituitary disorder or by adrenal or lung tumors, or by prolonged use of steroid drugs. Treatment consists of dealing with the underlying disorder.

The hypothalamus, which acts as the body's clock, sometimes initiates sexual development at a very early or late age. In addition, **delayed puberty** may arise either from failure of the pituitary to make sufficient amounts of gonadotrophins, or inability of the ovaries to respond. **Premature puberty** (precocity) can also occur because of a variety of hormonal abnormalities. Appropriate hormone therapy is usually effective in dealing with these problems.

Ovarian disorders sometimes result from tumors or cysts of the ovaries that cause secretion of excessive amounts of certain hormones and cause menstrual chaos or infertility. Some may also have a virilizing effect (producing male features such as increased body hair). Cysts arise when a developed follicle fails to burst and release the egg into the Fallopian tube. The follicle instead turns into a fluid-filled sac or a solid lump. Cysts usually disappear by themselves but, if discovered, are investigated to ensure that they are harmless. Weight loss, contraceptive pill taking and pituitary disorders may also result in menstrual irregularities. These can often be remedied with drugs to stimulate normal hormone output. Adolescent girls frequently have irregular periods, but unaccountable interruptions to a previously regular cycle should be investigated. The role of hormone imbalance in **dysmenorrhea** (painful menstruation), **premenstrual tension** and **postpartum depression** is complex. Administration of progesterone or the contraceptive pill seems to work for some women, but not all. Other drugs such as diuretics which reduce the symptom of premenstrual bloating, and bromocriptine which suppresses prolactin levels, may be helpful. Severe symptoms should be dealt with by a qualified specialist.

Hirsutism (excess body hair) is seldom attributable to hormonal imbalance, though if it occurs relatively suddenly it needs to be investigated. Most often there is an ethnic or hereditary predisposition. Traditional methods of hair removal (see p. 70) should be tried. Only very rarely will a woman need referal to an endocrinological clinic.

Immune disorders

There are two kinds of immune system disorder: the body's recognition of its own cells may become faulty, resulting in attack and inflammation or destruction of certain tissues (autoimmune disease); or an immune system component may fail, allowing infection to overwhelm the body.

AUTOIMMUNE DISEASE

Autoimmunity is thought to be a factor in many important diseases including **rheumatoid arthritis**, **endocrine disorders** and **diabetes**. It is not clear why the immune system should suddenly mistake body tissues as being foreign and therefore to be attacked. A genetic predisposition to certain autoimmune conditions has been established, but not everyone with a particular "tissue type" will necessarily develop the disease with which it is associated. Viral, environmental or dietary factors are also likely to play a part. Treatment may include corticosteroid drugs to suppress the underlying inflammatory process; and other symptoms are dealt with according to the disease's site and nature.

IMMUNE DEFICIENCY

Radiation, some viruses (such as HIV, the **AIDS** virus), and various toxic chemicals all have the potential to affect the immune system by destroying or deranging white blood cells. If stem cells are affected, the result may be complete loss of production (as in **aplastic anemia**) or overproduction of faulty, ineffective cells, as in **leukemia** (cancer of the white blood cells); or destruction of white cells. The end result, if untreated, is the same – inability to fight off infections. Normal stem cells can be restored by bone marrow transplant; and in leukemia, for example, treatment is directed at halting overproduction of abnormal cells.

Several other diseases also impair the immune system. **Hodgkin's disease**, for instance (a type of tumor of the lymph glands, known as a "lymphoma"), is probably caused by malignant transformation of lymphoid tissue. Principal symptoms are swollen glands in the neck, armpit, and groin; a fever, weight loss, and tiredness. If treated soon enough, it can often be cured by radiation theraphy or intensive anti-cancer drug therapy. **Non-Hodgkin's lymphomas** are, however, more difficult to treat and may result from malignant transformation of lymphocytes. A bone marrow biopsy and other investigations will determine which type of lymphoma is present, if any.

POST-VIRAL FATIGUE SYNDROME (PVS)

People who have suffered from a viral infection such as influenza may be subsequently afflicted with tiredness and depression which can last several weeks or even months. Not everyone who has had a particular virus will get PVS, and someone who has had PVS once will not necessarily suffer from it again after other viral infections. (PVS is not synonymous with benign myalgic encephalomyelitis.)

MYALGIC ENCEPHALOMYELITIS

Also known as ME, chronic fatigue syndrome, Yuppie flu, Iceland disease, this disorder affects twice as many women as men. At one time its existence was regarded with some scepticism by most doctors, but it is now widely considered to be caused by malfunction of the immune system in response to viral infection.

Very often the disease strikes people who have been particularly physically active or under prolonged stress, and it can last for many years. In many patients there is an imbalance of certain types of white blood cells, indicating faulty immune response, and excessive build-up of lactic acid in the muscles during exercise causing the characteristic symptom of severe fatigue.

There is as yet no general cure for ME. Symptoms vary, and one form of treatment may be quite effective for one person, but useless for another. The table below outlines some factors implicated in producing symptoms, together with treatments which some people have found to bring about an improvement in their condition, but it is by no means a full list. The holistic approach of alternative medicine has also been beneficial in some cases. Prolonged rest (around 6 months) and avoidance of stress may be recommended at the start of the disease; and recovery is likely to be slow with relapses, but ME is not fatal and most sufferers are eventually able to resume a "normal," if slightly restricted life.

Symptoms	Possible causes	Treatments
Physical fatigue	Lactic acid build-up	Rest
Mental fatigue	Disturbed sleep patterns	Rest, relaxation
Depression	Physical effects of virus Disruption of life style	Antidepressants Talking with other sufferers
Palpitations	Hyperventilating	Relaxation techniques
Dizziness	Hypoglycemia	Small, frequent meals
Intestinal problems	Food allergy	Elimination diet

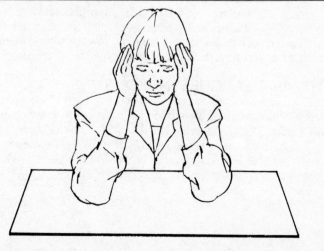

Allergies

About one woman in ten is born with an inherited tendency to develop an allergy at some time in her life. The allergy may be confined to one specific substance, such as a grass pollen, and cause irritating but purely seasonal discomfort or it may extend to a range of foods, cosmetics, animal scurf and dusts, resulting in disabling restriction on the sufferer's way of life. A vast array of symptoms have been attributed to allergic reaction. The most common and important are listed on this page.

Treatment mainly consists of identifying and, if possible, avoiding known allergens. Skin testing can help in the search for contact irritants, and elimination diets (the diet is at first restricted to "safe" foods and then expanded until allergy to a "new" food occurs) serve to identify dietary allergens. Desensitization (use of injections of pollens, etc) is effective in some circumstances but carries the risk of severe reactions; but if symptoms are serious (as with severe asthma), the risk may be justifiable. Antihistamine and corticosteroid drugs suppress the inflammatory processes that cause many allergic symptoms, but sometimes have unwanted side-effects. Sodium cromoglycate preparations prevent allergic swelling of the eye's mucous membranes and those of the respiratory tract. Bronchodilator drugs are also often prescribed for asthma.

SYMPTOMS
(Those in **bold** type require **immediate** medical attention)

Anaphylactic shock: (onset within a few seconds or minutes after exposure to allergen) nausea and vomiting, nettle rash, collapse, breathing difficulty
Asthma: breathlessness, wheezing (if severe)
Conjunctivitis (sore red eyes)
Coughing
Depression
Diarrhea
Dizziness
Headache
Indigestion
Migraine
Mouth irritation and swelling
Nausea
Rash
Runny nose
Sneezing
Vomiting

POTENTIAL ALLERGENS
(common forms are in *italic*)

Alcohol: *red wine, whisky*
Animals: *cats, dogs, horses*
Chemicals: *detergents, plastics*
Clothing materials
Cold
Cosmetics: *dyes, perfumes*
Dust: *house dust mite*
Emotional stress
Exercise
Foodstuffs: *cheese, chocolate, citrus fruits, coffee, eggs, fish, flavorings, maize, milk (especially cows'), nuts, preservatives, shellfish, strawberries, wheat*
Heat
Infections
Insects and their bites
Light
Medicines: *aspirin, penicillin, quinine*
Molds and their spores
Parasites
Plants and their pollens: *grass, poison ivy, primulas*

©DIAGRAM

Dangers to body and mind

Stress

Stress is nervous tension. It may be conscious or unconscious – that is, you may or may not be aware of feeling tense. It may be environmental or psychological: you may be reacting to a physical

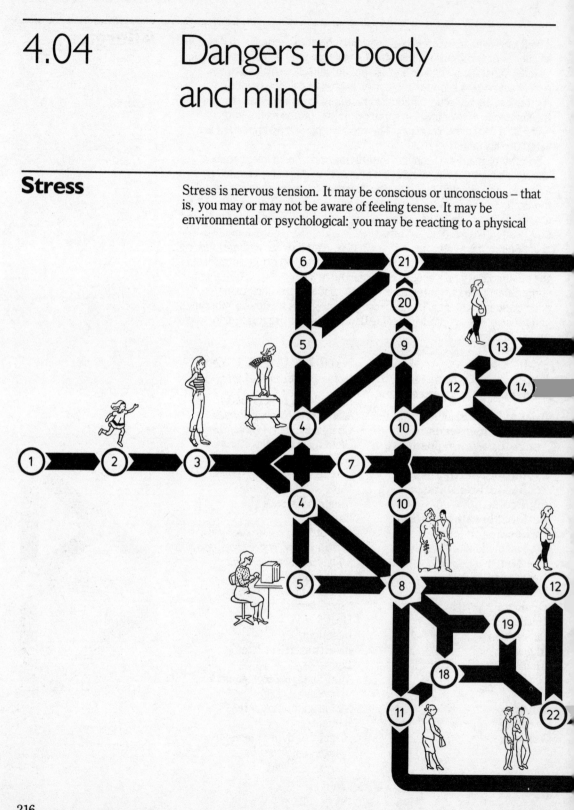

threat or a mental threat. And it may be acute or chronic (the threat may be a single event or a continuing situation). But whatever the cause, stress depends on your reaction, not on the outside event.

The life pattern of most women is dotted with potential stress points. Some of these, such as puberty, motherhood, and the menopause, are associated directly with the biological aspects of women as childbearers. And many women who follow a traditional role may find that such events create additional stress within the context of marriage and the family.

Today, an increasing number of women are choosing not to follow these patterns. But this decision can itself cause considerable stress, given the prevailing attitudes and arrangements of society.

Stress situations
1 Infancy
2 Childhood
3 Puberty
4 Leaving home
5 Job
6 Loss of job
7 Fertility
8 Marriage, cohabitation
9 Cohabitation
10 Conceive
11 Housewife, childless
12 Pregnancy
13 Abortion
14 New baby
15 Parenthood
16 Single parent family
17 Leave marriage
18 Divorce
19 Widow
20 Loss of partner
21 Living alone
22 Remarriage
23 Extra-marital affair
24 Mature student
25 Menopause
26 Child leaves home
27 Looking after elderly parents
28 Old age
29 Living with children
30 Institutionalized
31 Approach of death

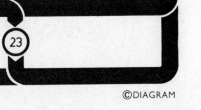

©DIAGRAM

Dependencies

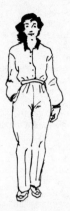

Stress threatens everyone to some extent: the conditions of our society make it hard to escape it. Despite this, many maintain an independent and intelligent approach to life, for stress need not be something that defeats us. But others seek refuge in some form of dependence, a false center around which their lives can revolve. Some of these patterns of dependence are encouraged by our society. Others are frowned upon, and yet others dismissed as superficial rather than treated as symptoms of an underlying escapism.

Socially acceptable female roles have traditionally encouraged dependency in women, a situation which can cause conflict both in women themselves and in their relationships with their partners and their children. Today some women are redefining these roles in terms of their own fulfillment. They have recognized that not only is suppression dangerous for themselves, it can also lead to too great a burden of dependence on and resentment toward their lovers, husbands and children. Without a sense of self, many women are also forced into the routine of using their sexuality for identity or as a weapon.

Drug dependence often has the image of an illegal and socially unacceptable addiction.

But far more common and socially significant is dependence on prescribed and legally obtainable drugs such as tranquilizers. Although **cigarette smoking** is more common among men, some 30-40% of adult women are dependent on cigarettes, and there is evidence that, despite the well-known dangers, they have greater difficulty in stopping smoking.

Alcoholism is currently the most serious form of drug abuse and its incidence among women is very much on the increase. Reasons for the dependency may include stress or uncertainty related to emotional or physical problems. Many women, bored or frustrated by the role of housewife, develop an extreme reliance on various time-wasting **displacement activities** or routine actions such as tea or coffee-drinking, or excessive housework.

Just as some women turn to alcohol, others turn to food for comfort, **eating excessively** to relieve stress or boredom. Others, by contrast, may react to emotional fears by **rejecting food** to an extreme degree.

Society's stereotype of the desirable woman as young and attractive has meant that many women become obsessed with maintaining their **youthful appearance**. For such women, the onset of middle age and the gradual process of aging may become increasing sources of stress.

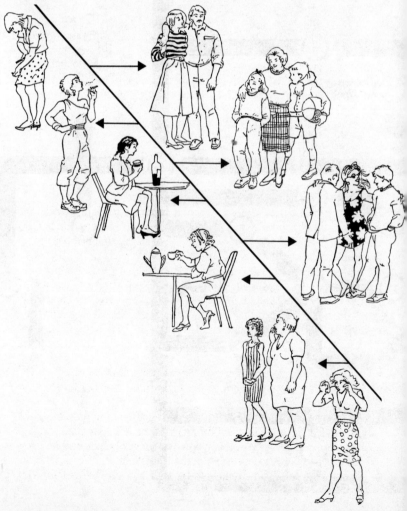

Smoking

By now we all know that smoking is bad for us, and that if we continue to smoke we are risking serious damage to our health. Smoking is also increasingly regarded as unattractive and antisocial. Many people are now deciding that the benefits of being a non-smoker far outweigh any difficulties they may encounter in giving up. But if you find it difficult to give up completely, there are still ways of reducing the amounts of tar and nicotine that you take into your body.

GIVING UP

Analyse your smoking habits Spend a few weeks keeping a record of every cigarette you smoke. Don't let yourself light up automatically. Work out why and when you need to smoke a cigarette.

Prepare yourself Really decide that you want to stop smoking. Think about all the benefits that not smoking will bring. Decide exactly on which day you are going to stop smoking. On the night before, smoke your last cigarette, clean out all the ashtrays and put them away, and dispose of any remaining cigarettes, lighters and matches. Then **stop** smoking.

Change your habits Your smoking record will tell you when you are tempted to smoke. Change your daily routine to keep away from these trigger situations. This might mean going for a walk after lunch instead of having a cup of coffee, for instance. You may also find that it will help if you give up smoking at a time when your routine will be different from usual – perhaps as you begin your vacation. Travel in non-smoking compartments, sit in non-smoking sections in theaters and restaurants, and so on. Keep as far away from smoking situations as you can. And if someone offers you a cigarette, tell them that you are a non-smoker.

Spoil yourself Save the money that you spend on cigarettes and use it to give yourself a positive reward by buying something you would not otherwise be able to afford. Remind yourself that you were able to afford this luxury because you have stopped smoking.

Give yourself time Remember that it takes six to eight weeks to break a habit. Don't be tempted back into smoking before you have really given your body a chance to get rid of all the toxins it has accumulated.

Extra help If you feel you cannot give up on your own, there is plenty of help and support available. Nicotine chewing gum may help to relieve any cravings you have; an anti-smoking group or clinic will give you moral support; and hypnotism or acupuncture may help to relieve any withdrawal symptoms.

CUTTING DOWN

- Change to filter-tipped cigarettes with a lower tar content.
- Even when you are smoking tipped cigarettes, use a cigarette holder that includes a tar filter.
- Buy cigarettes that are shorter in length than your normal brand. Never leave a cigarette in your mouth for more than one puff.
- Only smoke a cigarette halfway down its length before stubbing it out, as the last half is where most of the tar collects.
- Try smoking one cigarette less today than you smoked yesterday.

Benefits
These are some of the benefits you can expect if you give up smoking.
Feeling fitter
Fresher breath
Nicotine stains on fingers and teeth will disappear
Improved senses of smell and taste
Clearer skin
Less chance of wrinkles
Clothes and hair will not smell of smoke
Home will smell fresher
More spending money
Improved life expectancy
Less chance of developing lung cancer, heart disease, or other serious illnesses
Less risk to health of friends and family through passive smoking

©DIAGRAM

Women and alcoholism

Alcoholism was once thought of as primarily a male problem, but in recent years there has been a dramatic increase in the number of female alcoholics. Indeed, it is now estimated that as many as one-third of all alcoholics are women. Inveterate drinking accounts for some of these women alcoholics – young girls keeping boyfriends company or older women moving in the business world.

However, most women become alcoholics as a result of turning to alcohol in response to stress: and reasons for drinking often given by female alcoholics are physical troubles such as premenstrual tension, miscarriage, and infertility, as well as emotional difficulties associated with sexual roles, such as boredom, sexual problems or a divorce. But case studies show that alcoholism is often part of a general picture of depressive illness. In fact, many female alcoholics have emotional problems dating back to disturbed childhoods, often typified by the loss, absence, or inadequacy of one or both parents.

PHYSIOLOGICAL EFFECTS

The effects of alcoholism on the body include constant inflammation of the stomach and later the intestines, with severe risk of ulceration; malnutrition and vitamin deficiency diseases such as pellagra and beriberi, caused by neglecting diet for drink; cirrhosis of the liver – in which the organ shrivels, its cells largely replaced by fibrous tissues, and functions deteriorate; degeneration of muscles – including those of the heart; destruction of brain cells and degeneration throughout the nervous system – sometimes resulting in pneumonia, heart or kidney failure, or organic psychosis; or delirium tremens – a condition involving extreme excitement, mental confusion, anxiety, fever, trembling, a rapid and irregular pulse rate, and hallucinations, which characteristically occur when a bout of heavy drinking is followed by abstention.

TREATMENT

Treatments for alcoholism are similar to those used for other types of drug addition.

Detoxification treatment usually begins in a clinic or hospital. First the patient is deprived of alcohol (or the other drug to which she is addicted). This can produce severe withdrawal symptoms such as sweating, vomiting, body aches, running nose and eyes, convulsions, fits, and hallucinations. Sedatives are used to bring relief during this period but must be withdrawn before new addictions are formed. Any physical problems are treated, and the patient's health restored by good diet, exercise and rest.

After detoxification, attempts are made to identify and treat the underlying psychological reasons for addiction. The patient's motivation, self-confidence, and trust must be constantly supported. Treatment is often long-term, and success depends above all on the patient's desire to be cured. Meanwhile, organizations such as Alcoholics Anonymous provide group therapy led by former alcoholics, and can give very valuable support in rehabilitation and continued abstention.

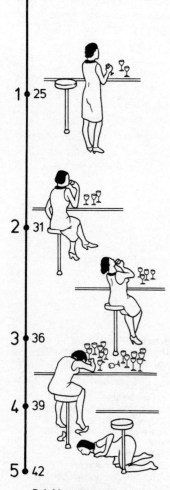

20 Years of age

1 • 25

2 • 31

3 • 36

4 • 39

5 • 42

Drinking patterns
1 Started drinking
2 Regular moderate drinking
3 First signs of alcoholism
4 Long periods of intoxification
5 Loss of control

Drugs

In the West, alcohol and tobacco are the principal drugs that are taken to alter mood. They are, of course, legal except that the sale of both is generally restricted to those over an age which varies from country to country. But some mood-altering drugs are prescribed by doctors. Tranquilizers and sedatives, for instance, are very commonly prescribed to women in a whole variety of circumstances. Indeed, it has been estimated that in most European countries as well as the USA, they may be taken by as many as 1 in 5 of the female population (as compared with 1 in 10 men). But many mood-altering drugs are strictly illegal, although it is as well to remember that drugs such as heroin, which we usually associate with addicts, also have important medical uses – to give pain relief, for instance.

The sections that follow outline the effects of certain drugs, among them caffeine, tranquilizers and a number, both legal and illegal, that are increasingly misused.

CAFFEINE

This stimulant of the central nervous system is found in coffee, tea, cocoa, and many cola drinks. Its action combats fatigue, but it is a comparatively mild drug. It is also a diuretic – that is, it increases the urine output of the kidneys. Medically, caffeine is also often included in headache pills to counteract the dulling effect of the painkilling ingredient. Abuse is unlikely because of the large quantities necessary, but those who drink considerable amounts of coffee probably have a mild psychological if not physiological dependence.

STIMULANTS

Amphetamines (also known as "speed", "pep pills" or "uppers") are commonly misused and are taken because they produce feelings of exhilaration and decrease the appetite generally.

The user experiences a sense of well-being and, with strong doses, euphoria. Alertness, wakefulness, and confidence are also accompanied by feelings of mental and physical power. The user often becomes talkative, excited, and hyperactive, too; and accompanying physical symptoms may include sweating, trembling, and insomnia.

Amphetamines are probably not physically addictive. However, psychological dependence is easily produced. Extra energy is "borrowed" from the body's reserves; and when the drug's action has worn off, the body has to pay for it in fatigue and depression. This creates a desire for more of the drug to counteract these effects.

Medical usage has become less common since realization of the dangers. But amphetamines are still prescribed for some purposes: to prevent sleep in people who have to be alert for long periods; to treat minor depression; and to suppress the appetite in a few cases of obesity – all, though, with increasing rarity.

Dangers include not only psychic dependence, but also physical deterioration due to hyperactivity and lack of appetite; induced psychotic conditions of paranoia and schizophrenia, resulting from prolonged overdose; suicide due to depression following large doses; and even death from overdose.

ANTI-DEPRESSANTS

These fall into two principal groups: **tricyclics** and **MAOIs (monoamine oxidase inhibitors)**. The latter are less often prescribed because of the possibility of harmful reactions with foods such as cheese, yeast extract spreads or alcohol. Most anti-depressants take a few weeks to begin to relieve symptoms; and side-effects may include blurred vision, lethargy and constipation. In spite of this, these drugs can be useful at times when psychotherapy may be unavailable or unsuitable to help a woman face the underlying problem and there is not a great risk of dependency. Be sure to check about any contraindications or foodstuffs to be avoided.

Lithium has been shown to be helpful in the treatment and prevention of manic-depressive illness; and because of certain serious side-effects that can occur, if your doctor has put you on this medication, you should see him or her at once if any unpleasant symptoms arise.

BARBITURATES

Barbiturates (once nicknamed "barbs," "candy," or "goof balls") are derived from barbituric acid. Like all depressants, they reduce the conduction of impulses in the brain. Because of this, they were medically prescribed for many years to relieve anxiety and tension and induce sleep; and some have also been used as anesthetics. But with greater realization of their dangers, they are now almost totally replaced by **benzodiazepines** which are thought to be far safer.

Barbiturates vary in their immediacy and duration of effect, depending on the rate at which they are metabolized and eliminated.

Someone who has taken barbiturates may well show signs of drowsiness, restlessness, irritability, irrationality, mental confusion, and impairment of coordination and reflexes, with staggering and slurring of speech. The pupils may constrict; sweating may increase. The person experiences initial euphoria, followed by depression. When an excessive amount is taken (an "overdose"), the depressive effect upon the nervous system is such that unconsciousness occurs, followed in extreme cases by death from respiratory failure.

Barbiturates create tolerance and physical dependence, and the effects of withdrawal in a chronic user can be worse than those of alcohol or heroin. They include irritability and restlessness, anxiety, insomnia, abdominal cramp, nausea and vomiting, tremors, hallucinations, severe convulsions, and sometimes death. Yet addicts are attracted by the possibility of escaping from emotional stress, through sedation; the feelings of euphoria on initial ingestion, when large amounts of the drug are tolerated; and the ability of barbiturates to counteract the effects of stimulants. (The cyclical use of "uppers" and "downers" can lead to dependence on both.)

The common prescription of barbiturates to induce relaxation and sleep once resulted in the largest group of dependent people being the middle aged, especially housewives. The same ready availability also made barbiturates a common suicide weapon, while the combination of their depressive effects with use of alcohol has brought many accidental deaths through taking barbiturates after heavy drinking.

TRANQUILIZERS

The **benzodiazepines** (such as Valium, Librium, Mogadon and others) are known as "minor tranquilizers" and are among the most frequently prescribed drugs to women for symptoms of anxiety (possibly following bereavement or during marital problems), and also as sleeping pills. Side-effects are often noticed (nausea and headaches, for instance); and concentration may well be impaired. Symptoms may be relieved, but tranquilizers do not, of course, make the cause of the stress disappear. In conjunction with psychotherapy, however, they may be more helpful.

Dependency can result: and adverse reactions may often occur if they are taken when drinking alcohol. Tranquilizers should also not be taken either by pregnant women or those who are breastfeeding. Your doctor should be able to recommend a satisfactory way of reducing any dose you are taking to tide you over a difficult period, and self-help groups are often a great support in suggesting means of coping while cutting down. ("Major tranquilizers" are sometimes prescribed for the severely anxious or psychotic.)

GLUE-SNIFFING

This is the breathing in of vapours given off by the fumes of certain solvents in order to get a "high." Common substances used include adhesives, gasoline (petrol), nail varnish, lighter fuel and paint-thinners.

The effects are very much like those of drinking alcohol. There may be slurred speech, confusion, dizziness and even hallucinations; and afterwards, a headache like that of a hangover.

Sniffing glue may not in itself be illegal, but in several countries it is now an offense to sell solvents to anyone under 18 if the vendor believes they are likely to be misused. Indeed, it is among school children that abuse of solvents is most usual: it is a cheap and easy substitute for alcohol, and often tried "for kicks" or out of boredom.

There is no evidence to show that solvent-abuse does direct permanent damage: but we do know that breathing in similar fumes day after day in a factory situation has sometimes resulted in damage to the liver as well as to kidneys.

A very real danger among young people, however, is the sort of accident that may occur while intoxicated.

CANNABIS

Otherwise known as marijuana, pot, hashish (or hash), resin or dope, cannabis (an illegal drug in most parts of the world although widely taken) is usually smoked in a cigarette or "joint" with some tobacco but can also be eaten, as part of the ingredients of a cake, for instance. The sensations it causes are those of relaxation and loss of inhibitions. There is some evidence of bronchitis and perhaps lung cancer after very heavy use: and during pregnancy, it has been shown to cause fetal damage in some cases. Research has also shown that regular use can cause psychological rather than physical dependence; and it is believed by some that it may also lead the individual to experiment with other more harmful drugs.

NARCOTICS

The opiates (or narcotics) are known in drug-taking circles as "the hard stuff." **Opium** itself and its derivative **heroin** are, in fact, the archetypal drugs of addiction. However, **codeine** and **morphine**, which are also derived from opium, are better known for their medical uses.

All depressants inhibit the activity of the central nervous system, impairing coordination and reflexes; but opiates especially affect the sensory centers, reducing pain and promoting sleep. As with alcohol, however, there may be initial excitement, as inhibitions are removed. In large doses, the opiates act on the pleasure centers of the brain, producing feelings of great peace, contentment and euphoria.

General effects of opiate abuse include loss of appetite, constipation, and constriction of the pupils. An overdose of an opiate is also likely to cause convulsions, unconsciousness, and death.

All opiates create physical dependence. The symptoms of withdrawal from abusive use begin with stomach cramps, followed by diarrhea, nausea and vomiting, running eyes and nose, sweating, and trembling. These are also accompanied by irritability and restlessness, insomnia, anxiety and panic, depression, confusion, and an all-consuming desire for the drug.

Opium is the dried juice of the unripe seed capsules of the Indian poppy. The plant is cultivated in India, Persia, China, and Turkey, and opium is then prepared in either powder or liquid form. The poppy possesses its psychoactive powers only when grown in favorable conditions of climate and soil. Poppies produced in temperate climates have only a negligible effect.

Opium is traditionally smoked, using pipes, but it can also be injected or taken orally.

Codeine (methyl morphine) is a less potent opiate. It is white and crystalline in form, and is often used with aspirin for treating headaches. Because of the inhibiting effect on nervous reflexes it shares with all opiates, it is used in many cough medicines, and sometimes in the treatment of diarrhea, since it reduces peristalsis (the automatic rhythmic contractions of the intestine). Risk of tolerance and abusive use is very small because of the large amounts necessary to produce pleasant effects.

Morphine is the basis of all opiate action and the main active constituent of opium. It was isolated from opium in 1805, and since then has been medically important as a pain killer. It is ten times as strong as opium, and must be administered with great care to avoid tolerance and physical dependence. However, instances of abuse are not too common, as drug users tend to prefer heroin.

Heroin (diamorphine) was first isolated in 1898. It is twice as strong as morphine, and has a quicker and more intense effect, though a shorter duration. Among drug takers, it is often known as "H," "horse," or "smack." In some countries, it may be used medically for pain relief. (**Pethidine**, for example, which is frequently used to reduce pain during childbirth, is also an opium derivative.) But production, possession, and use of heroin are all generally connected with drug abuse. A grayish-brown powder in its pure form, it is usually mixed with milk or baking powder to add bulk. This results in a white coloring. The high cost of the drug, and its necessity to those who have become dependent on it, account for the high crime rate associated with its users.

The powder is sniffed or smoked, but is usually injected, often into a muscle when use begins, but then into a major vein ("mainlining") as tolerance develops. Mainlining gives more immediate and powerful effects. Constant injection into the same vein causes hardening and scarring of the flesh tissue and eventual collapse of the vein. Unhygienic conditions and use of unsterilized needles can also cause infection, often resulting in sores, abscesses, hepatitis, jaundice, and thrombosis – and, more recently, the spread of HIV (the AIDS virus). Poor nutrition and self-neglect are also likely.

Almost immediately upon injection, intense feelings of euphoria and contentment envelop the user. The effect depends on the purity and strength of the heroin, and the psychological state of the user – the higher the previous tension and anxiety, the more powerful the subsequent feelings of pleasure and peace. In a chronic user, the ritual of injection is also important in the creation of pleasure.

Physical dependence on heroin can develop within a few weeks. Withdrawal symptoms will then begin four to six hours after the effect of the last shot has worn off.

If you have been abusing heroin or other opiates, you may be able to wean yourself off with gradually decreased doses: but best of all you should see your doctor or attend a drug center. You may be prescribed a substitute such as **methadone** which will help prevent dreadful withdrawal symptoms.

COCAINE

Cocaine (often nicknamed "coke" or "snow") is a white powder obtained from the coca plant found in South America. Synthetic derivatives are also available. It acts by stimulating the central nervous system, dispelling fatigue, increasing alertness, mental activity and reflex speed, and inducing euphoria. After an initial "rush," the effects become more steady. Accompanying physical symptoms include dilation of pupils, tremors, loss of appetite, and insomnia.

Opinions are divided as to physical dependence, but psychological dependence easily develops for the same reasons as it does with amphetamines. Cocaine is a short-acting drug and must be taken repeatedly to maintain the effects.

Abuse is the main use found for cocaine. As a powder, it is snorted, which eventually results in deterioration of the nasal linings and finally of the nasal septum separating the nostrils. Injection of the liquid form is an alternative, but using cocaine alone is unpopular, because of the sudden effects. So heroin and cocaine are often injected together.

Dangers of prolonged use include insomnia, paranoia, hallucinations in the sense of touch (known as "the cocaine bugs") and loss of weight and malnutrition through lack of interest in food. An overdose causes convulsions, and can result in death by respiratory failure.

Crack (also known as "wash", "base" or "rock") comprises small bits of "freebase" cocaine that are smoked in a pipe, on tinfoil, or in cigarettes. ("Freebase" refers to the process by which the cocaine is dissolved in water and then heated with a chemical to "free" the cocaine "base" from the salt.) It has been illegally available in the USA and in Great Britain for a number of years, and gives an almost immediate effect of euphoria which wears off after a few minutes. Long-term use of large amounts have been known to cause hallucinations, and common after-effects include extreme depression and feelings of paranoia. Use by a pregnant woman can also result in the birth of a baby who is addicted and suffers withdrawal effects.

HALLUCINOGENS

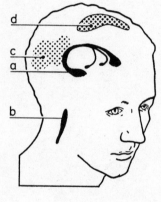

The most common of these is **LSD** (**lysergic acid diethylamide**), which can produce all manner of effects, among them visual and other sensory distortions and out-of-body experiences. Very disturbing reactions can also occur; and dreadful accidents have been recorded as a result of a "bad trip." Other hallucinogens include **mescaline** and **psilocybin**, and all are illegal in most parts of the world. Physical dependence is thought unlikely, and there is little evidence to show long-term damage other than the possibly fatal results of a bad experience while under the influence of such drugs.
Hallucinogens have strong effects on the limbic system (**a**), influencing mood and emotions, and on the reticular formation (**b**), making the user acutely conscious of sensory input. Visual centers (**c**) react by producing visions, ranging from flashes of light to complex scenes. Memory centers (**d**) are suppressed, together with other higher cerebral funcions such as judgment. The combination of effects on the limbic system, such as violent mood swings and loss of judgment, may prove highly dangerous to the user of these drugs.

DESIGNER DRUGS

These chemical substances are engineered to have similar effects to illegal drugs without being in themselves illegal at the time of manufacture, though they are usually rapidly scheduled.

Synthetic versions of heroin (such as MPPP and "China White") have been used as drugs of abuse, and each illustrates the dangers inherent in such designer drugs. In the case of **MPPP**, a substance similar to **meperidine** (**Demerol**), a contaminant (MPTP) was frequently also present. MPTP adversely affects nerve cells and has been linked to cases of Parkinson's disease in those who took contaminated MPPP. **"China White"** has also caused overdoses in heroin users because it is a more powerful substance.

MDMA (known as "Adam" or "Ecstasy") has features of both psychedelic drugs and amphetamines. It produces hallucinations in high doses, but the most usual effects are feelings of greater empathy and sensuality, euphoria, tension of the jaw muscles, nausea and dizziness, followed by fatigue and insomnia. Panic atacks may occur during a "high"; and adverse psychological effects (including dependence) and nerve damage may result from repeated use.

Dietary excesses

Overweight is almost always caused by taking in more food energy than the body uses up. Most is used to supply body energy needs, to maintain basic life processes and for all physical activity. Some people seem to get rid of surplus input because their bodies automatically speed up their metabolism and burn up any surplus rather than store it. This burning up process is called "thermogenesis." There is also a rise in the body's metabolism after every meal. Two people may eat exactly the same, but one will burn up more than the other if the food is taken in several small meals rather than two large ones. Food energy that is neither needed nor burned up is stored by the body in the form of fat.

ARE YOU OVERWEIGHT?

One way of learning whether you are among the overweight is to check your weight against a desirable weight table – such as the one given below.

But even without weighing yourself, it is possible to do a quick check for overweight. Start by asking yourself the following questions. Do you have telltale bulges? Do you look much fatter than you used to? Have your measurements increased appreciably? If you pinch your upper arm, thigh, or midriff, is there more than one inch (2.5cm) of flesh between your thumb and forefinger?

Height	Small frame	Medium frame	Large frame
4ft 9in (1.45m)	98lb (44.5kg)	104lb (47kg)	114lb (51.7kg)
4ft 10in (1.47m)	100lb (45.3kg)	107lb (48.5kg)	117lb (53kg)
4ft 11in (1.49m)	103lb (46.7kg)	110lb (49.8kg)	120lb (54.4kg)
5ft 0in (1.52m)	106lb (48kg)	113lb (51.2kg)	123lb (55.7kg)
5ft 1in (1.54m)	109lb (49.5kg)	116lb (52.6kg)	126lb (57.1kg)
5ft 2in (1.57m)	112lb (50.8kg)	120lb (54.4kg)	130lb (58.9kg)
5ft 3in (1.60m)	115lb (52kg)	124lb (56.2kg)	134lb (60.7kg)
5ft 4in (1.62m)	119lb (54kg)	128lb (58kg)	138lb (62.5kg)
5ft 5in (1.65m)	123lb (55.8kg)	132lb (59.8kg)	142lb (64.4kg)
5ft 6in (1.67m)	127lb (57.6kg)	136lb (61.6kg)	146lb (66.2kg)
5ft 7in (1.70m)	131lb (59.5kg)	140lb (63.5kg)	150lb (68kg)
5ft 8in (1.72m)	135lb (61.2kg)	144lb (65.3kg)	154lb (69.8kg)
5ft 9in (1.75m)	139lb (63kg)	148lb (67.1kg)	159lb (72.1kg)
5ft 10in (1.77m)	143lb (64.8kg)	152lb (68.9kg)	164lb (74.3kg)
5ft 11in (1.80m)	147lb (66.6kg)	157lb (71.2kg)	169lb (76.6kg)

Desirable weights
Desirable weight tables are based on statistics, usually collected by insurance companies, showing the correlation between different weights and health standards. This table shows desirable weights, according to height and body size, for women aged 25. Older women can expect to exceed these weights; but at age 45, for example, a woman probably should not be much more than 12–18lb (5.4-8.16kg) over the weights given for age 25.

EFFECTS OF OVERWEIGHT

Overweight people are not just more tired, and physically and mentally lethargic, with aching joints and poor digestion: they are also more likely to suffer from high blood pressure, heart disease, diabetes, inflammation of the gall bladder, arthritis, and varicose veins. They are more likely to die during operations, and have higher rates of mortality in general (including 3 times the mortality from heart and circulatory disease).

© DIAGRAM

a Overweight children often become overweight adults
b At puberty, female hormones increase deposition of fat
c Eating large meals on social occasions
d Excess gain in pregnancy
e Eating family leftovers
f Cutting down on exercise in middle age
g Using food as consolation when depressed

Slimming aids
There are many varieties available but not all are equally effective.
a Substitute low-calorie meals or biscuits (which do nothing to encourage new eating habits)
b Prescribed drugs (which, even if not addictive, will not be helpful long term)
c Reducing garments, saunas and Turkish baths (the effects of which are rapidly lost by drinking to replace water loss)
d Massagers and vibrator belts (reports on their effectiveness vary)
e Exercise (but it would take 12 hours of tennis to lose 1lb or .45kg)
f Joining a slimming clinic or club (many do find this helpful but expensive)

APPETITE CONTROL

Most people have an effective appetite control – or "appestat" – which prevents them from putting on too much weight.

Some people, however, ignore the messages from their appestats. Typical reasons are social habit or custom; excessive love of food in general or of certain foods in particular; habits of overeating acquired during childhood; and lack of exercise and eating for psychological support.

When physical activity falls below moderate levels, research has shown that appetite may actually increase – even though the body has no need for the extra food. Increasing the amount of exercise in such cases not only increases calorie output but also appears to put the appestat back into good working order. Of course, exercise above moderate levels will also increase the appetite.

LOSING WEIGHT

Losing weight is not easy. It demands controlled eating habits, discipline, patience, and a change of attitudes. There are special diets, too, that recommend cutting down on fats but maintaining a moderate intake of unrefined carbohydrate. There are no miracles; adopt a definite diet plan and stick to it; and if you need advice, get it from your doctor.

It is best to aim to lose weight steadily over a long period. Constant yo-yo weight changes are as bad for you as being overweight. Once weight is lost, keep a constant check, and deal with small gains as they occur. Three basic types of diet can work if you are sufficiently determined. Low-calorie plans set a numerical limit to daily calorie intake (usually 1000–1500 calories.) Constant reference must, of course, be made to calorie tables (see p.400). Low-carbohydrate plans also cut down calorie intake, but only by reducing consumption of carbohydrates (see p.104). No-count plans, simplified versions of the low-carbohydrate system, divide food into three categories: high-carbohydrate food that must be avoided; high-calorie, non-carbohydrate food to eat in moderation; and unrestricted foods.

DIETARY DEFICIENCES

When thinking about what you eat, it is important to look at the diet as a whole. An excess of one nutrient will not compensate for a deficiency of another.

Too much of certain minerals or vitamins can in fact cause deficiences in others by upsetting their absorption or storage. A deficiency of one nutrient can also lead to a deficiency of another by affecting the body's ability to make use of the second nutrient, even if it is present in the diet. Vitamin C deficiency can, for instance, lead to iron deficiency.

Interactions occur not only among vitamins, and between vitamins and minerals, but also between vitamins and proteins, vitamins and carbohydrates, and vitamins and fats; and there are many multiple relationships as well. Lack of protein can also be a problem in old people with little money, and in those following unusual diets.

Other than at times of stress, illness and during pregnancy, however, if you are following a normal balanced diet, vitamin and mineral supplements should not be necessary.

SEX EDUCATION

Young girls are frequently given little or no information about how their bodies function until they enter puberty, maybe not even then, and in many families discussion of such matters is kept secret or considered delicate. In some cases, girls may already have been sexually abused or be sexually active, with the attendant risks of infection and pregnancy. It is important that parents supply accurate information when it is required and are prepared to explain the dangers of promiscuity.

MENTAL AND EMOTIONAL DANGERS

Much mental ill-health in women results from conflict between other people's ideas of what "a woman" should look like, be, and do, and each woman's image of herself. The conditioning she receives from earliest childhood and the constant bombardment of society's ideas on how she should behave may make it hard for her even to form a consistent view of herself as an individual. Despite the efforts of those who promote equality between the sexes, stereotypical expectations of what girls and women are, and what they should do, are prevalent in all societies. Supposedly innate differences between the sexes are usually reinforced by parental handling, availability or type of education, and cultural influences such as religion or the media.

In general, women are seen as submissive, caring, and emotional rather than intellectual in nature, and girls are encouraged to regard such attitudes as essentially female and therefore to be aimed at in their growth toward womanhood. Aggressive behavior, which may be condoned in boys, is actively discouraged in girls so that learnt patterns of internalizing anger and frustration may later cause problems in adulthood. Indeed, constructively assertive behavior sometimes has to be relearned. Most children still grow up in a family unit where their immediate needs are met by a woman (either mother, relative or childminder) who puts other people's needs before her own. The low status that a male-dominated society still sometimes attaches to motherhood and caring thus reinforces the impression that women are, by their very nature, inferior.

Girls learn to be women largely by watching how their mothers relate to other adults and how they handle their children (although some make conscious decisions not to act in exactly the same way).

Difficulties in family relationships in childhood may thus form patterns of inappropriate or destructive behavior which tend to be lifelong unless treated.

Growing up female

©DIAGRAM

STEREOTYPE PRESSURE

Female stereotypes have been around as models of so-called womanly behavior from time immemorial. Virtuous, supportive wives and glamorous temptresses found in ancient literature are still stock characters in tv and movie dramas today. Yet now in industrialized countries there is an increasing tendency to divide women into groups according to age, sex, ethnic background, income and life style: and the emergence of "the career woman," "the single mother" and other categories and stereotypes challenges many traditional assumptions about the place of women as wives and mothers within family units. However, these new stereotypes have the potential to be equally as harmful as those which preceded them, since they completely disregard the features which make each of us an individual. They are also chiefly the tools of media pundits and marketing analysts, and are usually employed in an attempt to make us buy things which we otherwise would not want.

Evidence shows that most of us have some sense of belonging to a particular peer group, but that we aspire to the next rung up the ladder. Our reasonably objective view of ourselves is therefore flattered when the "typical" working mother in the soap-powder commercial is slim, elegant and totally unflustered by the myriad demands of her family, yet we must hold on to the fact that it is an unrealistic fiction.

Problems can arise when stereotype or peer group pressure forces us into harmful habits or into doing something which we do not really want to do. Schoolgirls may try fad diets, buy cheap cosmetics, take up smoking or even experiment with sex, alcohol and drugs because their friends persuade them that it is adult behavior. Young women whose friends all seem to be getting married and having babies may feel anxious that they have been left "on the shelf." Mothers who would rather stay at home with children may feel pressured into going out to work because it is a modern thing to do. In a society which values youth and beauty, older women are particularly vulnerable to the claims of plastic surgeons and cosmetic companies. At best, the stereotypes that are held up before us induce vague stirrings of envy: at worst, they may result in feelings of guilt, inadequacy and dissatisfaction with what we already are and goad us into inappropriate actions such as overspending or even theft.

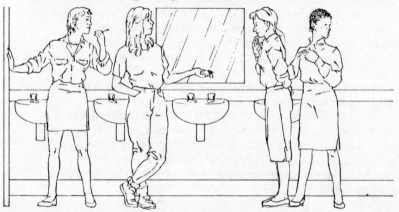

Role conflicts

Generalized views about the roles of women (and men) are, by their very nature, unhelpful and deny the existence of the personal resources which we all possess. Religion, culture, family and feminism all also produce points of conflict with which we must reach our own individual compromise.

Most women are familiar with classic role conflicts which put them in a no-win situation: just as men once liked to date sexually experienced girls but to marry virgins, so some still like their own wives to stay home and look after the family but admire the sophisticated "superwoman" who combines raising children with running her own company.

Depending on the vagaries of the economic climate, women may be told first that there are no jobs for them when they leave school and that they should therefore do what all "good" girls do – get married and raise children. When they have children, they may then be encouraged to go out to work and be "productive members of society." Such changes in attitude would be laughable were it not for the fact that they are often backed up by the opinions of selected "experts," creating a sense of guilt in those who are forced by circumstances not to move with the tide. Exhortations by governments and partners that women should work outside the home are seldom supported by proper childcare provision or help with household chores, adding to the emotional and physical burden.

In industrialized societies, with their emphasis on the value of employment and wealth creation, the role of carers is often undervalued. A society may appear to attach moral status to looking after children, the aged and the handicapped, but if this is not supplemented by appropriate levels of benefits and funding, those who provide care are bound to feel that their chosen role is of little public esteem, no matter how personally fulfilling.

Wide variations and conflicts in opinion about what women's liberation should entail have also created much confusion. Women who recognize the importance of caring and motherhood may have felt that feminists regarded them as unhealthily unassertive and undynamic. Yet women in high-pressure careers are now resisting the attitude which expected them to behave in the same ways as their male competitors and are exploiting their natural abilities in a commercial environment. Liberation should mean release from roles which are restrictive to each woman's personal growth and happiness: it should not deny the importance of relationships and responsibilities that are the emotional mainstays of our lives.

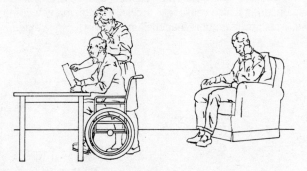

© DIAGRAM

Career pressures

It is not uncommon for it to appear that a woman's economic value to society is considered before her own and her family's welfare. In some parts of the world, maternity rights may not be legally encoded and fall to the discretion of employers, who can thereby adjust them according to economic trends. Encouraging noises about return to the workplace are only infrequently accompanied by real commitment to equality of opportunity and childcare provision. In addition to these problems, it is still not uncommon for women at work to face harassment, violence, poor or unequal rights of pay (especially for part-time work) and unsociable hours.

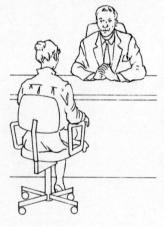

In all countries, women generally earn less, even when doing comparable jobs. Inequalities in employment opportunity begin before school-leaving age since girls do not generally pursue subjects that are seen as masculine or leading to male-dominated professions, such as engineering. Apparently glamorous occupations may, on the other hand, attract overqualified girls who are then disillusioned by the tedium and low pay of the work involved. Generally speaking, fewer girls than boys receive private education and enter further education on leaving school, reflecting the relative importance attached to their future careers. Young women entering the job market for the first time are often asked about their intentions regarding marriage, since most cultures still expect that women will marry and permanently or temporarily leave their profession. This may bar them from being accepted into occupations which involve lengthy or expensive training, however committed or well-qualified they may be. Discrimination on the grounds of sex, even if it is illegal, can be hard to prove.

Women who leave work because of family commitments often find it impossible to return to their occupation at the level at which they left. They may have to retrain at their own expense or accept a lower salary. Working mothers usually have to make their own childcare arrangements; company crèches are rare and are sometimes unfairly taxed in relation to other inducements. Sole parents may suffer high levels of stress in coping with the demands of work and family, particularly if they cannot afford after-school care or help with household chores. Women with partners, too, seldom find that the burden of looking after the home and children is equally shared, and this is often a source of resentment and family conflict.

"Burn-out" is a familiar syndrome in both women and men in high-powered jobs. Women who find that they are pressured into competing with their male counterparts on unequal terms and denying their own relative strengths and weaknesses may drop out or move into occupations which cause less stress, though many women do, of course, relish the stimulus that challenging work can provide.

Parenting and partnership pressures

Becoming a mother is something that many women hope to do at some point in their lives. Depending on a woman's background, it may be something that is expected of her automatically, or a decision that she must weigh against career or other commitments. In the case of a single woman, this decision may have to be given particularly careful thought. For those who would wish to spend time bringing up their children personally, motherhood, of course, entails loss of financial independence and a greater degree of reliance on a partner or upon the state. Given the long-term nature of parenting, this may be thought too great a price to pay.

Considerable emotional adjustments also follow the introduction of a child into a relationship, and so it is wise for partners to discuss at the outset what they would expect of each other in terms of emotional and practical support. But there may be problems, too, for those who have difficulty in conceiving. Infertility (see p.299) can itself create extra strains upon relationships: new techniques give hope but the procedures involved can be exhausting and may end in disappointment. Artificial insemination and adoption are sometimes alternatives, but the consequences of each need to be thought through.

Parenting is certainly a stressful activity. Pregnancy and childbirth usually proceed smoothly but there may be complications. Sadly, not every child is born completely healthy, and illness or handicap of a child places additional strain on parents and, possibly, on their relationship. Bonding between mother and baby may be hindered by prematurity or other complications, and postnatal depression sometimes adds to the anxieties most parents experience. Children pass through phases of exploration, with attendant accidents and mishaps, and self-assertion, with tantrums and rows. Ideas on raising children and the kind of education and discipline they require vary enormously, and differences in parental approach can lead to family tension. Adolescence, too, usually brings increased stresses within families as worries over academic progress, delinquency and experimentation with sex and drugs come to the fore. Ultimately, children require most to know that they are loved and valued – being brought up in a family that does not conform to the traditional nuclear norm need not matter.

Motherhood does not stop when children attain adulthood, and women tend to continue to worry about their offspring forever. However necessary, the process of letting go and being prepared to watch children make their own mistakes can be extremely difficult and cause great distress.

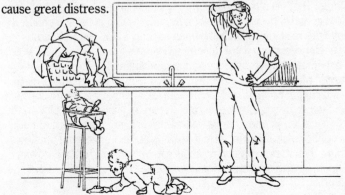

© DIAGRAM

Common partnership problems

a Possessiveness
b Extra-marital affair
c Arrival of new baby causing jealousy
d Quarrels over custody of child following separation

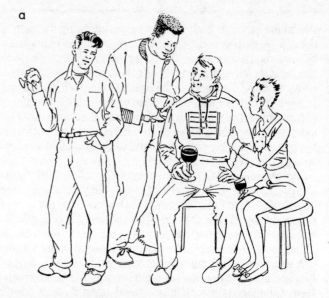

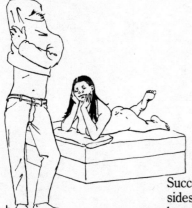

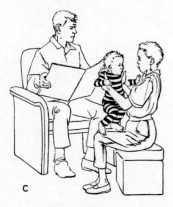

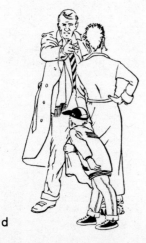

Successful relationships undoubtedly require give and take on both sides. On entering into a relationship, a woman may play down parts of her personality or behavior that she feels may not be acceptable to a loved one, and this pattern is normal. However, relationships can be in danger of becoming unhealthy when one partner's wants and needs are subjugated to those of the other. Women who have been brought up to be submissive and lack self-esteem may find it hard to be assertive and express their emotional needs, but inability to do so usually leads to stress and resentment. Possessiveness and jealousy are also aspects of manipulative behavior which put particular strain upon relationships.

Stress points commonly occur when children enter a partnership, changing the emotional framework of the relationship. Partners frequently find that they grow apart in many ways; and whether they stay together may depend upon the strength of their friendship and the viability of their life style as much as their love for one another. Sexual activity outside a partnership may be rationalized on the grounds that it keeps the relationship "fresh," but some loss of self-respect is usually incurred by one partner, with consequent strain upon the relationship.

Divorce, too, usually produces great stress because of the legal and financial complications. Quarrels over custody and access of children can involve damaging attacks on each partner's self- esteem; and reactive depression is a not uncommon sequel.

Bereavement and desertion, though fundamentally different situations, often provoke similar reactions. Anger is common, and the sudden disappearance of a close partner evokes persistent feelings of loss and grief. Living alone again after years of shaping one's life to the needs of another is one of the adjustments in a woman's life that may be hardest to make, particularly if she has not been working outside the home. But in time forgotten skills can be re-acquired, and new ones developed, as the compensations of a single life gradually become apparent.

POVERTY

Poverty is the most important factor contributing to physical and mental ill-health. It is not hard to see why. Lack of money affects access to such vital needs as housing and a healthy diet which are of principal concern to women. In developed countries, incidence of many diseases linked with stress, smoking and dietary factors is significantly higher in poorer socioeconomic groups, as is infant mortality. In developing countries, meanwhile, lack of resources for basic health care also leads to high mortality from preventable diseases. In addition, lack of money exacerbates the effects of other social pressures, listed *below*.

AGISM

In industrialized countries, the extended family has largely disappeared and with it has gone the respect and importance attached to the elderly as sources of traditional wisdom. Older people now frequently live alone or with an aging partner. Apart from the general effects of aging upon health, the elderly may suffer from lack of mobility and access to health care; insufficient money to ensure a varied diet; violence and, equally, the fear of it; and isolation.

RACISM

Women of minority racial groups may feel particularly vulnerable to harassment and assault. Immigration laws may also specifically discriminate against women by not allowing their husbands to join them or requiring extensive documentation from people who may be illiterate. Inability of immigrant women to speak the native language of their new home sometimes leads to extra problems in obtaining health care, education and legal assistance in the event of assault or family problems, too. Racial minorities are frequently among the poorest citizens of a given country: they therefore suffer proportionately more from bad housing, and poor diet and health care.

SEXISM

Women encounter discrimination on the gounds of their sex in many spheres of life. Religious or cultural dictates, for example, may produce physical or emotional stress in women (repeated pregnancy, fasting, or isolation during menstruation).

Although almost all forms of employment are now legally subject to equal opportunities legislation in developed countries, sexism remains as an unspoken influence, and discrimination in job or promotion opportunities can be difficult to prove. Lesbians, for instance, who reveal their sexual orientation have been shown to be more likely to face discrimination.

FATTISM

Women who are very overweight may also find that they are discriminated against on esthetic grounds, socially as well as in employment. What is more, they may be persuaded by social pressures which demand a certain shape to undergo procedures of unproven value to help them lose weight.

Social pressures

Disablism
Disabled women may suffer from a variety of problems, especially outside their home environment. Educational opportunities are sometimes limited by lack of access to buildings and equipment; and there may even be an assumption that disabled women are unlikely to seek work and do not therefore need to be trained. Physical handicap is also often confused with mental incapacity, resulting in inappropriately protective or dismissive behavior on the part of the able-bodied. Necessary medical facilities and equipment may be hard to obtain through public health care programs, and disabled women wishing to start a family have often faced distressing opposition from physicians and family members.

©DIAGRAM

Neuroses

The term "neurosis" is used to describe relatively mild forms of mental illness which, nonetheless, are very distressing to the sufferer and may result in the inability to lead a normal life. Neurosis generally represents a tendency to react excessively or abnormally to stress, and the level of anxiety felt appears inappropriate to the triggering factors and may seem to constitute a part of the sufferer's personality. Neurosis may take any of several forms indicating the presence of severe underlying anxiety which is expressed in a characteristic but inappropriate way. Each type of reaction is described separately *below*, but neurosis can manifest itself in a mixture of forms of unusual behavior.

ANXIETY STATES

These are the most common form of neurosis. Physical symptoms such as trembling, sweating, breathlessness and nausea are experienced. Panic attacks are also sometimes associated with a particular situation. For this reason they are also known as situational anxiety states or **phobias**. Agoraphobia, for example, is commonly defined as "fear of open spaces" and is usually characterized by the onset of symptoms when the sufferer attempts to leave her home, use public transport, or enter crowded public places such as stores.

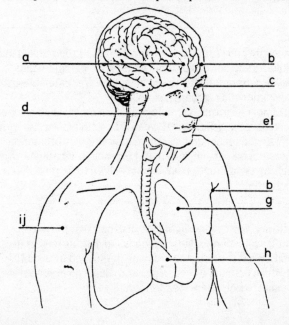

Effects of anxiety
An anxiety reaction may include any or all the following physical symptoms
a Tension migraine
b Sweating
c Dilated pupils
d Pallor
e Dry mouth
f Vomiting
g Breathlessness
h Irregular or rapid heartbeats
i Tremor
j Heightened muscle tone

HYSTERICAL OR CONVERSION REACTIONS

Sometimes, anxiety is "converted" into physical symptoms: for example, a person suffering from severe stress may become blind or lose the use of a limb, apparently without any physiological reason. The sufferer frequently appears relatively unconcerned by her disability, and symptoms disappear as the causes of anxiety are removed. Other types of hysterical behavior, in which the person shuts herself off from unbearable anxiety, include **sleepwalking**, **amnesia** and – rarely – **multiple personality**.

Types of neuroses
Neuroses are often classified into four main types.
a Anxiety neuroses consist of overreaction to an everyday event, such as seeing a particular animal or standing in a confined space.
b Hysterical neuroses involve the shutting down of some part of the body's system, such as one of the senses or motor control, so that the person does not have to confront the object of her fear.
c Obsessive neuroses involve inappropriate repetitions of certain thoughts or actions.
d Depressive neuroses involve inappropriately severe feelings of inadequacy in response to emotional stress or minor failures.

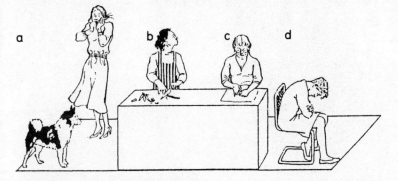

OBSESSIONAL NEUROSES

Many people occasionally worry about seemingly trivial matters: "Did I lock that door when I left the house?" or "How fresh were those eggs we had for breakfast?". It is not neurotic behavior to think back carefully to when those eggs were bought or even return quickly to make certain that door is locked. By these actions we reassure ourselves and abolish worry. Obsessive neurosis on the other hand is characterized by continuing feelings of unassuageable anxiety which surface in persistent intrusive thoughts or repetitive patterns of behavior which disrupt the patient's life.

TREATMENT

Treatments for neurosis vary widely according to practices prevailing within a particular country and the person who is first consulted by the sufferer. If the patient's behavior is very disturbed, specialist help is likely to be needed. If the causes of anxiety are immediately obvious, treatment will be directed at these.

In the USA and parts of Europe, **psychotherapy** (see p.248) is extensively used and deep-seated anxiety resulting from events in childhood may require lengthy psychoanalysis to help the patient recognize its causes and so come to terms with it. **Behavior therapy**, in which the patient is encouraged and supported in gradually confronting situations which cause anxiety, can be highly effective in dealing with anxiety states and phobias.

Obsessive and compulsive behavior may also respond to re-educative forms of treatment. If relationships within the family are thought to be the principal cause of anxiety, family counseling with a doctor or social worker may be most appropriate. Worries about health, money or the workplace may also require advice of an essentially practical nature.

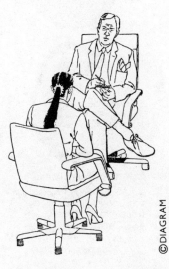

©DIAGRAM

237

Psychoses

More severe forms of mental illness than neuroses, psychoses have loss of contact with reality as one of their chief manifestations. In many instances, psychotic illness is thought to have an organic basis in the form of chemical imbalance within the brain or actual damage to a part of it. Drug treatment is often effective in controlling symptoms but the underlying illness may be long-lasting, perhaps for life.

Corpus callosum damage
Recent research into schizophrenia has suggested that some sufferers may have abnormalities of the corpus callosum, the bridge between the two halves of the brain. Scans and other tests on a small number of schizophrenics have revealed that each corpus callosum is thickened, damaged or non-functioning. If this proved to be the case with most schizophrenics, it would perhaps be possible in the future to provide screening before schizophrenic symptoms occur, so that preventative treatment could be given.

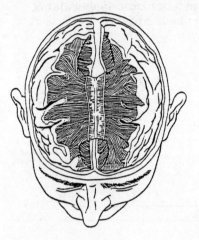

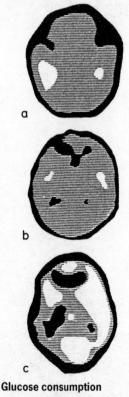

a

b

c

Glucose consumption
a Scan showing normal glucose consumption
b Scan of schizophrenic
c Scan of manic-depressive

 Glucose consumption

SCHIZOPHRENIA
The cause or causes of schizophrenia have long been sought, and some factors have been identified. The tendency to develop the disease is at least partly inherited, and pathological studies have demonstrated damage to the "corpus callosum" (the area of the brain linking the two cerebral hemispheres) in some patients. However, not every person genetically at risk will develop the condition, and environmental factors such as stress and family problems are also thought to play a triggering role.

Schizophrenia consists of retention of faculties such as intelligence and memory but disturbances of emotional responsiveness and perception, resulting in apparent "splitting" of the normally integrated processes of the mind. Some schizophrenics have the illusion that they are being persecuted; others may hear voices, telling them to behave in a certain way or suggesting false ideas. Sufferers may also become withdrawn or, if overstimulated, very excitable.

Drug treatment may help to "damp down" symptoms sufficiently for psychological and social therapy to be beneficial, but response is variable and schizophrenia is usually a long-term problem.

BRAIN SCANS
PET scans (*left*), used in tests on schizophrenics and manic-depressives, have revealed abnormalities in the brain's glucose consumption. The scans of schizophrenic patients showed decreased glucose consumption in some areas, while scans of manic-depressives showed increased consumption during the manic phases of their symptoms. Similar scans may enable neurologists to diagnose these confusing mental illnesses with greater accuracy in the future.

MANIC-DEPRESSIVE PSYCHOSIS

Everyone experiences fluctuations of mood – one day we wake feeling full of energy and optimism, the next despondent and sluggish. However, manic-depressive psychosis is an extreme disorder of mood swings; a phase of mania, with feelings of elation, restlessness and self-confidence in one's abilities (often misplaced and sometimes with disastrous consequences) alternating with deep depression during which suicide may be attempted. Imbalance of the brain chemistry which regulates mood is thought to be the main cause of the disorder, and closely-monitored treatment with lithium carbonate is often effective in suppressing symptoms. ˙

Psycho-somatic illness

Research into various physical disorders is increasingly implicating the role of mental stress in their development and progression. Health problems such as asthma, high blood pressure and stomach ulcers may be initiated or worsened by factors such as anxiety and overwork, although they can also have other causes and should always be medically investigated. In other important conditions, such as certain types of cancer and heart disease, the contribution of emotional factors is less easy to quantify and is controversial. Some doctors think that prolonged stress caused by an accumulation of adverse life events such as unemployment and family breakdown has the effect of lowering the body's resistance to illness. Statistics indicate that this may well be the case but the direct physiological effects of stress are harder to determine. People who suffer financial hardship or depression can understandably be less motivated to take interest in a limited diet or participate in regular physical exercise.

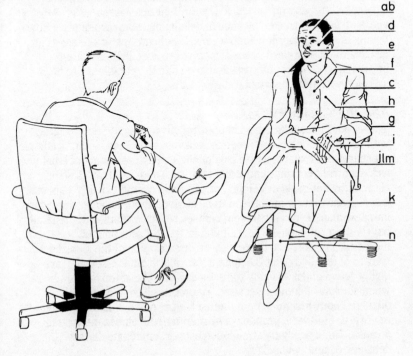

Effects of stress
Stress has been shown to contribute to, or aggravate, physical disorders such as:
a Headaches
b Exhaustion
c Excessive sweating
d Facial flushing
e Nasal catarrh
f Asthma attacks
g High blood pressure
h Heart disease
i Skin disease
j Stomach problems
k Vague aches and pains
l Diabetes
m Diarrhea
n Rheumatism and arthritis

©DIAGRAM

Eating disorders

Societies vary hugely in their perceptions of what is beautiful and desirable in a woman's appearance. At various times and in certain cultures, women's necks have been extended with necklets, their feet bound and mutilated, their lips and earlobes distorted by wooden plates – purely for esthetic reasons. Some cultures still value obesity in a woman, but in developed countries today the pinnacle of female glamor is considered to be that of a slender, lightly boned, young woman. This "ideal shape," widely promulgated through fashion, advertising and the media as being the key to attractiveness to the opposite sex, can lead not only to dissatisfaction that one is not, or can never hope to be, that shape but also to lack of confidence and self-esteem, particularly if there are other factors in a woman's life that reinforce these feelings.

Anorexia nervosa (see *below*) is probably the best-known eating disorder, but it constitutes the severest end of a wide spectrum of problems that many women suffer in dealing with eating and food habits. Eating can be a comfort in the face of stress and certain foods an "addiction," leading to unhealthy obesity. At the other end of the spectrum, anxiety to maintain control over food intake and body shape can become an equally undesirable, even fatal, obsession. Women who are prone to develop eating disorders may eat compulsively during early adolescence, suffer later from prolonged or eccentric dieting, and eventually develop **bulimia nervosa** (see p.241).

Treatments for eating disorders have varied from wiring up obese women's jaws to forcing anorectic patients to stay in bed until they have put on weight. Amphetamines were also prescribed as a slimming aid until the problem of addiction became apparent. Diet plans relying on the efficacy of wonder substances are still widely advertised, relying on our gullibility for their financial success. After years of distress caused by such manipulation, many women are now finding more appropriate support in self-help groups where they can discuss the emotional and social factors involved in their eating problems with other sufferers and even find the confidence to be satisfied with their figure just the way it is.

ANOREXIA NERVOSA

This condition usually arises in teenage girls and is often associated with pre-existing stresses such as tensions within the family, academic pressures or sexual abuse in childhood. The sufferer may feel that she lacks control over anything except her own body, and may also be alarmed by her rapid development of female characteristics, especially if she already has some reason to be anxious about turning from a girl into a woman. Typically, the girl refuses to eat, or eats with the family but then secretly makes herself vomit. As she gets thinner, menstruation halts and there may be discoloration of the skin and growth of fine body hair. Despite a low calorie intake, she appears highly active and is unlikely to recognize that she is too thin, even when she has become emaciated. Anorectics have a detectably distorted body image, seeing themselves as much bulkier than they really are, but this is probably a symptom of the illness rather than a cause. Emergency treatment consists of remedying dietary deficiencies and counseling.

Distorted views
All people have a distorted view of their own body proportions, but the anorectic grossly overestimates even when severely emaciated.
a Normal reflection
b Average-sized girl
c Anorectic reflection

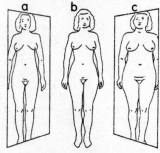

Degree of distortion in the perception of body size

	Normal %	Anorectic %
Face	94.7	157.6
Chest	95	134.2
Waist	100.2	146.6
Hips	96.6	128.8

(100% equals actual size)

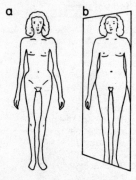

a Chronic anorectic
b Anorectic reflection

BULIMIA NERVOSA

This is characterized by bouts of grossly excessive eating, usually of any foodstuff that happens to be available, followed by self-induced purging through vomiting or laxatives. The condition sometimes co-exists with anorexia nervosa and can endanger long-term health or even be immediately fatal. Frequent binges irritate the esophagus and intestines, disrupting the normal workings of the digestive system, and life-threatening electrolyte imbalance may result from severe, prolonged vomiting after a huge intake of food.

COMPULSIVE EATING

This is a common problem among women and the resulting obesity can cause considerable distress. Many women indulge in occasional bouts of "stuffing" but these are rarely significant. The compulsive eater, however, is addicted to food. She may use it to relieve feelings of loneliness, isolation and frustration, dissatisfaction or boredom. She may also use it to comfort herself if she feels guilty, depressed or unattractive. During adolescence she may overeat to stifle her emerging sexuality, and later in life she may use her obesity to avoid contact with the opposite sex. Overeating – a secret and solitary activity – needs handling with sensitivity and understanding. To help overcome the problem, a woman should avoid being alone for longer than necessary, ensure that only low-calorie snacks are kept in the house, and divert herself with physical activity when the craving for food starts. Severe cases often need clinical help. Reasons for compulsive eating vary, but the vicious circle illustrated (*right*) is common to many women.

PROLONGED, REPEATED OR ECCENTRIC DIETING

It is tempting to believe, when confronted with wondrous claims of rapid weight loss, that a new diet will be the one that finally helps us to achieve a sylph-like figure. For those who have not dieted before or are more than 28 pounds (13kg) overweight, any reasonable diet plan is likely to produce some pleasing short-term effect. However, evidence is growing to show that prolonged or repeated low-calorie dieting merely alters the body's metabolism, slowing it down and making it more energy-efficient. When dieting stops, the body has a greater tendency to store fat than it did before. Worse still, in a very calorie-restricted diet or fast, weight loss will consist largely of lean tissue such as muscle. Hunger pangs may lead to bingeing on fatty, unhealthy foods and ultimately to eating disorders such as bulimia.

Any diet plan should permit enough calories to maintain sufficient intake of nutrients such as protein and vitamins – at least 1200 calories are required. Fiber is also important if you are to avoid constipation and other digestive problems.

If it is important for health reasons to lose some weight, long-term changes in eating patterns are often necessary and weight loss is more likely to be lasting if it takes place slowly in the context of a healthy, well-balanced diet. Compulsive eaters may benefit from keeping a food diary which helps to show up when binges are likely to occur so that avoidance measures can be taken in future.

The vicious circle
1 I feel miserable
2 I'll eat to comfort myself
3 I look fat
4 I feel guilty/I look ugly

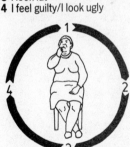

Obesity
This well-known consequence of compulsive eating results in external bodily changes, and the increased risk of diseases.
a Respiratory disease
b Heart disease
   High blood pressure
c Diabetes
d Kidney disease
e Varicose veins
f Double chins
g Flabby upper arms
h Drooping breasts
i Bulging stomach
j Fatty deposits on thighs
k Flat feet

©DIAGRAM

241

Depression

The word "depression" is used by almost everyone to cover a wide range of feelings of unhappiness, from the brief but intense sadness following a domestic row or disappointment to the prolonged misery that descends, often apparently without immediate cause, to blight the sufferer's life. Medical statistics indicate that far more women than men suffer from depression. Some doctors divide depression into two categories – **exogenous** or **reactive** (that is, arising from external causes) and **endogenous** (coming from within). This distinction is useful in comparing, say, the "excessive" grief of a person following a bereavement against sudden onset of mental symptoms due to chemical imbalance within the brain and responding well to appropriate medication. However, in many instances, there is no clear-cut cause: feelings of loss and anger suppressed successfully for many years may surface in response to a seemingly trivial trigger or physical illness. Postnatal depression ascribed to hormonal imbalance may also be contributed to by resurgence of emotional conflict felt by the mother during her own early childhood, or her feeling that control of her previously well-ordered life seems to have passed to the unfathomable whims of her baby.

There are well-defined factors known to contribute to the development of severe reactive depression. Statistically, women are most likely to be affected if they are poor, belong to a racial or other discriminated against minority, have young children and marital difficulties, and – crucially – if they have suffered the loss of their mother at an early age. Why women become depressed more often than men in such circumstances is controversial. Freudian psychology holds that the depressive tendency arises in unresolved emotional conflicts during the oral stage of development during infancy, but these "conflicts" should, in theory, affect women and men equally. Feminists point out that society generally holds women in lower esteem than men, and women are often encouraged to see themselves purely as providers of services for other people, especially members of the family, repressing their own wants and ambitions. Girls are taught not to express anger or aggression, lest they appear "unfeminine." The ultimate result is that women tend to feel powerless to change aspects of their lives which cause unhappiness. Anger and resentment, if they are not to be inflicted on other members of the family, are directed inward and result in further misery.

Severe depression
Situations involving emotional stress often act as catalysts in the development of severe depression.
a Postnatal depression may be mild or severe
b The death of a spouse or close relative is extremely stressful
c The emotional and social upheaval of divorce may lead to severe depression
d Retirement can be a severe shock to the system of career-minded people.

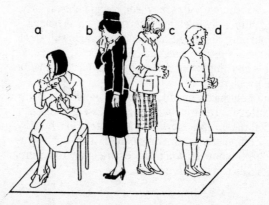

SYMPTOMS AND TREATMENT

When severe, depression causes symptoms such as disturbance of sleep patterns, disruption of the menstrual cycle and loss of sex drive. However, the most characteristic feelings experienced include tension and irritability, loss of motivation and energy for daily activities to the extent that the sufferer just wants to stay in bed, and a sense of hopelessness and lack of self-worth so deep that suicide may be contemplated or attempted.

The first, and most urgent, need is for a sympathetic listener. Even if friends cannot change what is causing the distress, they can aid a sufferer simply by being prepared to listen. A family doctor may be able to help in several ways: she or he may not have much time to discuss the problem but should be able to offer referral to a specialist or counseling service.

Depression is occasionally attributable to a physical ailment, and medical treatment may then be necessary. In severe cases there is a role for drug treatment, either in the form of anti-depressant drugs which can be highly effective but may take several days to start working, or the short-term use of tranquilizers, though these may in themselves create problems of dependence and only delay the essential process of coming to terms with what is really causing the depression. Helplines such as the Samaritans offer a listening service, and women's support and self-help groups may be able to advise on the availability of specialist help or even provide services such as co-counseling.

Depression often occurs in bouts which alternate with periods of relative normality, and some sufferers find that they are able to use these respites to formulate ways of detecting and dealing with the onset of depression. Although each person becomes depressed for different reasons, and one person's remedies may not work for another, much can be gained from discussion within a self-help group, including the sympathetic support that fellow sufferers can offer.

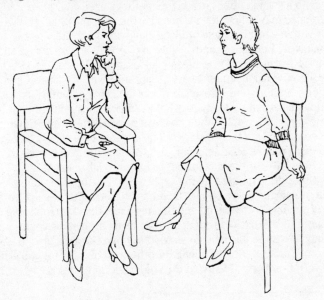

Support for the depressed from a friend or through a self-help group can be vital.

©DIAGRAM

243

SELF-MUTILATION

Emotional distress sometimes shows itself in the urge to harm oneself physically. This may be a manifestation of guilt and self-hatred or result from the desperate need to have someone take notice of the distress and do something to help. Because women are conditioned not to give vent to aggression and anger as men do, they are particularly likely to suppress these feelings and inflict damage on themselves instead of other people or their surroundings.

Self-mutilation can be severe in those who are suffering from undiagnosed or improperly treated mental illness, but more often it takes the form of skin complaints and other minor "ailments" which can often be difficult to differentiate from purely physical conditions. Self-inflicted injury requires careful and sympathetic investigation – friends, partners or parents are frequently in a better position than a doctor to detect self-mutilation and to have some idea of the stresses to which the sufferer is being subjected.

Treatment is related to determining the underlying causes and the end of a short-term worry such as academic examinations may result in the disappearance of a dermatitis-like rash.

SUICIDE

Suicide is the action of last resort – it represents the only means left to escape from or draw attention to unbearable pressures such as loneliness, depression or difficulties in relationships. In many developed countries, the rate among young people is increasing as highly competitive academic or employment conditions produce harmful levels of stress and heightened fear of failure. Suicide most often results from lack of self-esteem – feelings that life is not worth living because the person has nothing of worth to offer. Adverse life events like unemployment and divorce are therefore associated with increased risk of a suicide attempt as a situational reaction.

There are striking differences between men and women when it comes to a suicide attempt, and the methods used and these differences may reflect the reasons for the attempt. Statistically, elderly men who are single or living alone are most likely to kill themselves. Loneliness and despair may lead to a determined effort to end a life which seems relentlessly miserable and purposeless. On the other hand, it has been postulated that those who are closely involved with other people and whose emotional difficulties stem from that relationship are more likely to attempt suicide as an effort to get help by showing the extent of their distress or as a form of punishment to the person causing their distress. The impetus may simply be to find immediate relief from mental anguish, perhaps in an overdose of narcotics, without there being actual intent to kill oneself.

However determined someone appears to be, there is almost always some remaining desire to live. Depression frequently results from the lack of anyone to confide in, and the mere fact that someone else is prepared to listen can be enough to persuade against a suicide attempt. Most people who do survive say that they are glad to have done so. Subsequent counseling (or other treatment if mental illness is involved) is important to avoid the risk of another attempt.

Therapies

DRUGS

Minor tranquilizers, such as the **benzodiazepines**, are regularly prescribed for women by doctors, usually for symptoms like anxiety and often in response to problems arising from bereavement or difficulties in relationships. They can be effective in relieving anxiety or providing a few nights' good sleep in the short term, and this may be all that is required to help a person feel better able to cope with life again. However, in the case of benzodiazepines, the beneficial effects are of limited duration and, as with barbiturates, drug dependence may develop with long-term use (see p. 223). Although the more commonly prescribed tranquilizers have few serious immediate side-effects, there is a possibility that, by dulling pain and other symptoms of misery, they let the person continue in an inappropriate life style without taking action to resolve real problems. The mood-dampening effects may even worsen existing depression. Symptoms of withdrawal are often mistaken for return of the condition for which the tranquilizer was first prescribed, and it is important for long-term users to consult their doctor for advice on tapering off the dosage.

Major tranquilizers and anti-psychotic drugs are used chiefly to sedate very disturbed patients, such as those suffering from schizophrenia or other psychoses. They are usually administered under hospital supervision, and it is important that patients released into the community should continue to take their medication as prescribed to avoid recurrence of symptoms. However, any apparent side-effects should be reported to a doctor.

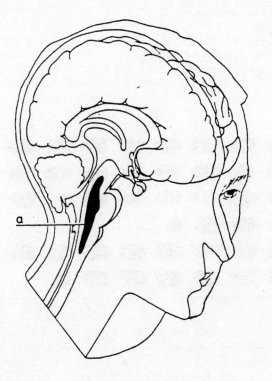

Psychotherapeutic drugs
Drugs are used to treat a wide range of mental conditions as they are usually effective in alleviating symptoms. They do not always, however, help to cure the underlying illness. Most drugs work by affecting the transfer of messages between neurons: sedatives, for example, slow down the brain and so may calm patients with schizophrenia or anxiety neurosis. Some drugs affect the reticular formation (**a**) which helps to regulate consciousness and the level of activity in the rest of the brain.

©DIAGRAM

Anti-depressants, as their name implies, are prescribed for sufferers from depression. They act upon the brain's internal chemistry, helping to maintain levels of certain neurotransmitters within the centers governing emotional responses. For this reason, they are most effective in treating endogenous depression, where there is presumed to be some pre-existing disturbance of brain chemistry. People who are highly agitated are less likely to respond to anti-depressants and may even become manic.

There are two main kinds of anti-depressant – **tricyclic anti-depressants** and **mono-amine oxidase inhibitors (MAOIs).** Both react with certain other kinds of drugs, and takers of MAOIs should receive from their doctor or pharmacist a list of drugs and foodstuffs – such as cheese or alcohol – that can cause a dangerous rise in blood pressure if taken in combination with their medication. Both types of anti-depressants take a while before they have a noticeable effect – around 2 weeks for the tricyclics and as much as 6 weeks for MAOIs. Side-effects are common with both types and should be reported to the doctor.

Side-effects of anti-depressants
Rapid heartbeat
Mania
Dry mouth
Tremor
Constipation
Insomnia
Fatigue
Excessive sweating
Headache
Confusion
Dizziness on standing or sitting
Skin rashes

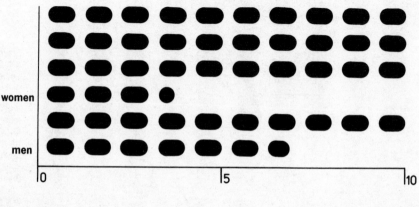

women

men

|0 |5 |10

Mood-altering drugs
50 million prescriptions are issued each year in the UK alone for mood-altering drugs. Two-thirds of them are for women.

⬤ = 1 million

L-tryptophan is an amino acid sometimes prescribed as an adjunct to treatment together with certain MAOIs and has also been used as an over-the-counter remedy for depression. It is able to enter the brain and undergo conversion to a neurotransmitter substance. However, at the time of writing, L-tryptophan has been withdrawn from sale in health shops and pharmacies in the USA and UK because of concern over adverse effects.

Lithium carbonate is used to treat mania, the highly optimistic and hyperactive state which alternates with depression in manic-depressive psychosis and rarely occurs by itself. Regular intake helps to prevent subsequent mood swings, and lithium is also sometimes prescribed for recurrent depression. Treatment is frequently started under hospital supervision since blood levels of the drug have to be monitored to be sure that the dose is neither too low nor too high. Possible side-effects include tremor, visual disturbances, slurred speech, vomiting, and diarrhea.

ELECTROCONVULSIVE THERAPY (ECT)

This is a controversial method of treatment for severe depression. It is only employed when other methods have failed or the patient is considered to be in danger of taking her own life. Despite the "convulsive" element of the name, no violent convulsion occurs as anesthetic and muscle-relaxant drugs are given. An electrical current is passed through the head between electrodes, creating patterns of brain cell activity similar to those of an epileptic seizure. Up to 3 or 4 sessions may be needed to obtain relief of symptoms. While ECT can be very effective in the relief of depression, there is concern that its effects on the brain are not clearly understood, and there may also be some subsequent memory loss.

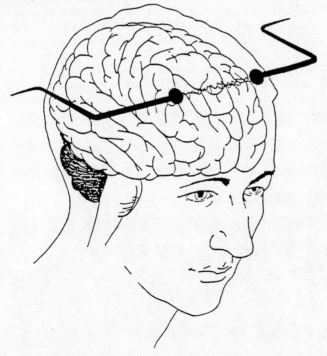

Electroconvulsive therapy (ECT)
Some doctors consider ECT to be helpful in the treatment of severe depression. The patient is given a drug to relax the muscles, and a general anesthetic. An electric current is then applied to the brain through electrodes taped to the scalp. This results in furious electrical activity in the brain. The patient wakens soon after and may suffer from a temporary loss of memory. The treatment is repeated over a few weeks.

© DIAGRAM

PSYCHOTHERAPY

Counseling and co-counseling aim to help the sufferer find out what she thinks is wrong in her life and assess how it can best be changed. Some counselors operate in specific fields such as bereavement or student problems, while others perform more general psychotherapeutic work. The kind of training that counselors receive also varies widely. Some family doctors are able to offer counseling themselves or they may have to refer their patients to an appropriate source, either privately or as part of a public health service. Women's groups may provide self-help facilities for those who suffer from eating disorders or depression. They can also sometimes make referrals and may have a list of therapists known to be sympathetic to women's problems. In co-counseling, participants have a short training course and then work together as both "client" and "counselor."

Women who are not deeply disturbed and who can easily talk about their emotions may find counseling and co-counseling particularly useful because these techniques acknowledge to some extent the contribution of social factors to mental illness. The emphasis is more on learning to help oneself than being a patient directed by a doctor, and the aim of this approach is to create greater confidence and independence. Counseling is most often short-term, lasting just a few weeks or months.

Analytical and reconstructive psychotherapy is a long-term form of therapy which requires regular uninterrupted sessions in order for the client and analyst to build up a trusting and productive relationship. It may not be available in a public health care program because it demands one-to-one treatment over a considerable period and is therefore expensive. Psychiatrists and clinical psychologists are trained using the psychological tenets of Freud, Jung, or others, but some clients report that they may make a "diagnosis" which appears to take little account of the influence of practical circumstances on a woman's life. Treatment is often directed at detecting the reasons for current emotional problems in what happened in the past, often in childhood. The close relationship which builds up between patient and therapist parallels other relationships in the patient's life, enabling discovery of where problems might lie.

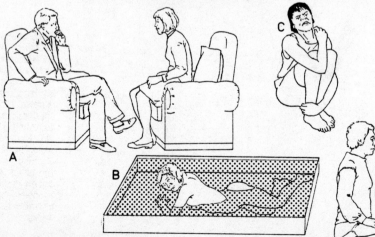

Freudian techniques are also the basis of **rebirthing** and **primal therapy**, which recognize the importance of earliest experiences in producing tension and pain.

Behavioral therapy is a more specific form of therapy aimed at changing a person's behavior in the context of a situation which causes emotional difficulties, particularly anxiety. It does not explore why the problems might have arisen and is therefore of limited scope, but it has proved useful in treatment of neurosis, phobias, and anxiety attacks.

Humanistic psychology comprises techniques such as **transactional analysis (TA)** and **Gestalt therapy**. TA analyses human emotional response and communication in terms of three "voices" – child, adult, and parent. Learning to recognize which voice is speaking, and what it signifies, can help patients to realize what their needs are and express them more clearly. Gestalt therapy aims to enable patients to re-discover elements of their personality that may have been suppressed and utilizes creative activities to bring these out. It also emphasizes learning the ability to assume control over one's life.

Family therapy is used to explore psychological problems which are concerned with relationships between family members. It aims to help partners and children to understand each other better and find ways of living together that are less stressful. **Self-help therapy groups** often have limited aims, such as discussion of eating disorders, but they can be useful in enabling sufferers to share experiences and provide support. Experience of **encounter group therapy** may be combined with another form of therapy or it may be sought separately. Participants explore problems in their dealings with others by talking, and gain insight into how they themselves appear to others. The choice of a group should be made carefully, and it is important that it is led by an experienced therapist.

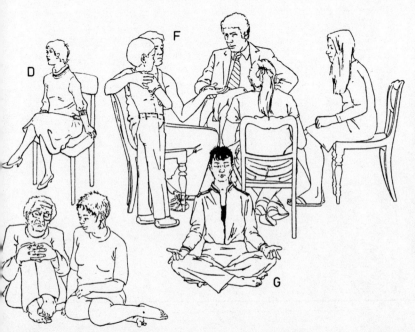

Freeing the mind
The illustration (*left*) portrays some of the most widely used psychotherapeutic techniques. In (**A**), a patient lets her thoughts roam freely while the therapist listens for clues to causes of conflict. The rebirth technique (**B**) and primal therapy (**C**) are developments of Freud's pioneering techniques. Reeducative therapy (**D**), group therapy (**E**), and family therapy (**F**) all work on the basis of a free discussion of problems in which the therapist takes a counseling role – helping a patient to understand her own emotions and problems and so come to terms with them. Self-suggestion and self-hypnosis methods (**G**) are still rather more experimental but have their adherents.

©DIAGRAM

SEXUALITY

Today in the West as never before, a woman may opt to reject repressive social attitudes if she wishes, and can choose the nature of her sexual experience with a completely new freedom.

But truly satisfying life-long sexual pleasure undoubtedly requires thorough understanding of the physical processes involved. For some women, too, certain alternatives may be preferable.

How safe are oral and anal sex? What can be done about vaginismus? And who may need sexual counseling? These and many other aspects of sexuality – including the handling of abuse and violence – remain major concerns for all women.

Chapter five

Anatomy of sex

Female sexual organs

Most women are actually rather vague about the appearance and function of their sexual and reproductive organs – perhaps because, unlike those of a man, those of a woman are almost entirely hidden, so that in a standing position the only obvious sign is the pubic hair. Collectively, the female external sex organs or genitals are known as the **vulva**. At the front, is the **mons veneris** (**mount of Venus**) or **mons pubis**, a pad of fatty tissue over the pubic bone. From puberty, this is covered with pubic hair. Extending downward and backward from the mons veneris are the **labia majora** (outer lips), two folds of fatty tissue which protect the reproductive and urinary openings lying between them. These outer lips change size during a woman's life; and from puberty their outer surfaces are also covered with hair. Between them lie the **labia minora** (inner lips). These are delicate, hairless folds of skin, quite sensitive to touch. During sexual arousal, they swell and darken in color. Below the mons area, the labia minora split into two folds to form a hood under which lies the **clitoris**. This is a small, bud-shaped organ and the most sensitive of the female genitals. The clitoris corresponds exactly to the male penis and is also made up of erectile tissue. During sexual excitement, the clitoris swells with blood, and for most women is the center of orgasm.

Just below the clitoris are the **urethra** – the external opening of the urinary passage which leads direct to the bladder – and the vaginal opening, the outside entrance to the **vagina**. The **hymen**, or **maidenhead**, is a thin membrane just inside the vaginal opening. It varies greatly in shape and size; and in a virgin, it may be stretched or torn during the first experience of sexual intercourse, but quite often has already been stretched, perhaps by the use of tampons or strenuous activity such as horse-riding. If torn during intercourse, there is usually some bleeding and possibly pain. But it has a small perforation even in a virgin to allow the flow of menstrual fluid.

Bartholin's or **vestibular glands** lie either side of the vaginal opening. Contrary to previous belief, these glands play little part in vaginal lubrication, but may occasionally become infected (as in gonorrhea). The **perineum** is the triangular area of skin lying between the end of the labia minora and the anus. Below its surface are muscles and fibrous tissue that are stretched during childbirth. The **anus** lies below the perineum and is the external opening through which feces pass out of the body.

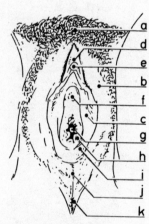

External sex organs
a Mons veneris
b Labia majora
c Labia minora
d Clitoral hood
e Clitoris
f Urethra
g Vaginal opening
h Hymen
i Bartholin's glands
j Perineum
k Anus

THE BREASTS

The breasts undergo great changes during a woman's life. Before puberty, the breast is simply a nipple projecting from a pink area – the **areola**. By the 11th year or thereabouts, however, the areola begins to bulge, the nipple still projecting from it. Secretions of the hormones **estrogen** and **progesterone** then stimulate breast development. The milk ducts develop from the nipple inward, and fat accumulates around them so that by the age of 13–15, the breasts are prominent.

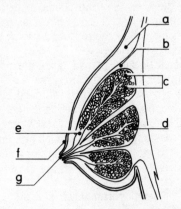

The breast
a Fat cells
b Fibrous tissue
c Alveoli
d Lobes
e Main duct
f Areola
g Nipple

The adult female breast, or mammary gland, consists of 15–25 lobes that are separated by fibrous tissue, rather like the segments of an orange. Each lobe resembles a tree and is embedded in fat. After childbirth, milk produced in the **alveoli** of each lobe (the "leaves" of each "tree") travels along small ducts into the main "trunk" or milk duct. This duct is enlarged to form a reservoir just below the areola. A narrow continuation of the duct links this reservoir with the nipple's surface. Each of the breast's 15–25 lobes has its own opening on the nipple.

Early signs of pregnancy often include swollen areolae, breast tenderness, and a marbled appearance produced by prominent veins in the breasts. In the first three months, changes in blood supply and growth of milk ducts and alveoli enlarge the breasts by 20–25 percent, so that toward the end of pregnancy, they are about one-third larger than normal. Breastfeeding triggers further development but the breasts resume their former shape once breastfeeding ceases.

Around the menopause, the breasts begin to droop and become less firm, as fibrous tissue slackens and milk ducts and alveoli shrink.

Changes in the breast
1 Pre-puberty
2 Puberty
3 Maturity
4 Pregnancy
5 Later life

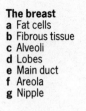

©DIAGRAM

253

SHAPE AND SIZE

The shape and size of breasts vary enormously from woman to woman. Though their size often corresponds to the overall body size, many slim women have large breasts and many obese women have comparatively small breasts.

Large breasts can occur because of fluid retention, obesity, or excessive hormone stimulation. Breasts also tend to become larger during pregnancy and lactation, and many women find that their breasts enlarge after the age of 35. A firm supporting bra will help, and extreme enlargement can be corrected by hormone treatment, or by cosmetic surgery which involves the removal of some of the pads of fat which give the breasts their size.

Small breasts can occur because of inadequate hormone stimulation or just because a woman is slim. Cosmetic surgery may help. Surgeons can insert silicone, or bags filled with fluid, between the breasts and the pectoral muscles but there is a danger that the breasts may become infected later as a result. For most women who are anxious about small breasts, however, a padded bra, upright posture, and perhaps exercises to strengthen the underlying pectoral muscles are all that is really necessary. Small breasts are in fact quite adequate for breastfeeding.

The need for a bra has been overemphasized in the past; but women who are in late pregnancy or breastfeeding are generally advised to wear one to avoid stretching supporting tissues.

ABNORMALITIES

Naturally **inverted nipples** are a development fault, sometimes making breastfeeding difficult unless a special shield is used and nipple-rolling exercises carried out although they often become protruberant naturally during the pregnancy. But retraction of previously normal nipples may sometimes be a sign of breast cancer; and so if this occurs, it will be wise to see your doctor immediately. **Discharge** from the nipples of women who are not breastfeeding can sometimes be due to excessive stimulation in lovemaking, the effect of certain drugs, glandular disorder or a tumor, either benign or malignant. **Extra nipples** sometimes also occur, usually below the breast, and advice can be sought about removal by surgery.

Exercises to strengthen the chest muscles
1 With both arms horizontal at shoulder level, push your palms against each other for 10 seconds or so
2 With arms horizontal, link the fingers of one hand over the other and pull for about 10 seconds. Relax. Repeat several times
3 Stand with your arms bent and hands at waist height for a few seconds. Then have your forearms at right-angles to your upper arms, and again hold for a few seconds. Keeping your shoulders relaxed, stretch both arms above your head in a 'V' shape. Hold for another few seconds. Relax. Repeat 3 times

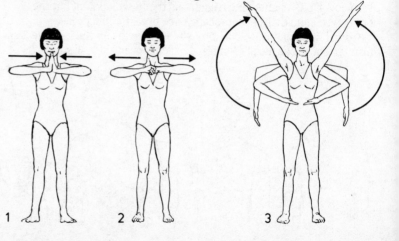

1   2   3

254

Sexual response

Important changes take place in the body during lovemaking, as a result of muscular tension and the swelling of certain tissues with blood. These processes were first described in detail by William Masters and Virginia Johnson, in their book *Human Sexual Response*. The act of lovemaking can be divided into four stages: the excitement phase, the plateau phase, orgasm, and the resolution phase. The duration of the **excitement phase** varies according to the amount and effectiveness of the stimulation.

Early in the excitement phase, the breasts' nipples become erect. Later, increased definition of the vein pattern in the breasts becomes obvious, too, and there may be an increase in the size of the breasts themselves. There are other external genital changes, too. The clitoris, for instance, increases in length and diameter. The labia majora open and spread flat, while the labia minora swell and extend outward. General muscular tension begins, and heart rate and blood pressure start to increase.

The **plateau phase** is an extension of the excitement phase – the breasts continue to enlarge by as much as 25 percent, particularly in women who have not breastfed, and the areolae become prominent. A pink mottling, known as the sex flush, may also appear on the breasts. The labia majora swell further, and the labia minora change color from pink to red, or from red to deep red in a woman who has had children.

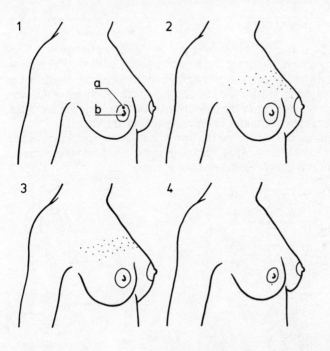

Changes in the breasts during lovemaking
1 Excitement
2 Plateau phase
3 Orgasm
4 Resolution
a Areola
b Nipple

© DIAGRAM

The **orgasmic phase** usually lasts only a matter of seconds. Orgasms do, however, vary in intensity and duration from woman to woman and occasion to occasion. When orgasm is over, the **resolution phase** begins. The areolae subside, leaving the nipples prominent for a while, and the breasts gradually resume their normal size. If effective stimulation continues, sexual tensions increase and the desire for release of tensions through orgasm is intensified. There is gradual muscular and physiological relaxation, and within 30 minutes the body returns to its unstimulated state.

External female genital changes during lovemaking
1 Excitement phase
2 Plateau phase
3 Orgasm
4 Resolution phase
a Clitoris
b Urethra
c Vagina
d Labia minora
e Labia majora

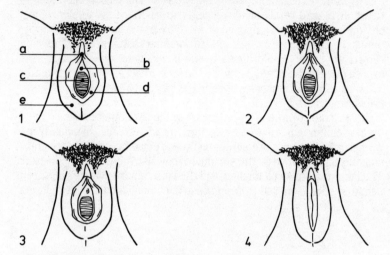

Internally, during the excitement phase, the vagina becomes moistened with a lubricant "sweated" through its walls. The uterus and cervix pull away from the vagina, and the inner two-thirds of the vagina expands. During the plateau phase, the expansion of the inner vagina continues, while the outer third contracts, gripping the penis. The uterus also continues to move away from the vagina.

At orgasm, the uterus and the lower third of the vagina experience a wave of contractions. Afterward, during the resolution phase, the uterus, cervix, and vagina return to normal.

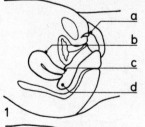
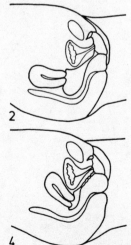
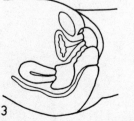

Internal female genital changes during lovemaking
1 Excitement
2 Plateau
3 Orgasm
4 Resolution
a Clitoris
b Uterus
c Cervix
d Vagina

EROGENOUS ZONES

Erotically-sensitive areas of the body vary quite considerably from individual to individual; and stimulation by hand or mouth (or other light object) of any of these sensitive areas is not only an important part of lovemaking but can also be sexually satisfying in itself. It can lead to mutual masturbation or oral-genital sex, even though in the West lovemaking usually follows a pattern of foreplay, intercourse, and orgasm. Many people – women and men alike – prefer sexual activity to end with the particular closeness of intercourse, and indeed many believe that lovemaking *must* always finish with vaginal intercourse: but to consider that stimulation of the erogenous zones of the body is only a prelude to, or substitute for, orgasm through vaginal intercourse, or even oral-genital sex-play, is to limit the pleasures that it can bring.

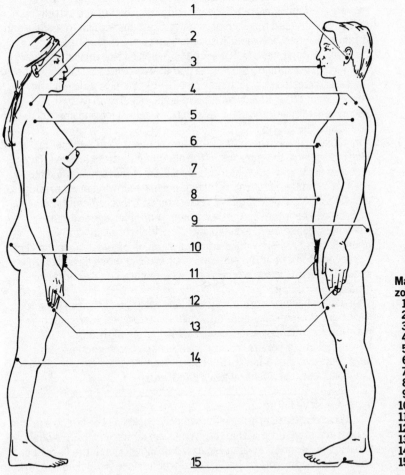

Male and female erogenous zones
1 Ears
2 Cheeks
3 Mouth
4 Neck (front and back)
5 Shoulders
6 Breasts and nipples
7 Waist
8 Navel
9 Base of spine
10 Buttocks
11 Genital area
12 Hands
13 Insides of thighs
14 Back of knees
15 Soles of feet

©DIAGRAM

ORGASM

The female orgasm has possibly been the subject of more debate and literature than any other area of human sexuality. But fortunately, since the work of Masters and Johnson in the 1960s, many of the myths and mysteries surrounding it have gone. It is now known that, although the experience and intensity of orgasm may vary considerably, the actual physical process of orgasm is always the same.

Women vary greatly in what they respond to sexually, but the mons pubis, labia minora, clitoris, and vaginal entrance are almost always important. The clitoris is the most sexually responsive part of a woman's body, and in most cases fairly continuous clitoral stimulation is needed for orgasm. However, as the tip of the clitoris is extremely sensitive, constant direct touch can become painful. So for the majority of women, caressing of the whole genital area of the mons pubis is more pleasurable. During intercourse, movement of the penis in and out of the vagina provides continual clitoral stimulation by moving the labia minora backward and forward over the clitoral tip.

The time needed to reach orgasm varies from woman to woman and from occasion to occasion. Just before orgasm, there is a feeling of tension, lasting possibly 2–4 seconds, when all the small muscles in the pelvis surrounding the vagina and uterus contract. This is followed by the orgasm itself, which may last 10–15 seconds. It is felt as a series of rhythmic muscular contractions, occurring every 0.8 seconds, firstly around the outer third of the vagina and spreading upward to the uterus.

In a mild orgasm, there are 3–5 contractions; in an intense one, 8–12. During orgasm, the muscles of the abdomen, buttocks, arms, face, legs and neck may also contract. Breathing is more rapid, and blood pressure climbs. All these return to normal following orgasm which is usually followed by feelings of relaxation and peace. Sometimes orgasm can be intense; at other times, more like a gentle ripple.

Women, unlike men, are capable of multiple orgasm: that is, immediately or shortly after a first orgasm, if a woman maintains her sexual excitement at the plateau level, she can move directly into a second orgasm. Some women can even experience 3–5 orgasms within a few minutes.

Virtually all women are physically able to attain orgasm. But some never do. Women also generally take longer to reach orgasm than men (fifteen minutes as opposed to an average of three). Nevertheless, it seems that the vast majority of women prefer intercourse to any other form of sexual activity, perhaps, because of the closeness and affection associated with it.

THE G-SPOT

The **Grafenberg spot** (also known colloquially as the G-spot) is said to be a sensitive area within the vagina, on its front wall. Although still a matter of debate, certain research has shown that if the G-spot is stimulated during intercourse, some women lose body fluid in a form of ejaculation at the point of orgasm, which it is claimed intensifies the sensation, but this is by no means a universal experience.

INTERCOURSE IN PREGNANCY

For women who have had a previous miscarriage, intercourse in the first three months of a pregnancy can sometimes be unwise. A doctor will advise on this when the pregnancy is first confirmed. Later in pregnancy, the woman's thickening waistline may also make intercourse in more conventional positions uncomfortable, if not impossible.

A variety of positions can be adapted for use during pregnancy. Among the most suitable are rear-entry positions and those in which the woman can control the depth of penetration. Illustrated here are a rear-entry position with both partners kneeling; a face-to-face position on a chair, the woman seated above the man, allowing her to control the degree of penetration; and a suitable position for the final months of pregnancy in which pregnant woman's body and feet are supported and there is no pressure on her abdomen.

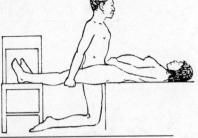

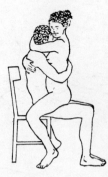

POSITIONS FOR BACK PAIN SUFFERERS

People subject to back pain may suffer excruciatingly in the conventional positions for intercourse. But there are often less usual positions that the victim can enjoy or at least tolerate. A considerate partner will try to find what these are. Four positions that are safe for most people with back pain are pictured here. In each case, the pelvic thrusting should be left to the pain-free partner.

1 He lies on a bed while she sits astride leaning forward. (He is the one with the pain.)

2 He stands for rear-entry as she kneels face down on a bed. (He is the one with the pain.)

3 She lies on a bed while he leans forward between her legs. (She is the one with the pain.)

4 They sit face-to-face on a chair, she on his lap so she can do all the thrusting. (He is the one with the pain.)

4

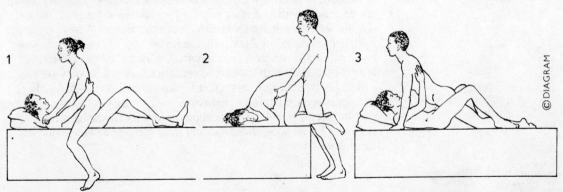

©DIAGRAM

POSITIONS FOR VIRGINS

Many first-timers adopt the well-known missionary position (**1**). But for male and female virgins, the position matters less than the approach. This should be slow and considerate. Foreplay will also stimulate lubrication of the vagina so that a woman should feel little discomfort, especially if past petting has stretched or torn her hymen.

POSITIONS SUGGESTED FOR PEOPLE WITH PROBLEMS

A squatting position (**2**) helps full penetration of women with tight vaginas. Side-by-side, facing (**3**) helps the ill, old, tired, tall-and-short. A side-by-side, rear-entry position (**4**) is recommended for men with a weak erection. A woman-on-top position (**5**) is used in the treatment of male impotence and premature ejaculation. It is also used as a preliminary position in therapy for non-orgasmic women. A side-by-side position (**6**) make uncontrolled hip movements easier for the woman and helps her reach orgasm.

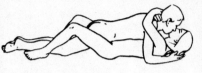

1

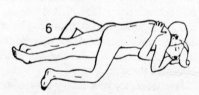

2

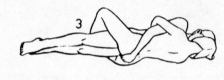

3

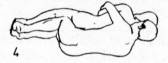

4

5

6

SEX AND THE HANDICAPPED

Several physical conditions have implications for continuing sexual activity and certain forms of medication cause diminution of sex drive and response: for example, there may be pain because of joint stiffness, or reduced or altered sensation if nerves are involved. Pain and spasm are best dealt with by finding different positions and support, and a physiotherapist will usually be able to offer guidance. Women suffering from nerve injuries or disorders which affect the nervous system may find that greater stimulation is required, perhaps with a vibrator, yet areas of the body with unaffected sensation may still be very sensitive.

Mentally handicapped women are vulnerable to sexual exploitation, but sex is equally vital as an expression of a loving relationship. Advice on contraception and the implications of fertility should be given by a person who has good understanding and experience of the individual's capabilities.

Alternatives

Lovemaking does not have to include penile-vaginal penetration. Many couples derive just as much pleasure from the other sexual activities described here. These can be enjoyed as specific alternatives to intercourse or may be incorporated into lovemaking before or after intercourse. Used as alternatives, some have the obvious advantage of avoiding conception, and are therefore sometimes recommended to couples using the rhythm method of birth control. But certain alternatives described may be distasteful to some couples.

In a great many parts of the world, **anal** (as well as **oral**) **sex** is illegal, although prosecutions are unlikely. Many women also find even the thought of anal sex totally abhorrent. Others, however, find it a stimulating part of lovemaking, and in many countries it is widely used as a form of contraception, although pregnancy is still a risk if any seminal fluid comes near the vagina. Although condoms do reduce the risk of becoming pregnant and catching a sexually-transmitted disease, they can, of course, tear or even come off completely. However, because the anus is not designed to accommodate the penis, some kind of lubrication is invariably needed and a strong condom should always be used to reduce risk of infection.

Anal intercourse should never be followed by vaginal intercourse without thorough washing as bacteria can easily lead to vaginal infections. There are other dangers, too. If anal intercourse is practiced regularly over a long period of time, the anus can become over-dilated, leading to permanent damage. Because the walls of the rectum are particularly thin, they are very susceptible to damage, so you may be more at risk from catching AIDS from an infected partner. The virus can be transmitted in either blood or semen through small tears in the skin. Anal intercourse should definitely be avoided with anyone you consider to be a high AIDS risk.

Oral-genital sex is of two kinds. In **cunnilingus**, a man uses his mouth to stimulate a woman's genitals; in route for a woman uses her mouth to stimulate a man's genitals.

Techniques for each include kissing, licking, sucking and, in the case of fellatio, friction of the penis inside the woman's mouth. Oral-genital sex is sometimes disapproved of on the grounds that it is unnatural, unhygienic or simply "wrong." Its practice remains an offense in some statute books but prosecution is extremely unlikely and many people now accept oral-genital sex as a perfectly natural and enjoyable form of sexual activity. Women in particular can reach orgasm very easily in this way. But there is reason to believe that there could be risk of infection from a partner who carries the AIDS virus if there are bleeding gums or mouth sores. Menstrual flow from an infected woman entering the site of a mouth ulcer might also provide a **fellatio,** transmission of the virus.

Mutual **masturbation** is a common sexual activity among couples, and involves the erotic stimulation of the genitals by means other than sexual intercourse. Frequently used as an arousal technique, masturbation by one partner of the other can also be continued to orgasm. For maximum pleasure, each partner should be aware of the

©DIAGRAM

other's preferences. For instance, a woman manually masturbating a man should be aware of the speed of stroke and degree of pressure that he prefers; while he should remember that most women prefer pressure to be applied to the side of and around the clitoris rather than directly to it.

Masturbation positions

1 She sits on the floor, legs gently apart. He kneels facing her so that each of them can at the same time masturbate the other.

2 He lies back: she sits astride to masturbate him.

3 The couple lie in an embrace and he masturbates her.

Interfemoral sex positions

In these, the man's penis is masturbated by the woman's thighs. Note that these positions are not effective in avoiding conception; sperm may enter the vagina from the vulva.

4 The couple lie side by side.

5 The couple stand to embrace.

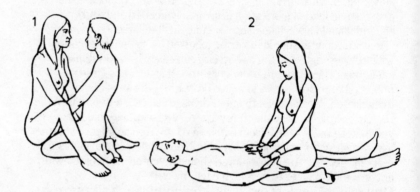

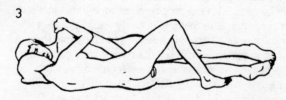

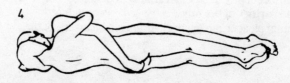

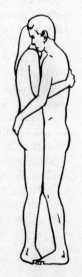

Lesbian lovemaking

Lesbian lovemaking has always been seen in two completely different lights. On the one hand, there is considerable ignorance and fear among the population generally about lesbian activities; while on the other hand, distorted presentations of lesbian activity have long been accepted as a source of erotic arousal in classical art, and even contemporary pornography. Both views incorrectly assume that lovemaking between women is a preliminary to, or a substitute for, heterosexual intercourse. In fact, the reverse seems to be true. What is notable is that lesbians claim they can achieve far greater sexual satisfaction with each other than many other women achieve in their heterosexual relationships. Nearly all lesbian lovemaking brings orgasm for both women, which may explain why men have sometimes tended to feel threatened by lesbianism.

Many sexual activities are common to both lesbians and heterosexuals. In both, there is mutual kissing and caressing, particularly of the breasts and genitals, and the general giving of affection. By its very nature, there is no pre-intercourse foreplay in lesbian lovemaking, and most activity centers around clitoral stimulation. The main techniques used are mutual masturbation, and cunnilingus (kissing, sucking, and licking of the clitoris). Vibrators are commonly used for clitoral stimulation; but the dildo, or artificial penis, is not used. By definition, lesbians are attracted to other women and their lovemaking does not center on penis-substitutes. One additional practice which is sometimes used, however, is that of tribadism – where one woman lies on top of another and moves in such a way as to stimulate the clitoris of each other.

A common myth is that each partner takes an exclusively "butch" (active male) or "femine" (active female) role. In practice, if such roles are assumed, they usually alternate. A further myth is that all lesbians are first and foremost sexual beings, whereas they are no more sexually active or sexually obsessed than are most people. In fact, by comparison with male homosexuals, sexual promiscuity is rare among lesbians, as is prostitution. At the same time, promiscuity is neither more nor less frequent among lesbians than among heterosexual women.

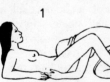

1

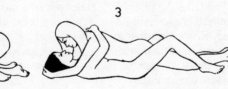

3

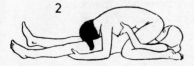

2

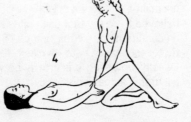

4

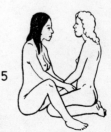

5

Lesbian lovemaking
1 Receiving oral-genital sex
2 Mutual oral-genital sex
3 Body rubbing (tribadism)
4 Being masturbated by partner
5 Mutual masturbation

©DIAGRAM

There have been few studies investigating the nature of lesbianism. Physical explanations, such as hormone imbalance or congenital defects, have been put forward, but findings are ambiguous and not generally accepted. In the past, lesbianism has also been defined in terms of neurosis or of immature development, but these are generalizations based on lesbians who have sought psychiatric help. One of the most sympathetic theories is that of the psychiatrist, Dr Charlotte Wolff. She has emphasized the bisexual nature of lesbianism, seeing an essentially bisexual element in the female's clitoris, and has explained lesbianism as a recognition, and rejection, from early childhood of "second sex" attitudes that debase the social position of women. Because of this, she has also said that lesbians are ideally suited to lead a move for the equality of women and the rejection of female/male stereotypes.

Female homosexuality has been regarded as a deviation by some, while it has also often been ignored or just ridiculed. These last attitudes, which reflect the approach of male-orientated societies toward women, have meant that female homosexuals have significantly escaped the same degree of legal persecution suffered by males. Lesbianism was generally accepted in ancient Greece and Rome; and it is also known that the Mohave Indians of North America openly recognized and accepted a class of homosexual women.

But references to lesbians have been scanty throughout history, even during the Middle Ages when persecution of homosexuals reached fanatical proportions. In most European countries, homosexuality was once a capital offense; but significantly more sentences were carried out on males.

During the 20th century, lesbians have therefore had to fight two battles: one for basic recognition and one for acceptance. Today, lesbianism is out in the open for the first time. Despite its relative legal freedom, lack of understanding about lesbians and discrimination against them – socially and economically – are still widespread.

As a result, a woman who feels attracted to other women may fear the opinion of others, both within the family and society, and may even have difficulty in admitting her sexual preference to herself. There has been extensive liberalizing of attitudes in society recently, however; and with the development of the women's movement, some have felt a commitment to lesbianism as part of a rejection of a prime need for the male. However, other lesbians still feel the need to repress ordinary expression of their sexuality, and perhaps to play a token part in heterosexual relations. (In some cases, such activity may be part of a genuine bisexuality.)

Bisexuality

Most of the confusion and disgust surrounding bisexuals exists because it is too frequently assumed that they deviate markedly from normality. There is very little evidence to support this. Instead, it is believed by many that each of us is inherently bisexual; and depending on conditioning, we may choose a partner from the opposite sex (heterosexuality,) our own sex (lesbianism) or both (bisexuality). Usually, however, it is utterly bewildering to discover that your partner is actually bisexual.

MASTURBATION

Lone sex and celibacy

Masturbation refers to stimulation of the genitals by hand or with some other object, usually to attain orgasm. It generally refers to self-stimulation, although mutual masturbation is common in both heterosexual and homosexual activity. At least 1 in 6 women masturbate at some time in their lives, and for many it is the most direct and successful means of achieving orgasm. In our society, masturbation has long been a taboo subject; and traditionally the attitude has been one of disapproval. To some extent, attitudes toward masturbation have reflected those of society toward sexuality in general, but with an additional dimension: whereas interpersonal sex could be "justified" on grounds of love and marriage, masturbation by its very nature was too blatantly an expression of an individual's inherent sexuality.

In recent years, however, masturbation has become recognized for what it is: a part of normal sexual experience and one that causes no particular physical or mental harm. In fact, the reverse may be seen as true. Not only does masturbation release acute tension due to an unsatisfactory sexual life or absence of a partner, but it also can be used by a woman as a learning process for a better understanding of her sexual responses, leading in turn to greater fulfillment with a partner.

But despite more enlightened social attitudes, recent studies show that most women still suffer guilt and anxiety about masturbation.

Techniques

Women have various ways of masturbating, although the most commonly used rely on stimulation of the clitoris. Over 80 percent of women who masturbate regularly concentrate on direct stimulation of clitoris or labia. One or more fingers can either be rubbed over or around the clitoris, or the whole hand may be used to apply steady and rhythmical pressure. (Few women masturbate by actually rubbing the clitoral glands; more commonly they massage the shaft or general clitoral area.) A pillow, vibrator, or continuous stream of water from a faucet may be used instead of the hands. Alternatively, some women masturbate by crossing their legs and applying steady pressure from their thighs onto the genital area. In addition, while using any of these techniques, a finger or similar object may be inserted into the vagina, although few women rely on vaginal insertion alone.

Slightly different from these methods is a technique used by about 5 percent of women. In this, a woman assumes a position similar to that of the woman-on-top position in intercourse. Although there may be some direct stimulation of the genitals, possibly with a pillow, it is usually very slight, and a climax is achieved by rhythmical pelvic thrusting combined with a build-up of muscular tension similar to that experienced during intercourse.

In most women, the breasts and nipples are highly sensitive and, in a few cases, their stimulation alone is sufficient for orgasm. Likewise, a very few women find they can achieve orgasm simply through fantasy.

©DIAGRAM

Exercises to improve your love life

Sexual intercourse is itself an excellent form of exercise: and it is certainly true, too, that if you are physically fit, you are likely to enjoy lovemaking all the more. Research has shown that the heart rate can increase to 180 beats per minute just prior to climax, and this equates with the rate experienced by professional runnners during a race. Making love is known to be a relaxing activity, too, as shown by the fact that people usually sleep far more soundly afterwards, and for a longer period.

You do not need to be a top class athlete in order to give pleasure and also achieve orgasm yourself, however. But there are a number of simple exercises that a woman can practice in order to increase sensation for both partners.

To help you relax
Perhaps try this exercise together with your partner.
1 Lie down on a firm bed.
2 Now spend a couple of minutes waving your arms and legs about, and making angry child-like noises to release the tension of the day.
3 Lie still and breathe deeply for two more minutes.

To strengthen the vaginal muscles
This exercise was first developed by Dr Arnold Kegel in the attempt to help women relieve backpain during pregnancy; but he also found it stengthened their internal muscles and sexual function. It can be done anywhere, and at anytime.
1 Imagine you need to find a lavatory but there is not one nearby.
2 Contract the muscles that you use to control both urination and a bowel movement.
3 Contract your vaginal muscles, too. (With practice, you should find that you can soon do this without first involving the other muscles.)
4 Contract and relax the vaginal muscles in this way ten times. Repeat intermittently throughout the day, and use the technique during intercourse.

To exercise the pelvic area
1 Lying on your back, bend your knees and have your legs apart. Keep your feet flat.
2 Breathing in, try to move the pelvis area upward a little. Do not expect to be able to do this to any great extent: only a small amount of movement is possible.
3 Breathe out as you lower the pelvis.
4 Relax and repeat.
5 Standing, have your feet apart and facing forward. Relax your knees.
6 Swing your hips in a clockwise circular movement but keep your upper body still.
7 Repeat in an anti-clockwise direction.
8 Now move your pelvis backward and forward.

Emotional needs

Close, caring relationships are not just about sex – they are also about emotional needs. In 1987, the American feminist Shere Hite published a major work called *Women and Love* – a detailed survey into the emotional needs and experiences of 4,500 women of all ages and backgrounds. It caused an enormous stir because it showed clearly that, despite other changes, most women today feel that their emotional needs are not being met by men.

Only 17 percent of the women interviewed said that communications within their relationships with men were good or made them happier. By far the majority felt that they received much greater emotional support and understanding from other women, and that they were emotionally deprived in relationships with men. In particular, many women feel that their male partners do not listen to them, that their opinions are undermined or trivialized; and, perhaps most importantly of all, that their male partners are often either unwilling or unable to discuss deep emotions. It seems that men are unwilling or unable to find a means of expressing intimacy, sensitivity and love. And for most women, if some means of meeting emotional needs is not included in a relationship, a satisfactory sexual relationship cannot be sustained.

Statistics show that the majority of heterosexual women today still want to marry or to share loving relationships with men. But in practice many women find that, although there have been social changes and greater moves toward equality outside marriage, within marriage a woman's role has remained the traditional nurturing one of providing emotional support for men – not the other way around. Many women feel too that their attempts to ask for a greater degree of shared emotional intimacy often leads to misunderstandings and a reluctance on the part of men to talk which in turn can lead to sexual problems, arguments, and sometimes violence. As a result, many women separate themselves emotionally from their men, find satisfaction in work, children, and friends, and many have extra-marital affairs, or may leave the relationship.

Many women today are turning to counseling and couple or group therapy in order to find a solution to the problem. Evidence shows that this can be successful. But many women also feel that this, once again, leaves the responsibility for change with them.

Increasingly, many women are saying that for their emotional needs to be met, men themselves have to make changes and break away from the traditional conditioning that has made it difficult for them to express their feelings in a non-sexual way. Many women argue that for relationships to improve, men have to learn to express the so-called "feminine" skills of sensitivity, warmth and sharing, without being asked. Basically, women are asking men to learn how to love, not only sexually, but emotionally as well.

©DIAGRAM

Sexual problems

A wide range of problems can affect a woman's enjoyment of her sexuality. They may be physical or psychological in origin, but the result usually is the same – distress for both partners.

A very few women are truly frigid – that is, incapable of responding to any kind of sexual stimulation. But there are many who are temporarily unable to achieve orgasm. Some women find penile penetration or intercourse painful or even impossible; while others have a partner with some kind of sexual difficulty. The purely physical problems are usually easy to identify: psychological problems can also be treated but the origin of the problem must be traced first. Common underlying causes of psychological problems are feelings of fear, shame, or guilt about sexual response, or anxiety connected with pregnancy. Important in the treatment of such problems are a number of sexual therapy techniques, as first developed by Masters and Johnson. Consultation with a specialist sex therapist can be very helpful.

FRIGIDITY

This is a complex female complaint in which a woman derives little or no erotic pleasure from sexual stimulation. Treatment often takes the form of sensate focus therapy, in which the couple refrain from intercourse and orgasm for a period. During this time, they learn to caress each other's bodies until the woman is sufficiently aroused to initiate intercourse.

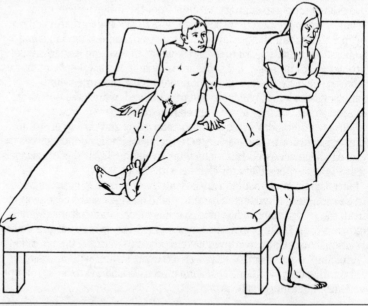

Lack of response
Self-consciousness and fear of failure are among several possible causes of frigidity

FIRST INTERCOURSE

In a woman who has not previously experienced intercourse, the hymen may be intact and unstretched. On the first few occasions intercourse takes place, there may be a little pain or even slight bleeding as the hymen is stretched or torn to accommodate the penis Only a very few women have tough hymens which may necessitate minor surgery.

VAGINISMUS

This is a comparatively rare disorder in which the muscles surrounding the vaginal entrance go into spasm when penetration is attempted. Treatment involves the woman learning, over a period of time, to insert first one, then two fingers into her vagina without experiencing muscular spasm. Her partner takes part in this; and when the woman's confidence is established, intercourse can take place.

PAINFUL INTERCOURSE

This may be caused by several factors. Vaginal infection and irritations can be exacerbated by the friction of the penis moving in the vagina. Insufficient vaginal lubrication can also cause pain. During normal stimulation, the vaginal walls secrete a lubricating fluid which facilitates entry by the penis. But pain results if the man attempts entry before the woman is sufficiently aroused. A lubricating jelly, or even saliva, may also help solve the problem.

Another common cause of pain in the pelvis is the penis hitting the cervix during particularly deep thrusts. Alternatively, pelvic pain can also be caused by infections of the uterus, cervix, or Fallopian tubes, cysts or tumors on the ovaries, or tears in the ligaments supporting the uterus following childbirth.

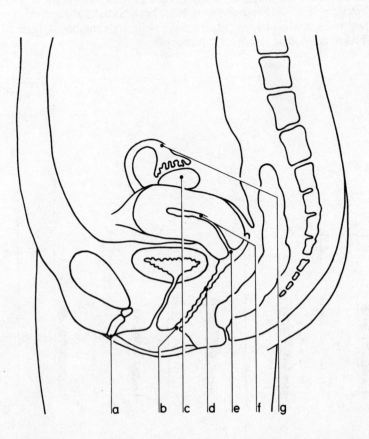

Pain in women on intercourse
Common sites and conditions include the following:
a Clitoris: pain due to infection, or injury as when a man directly rubs the clitoris
b Vaginal outlet: scars or tears linked with first intercourse, IUD strings, rape, abortion or childbirth; or atrophy due to aging
c Ovaries: inflammation, displacement, or cysts
d Vagina: poor lubrication due to lack of estrogen: or infection due to a lowering of vaginal acidity caused by douching or invasion of germs via fingers, penis, etc; or sensitivity to rubber devices
e Cervix inflamed by infection or "spilt" bits of womb lining causing fibrous growths in the genital system (endometriosis)
f Uterus inflammation (as **c**), displacement, or torn ligaments
g Fallopian tubes: (as **e**)

© DIAGRAM

273

Improving sexual response

Sexual inadequacy among women chiefly takes the form of failure to reach orgasm. Some societies do not recognize that women need this sexual climax. But repeated congestion of genital organs without relief via orgasm can bring discomfort, frustration and psychological damage.

Sometimes the cause is the man's impotence or ineptitude. If the trouble lies in the woman, it may be organic. There may be defects of the sexual system, imbalance of hormones, or injury or inflammation affecting the genitals. Certain nervous disorders, excessive drinking or drug-taking, stress or aging may also be to blame.

Psychological causes are by far the commonest, however. The woman may find the man sexually unattractive or selfish. Mentally, she rejects him as a mate and makes this evident by her lack of sexual response.

Some "frigid" women were taught as children that sex is bad, wrong and dirty. Such notions can warp a woman's attitudes to sex so that she views with guilt, fear and shame her own sexual feelings and tries to suppress them, remaining sexually unresponsive.

Other (often related) psychological blocks are emotional ties with the father; subconscious hatred of men; fear of pregnancy; and fear of pain on intercourse. But some women fail because they are actually over-eager to succeed, and so too tense to reach orgasm.

Treating the non-orgasmic woman involves considerate, stimulating sex play when she is relaxed and both partners are in harmony. Techniques such as those shown *opposite* have brought orgasm to many women who had never had it and a very large number of those who had previously lost orgasmic ability.

Unconsummated marriage
One survey of 1000 women with unconsummated marriages revealed the following reasons:
a Sex too painful (20.3%)
b Sex considered nasty (17.8%)
c Husband impotent (11.7%)
d Fear of pregnancy or childbirth (10.2%)
e Other factors, such as vagina too small, ignorance, lesbianism, or penis phobia (40%)
Early sex education would have stopped most problems arising.

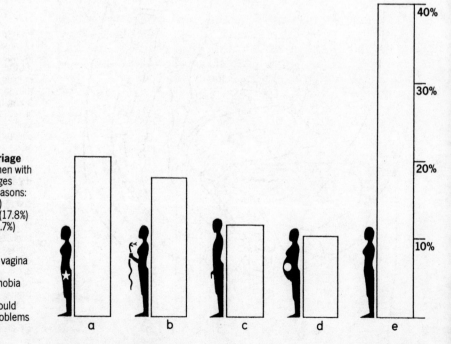

STIMULATION TECHNIQUES

1 a Considerate caressing by the man when the woman is feeling relaxed may help to arouse her. He should find which areas she most likes to have stroked, and periods of rest should punctuate attempts at arousal. Tenderly telling the woman he loves her will usually make her far more responsive than roughly seizing and manipulating her.

b A non-orgasmic woman seeking arousal sometimes finds it helpful to concentrate her mind upon some sexual fantasy. Reading erotic books and looking at erotic magazines may assist her. Meanwhile, the man can encourage her with words of endearment to show that she gives him pleasure. Talking about sexually stimulating topics can also help.

c Masturbation by vibrator or by hand may help to stimulate some women who can be aroused yet are sexually less sensitive than most. Other physical aids include deep penetration by the penis, and oral-genital contact. The man can again reinforce physical efforts with encouraging words. Any method that brings orgasm once makes it easier for a woman to achieve orgasm later.

SENSATE-FOCUS THERAPY

2 a The couple sit nude on their bed – the man, legs apart, propped up by the headboard; the woman seated with her back to his chest and her legs on his. She guides his hands briefly over her inner thighs, vaginal lips and clitoral region. In this way, she can control her sexual sensations and stop them becoming too intense for her.

b In subsequent sessions, the couple eventually work up to the point where the woman kneels astride the man and finds pleasure in keeping still with his penis inside her vagina. She can then try slowly moving her hips to and fro, thrusting faster and harder when she finds that she wants to. Next she has him join in with his own thrusting hip movements.

c The last form of therapy involves both partners lying sideways, so she rests largely on his chest, stomach, one leg, and the knee of the other leg. This position makes uncontrolled hip movements easier and orgasm more likely for women than positions where they can consciously control the movements made by their bodies.

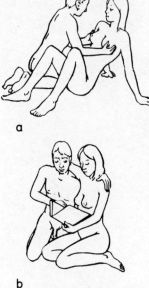

1

a

b

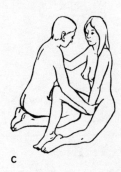

c

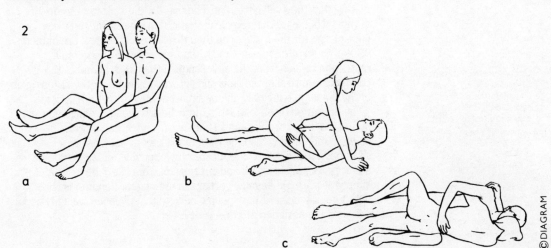

2

a

b

c

©DIAGRAM

Sexual aids

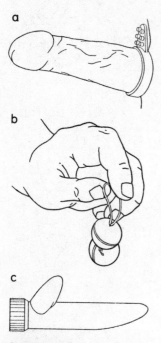

Sexual aids
a Clitoral stimulator condom
b Chinese balls
c Vibrator

The use of stimulators for love-making goes back centuries, and some early Eastern devices are still popular today. Many women find them an exciting and often beneficial part of their sex lives.

Perhaps the most widely used aids are various forms of erotica, ranging from visually-stimulating clothing and underwear to explicit magazines and videos. Another very popular aid is the dildo or vibrator, which is penis-shaped with an optional vibrating mechanism. Usually battery-powered, it may also have speed variations and a selection of attachments which can stimulate the clitoris at the same time as the vagina.

Some women find they are able to reach a climax with a vibrator when this is difficult through intercourse alone. It can also be used as a masturbation aid, particularly by women who do not have a partner. Some form of lubrication is often necessary with vibrators and other sexual aids, particularly at certain times of the menstrual cycle.

Many couples also enjoy using brightly coloured and textured sheaths, which can be put on the penis or on a vibrator. Condom-like attachments can also be put over the penis to enlarge it. This may be particularly stimulating for women who enjoy deeper penetration. If the man has difficulty maintaining an erection, a ring can be placed around the base of the penis to prevent the blood escaping.

Local anesthetics in the form of sprays and creams are supposed to delay a man's ejaculation, although there is no evidence to suggest that they have any real physical effect. Chinese balls, meanwhile, are designed to stimulate the vagina over longer periods of time. When inserted, they vibrate as the woman moves and can be left in for some time.

Most sex aids are perfectly safe if used correctly. Not only do they enhance pleasure, but they can be a great help in treating many sexual problems for both men and women.

Female circumcision

Female circumcision is a traditional custom practiced on thousands of women each year, principally in Africa. Although women themselves often resent having had it done, they still subject their daughters to it, fearing that they will fail to find a husband if they are not circumcized.

It is still believed that female circumcision makes intercourse more pleasurable for the man, even though as a result women are denied pleasure and often find sex excrutiatingly painful. The genital mutilation ranges from the severence of the clitoral hood to the complete removal of the labia and clitoris, followed by the stitching up of the vulva, leaving only a very small opening for menstruation.

The operation often leads to serious health problems including
1 hemorrhaging, chronic vaginal and urinary infections, cysts and incontinence. Many also die from blood loss or septicemia.

Although many governments are now opposing female circumcision as a form of sexual abuse and oppression, this often means that it is simply performed illegally, perhaps in unhygienic conditions and without anesthesia. Many people believe that changes will only occur if a campaign is aimed at grass root level.

The world of male sexual fantasy is well known. Pornographic magazines, videos, postcards, and even advertising have pushed male sexual fantasy into the public eye where they have dominated images of sexuality for many years. But women, too, have sexual or erotic fantasies; and it has even been estimated that the majority of women fantasize during masturbation, and probably well over half of all women also fantasize when making love with a partner.

In the past, and even today, many women have felt guilty or worried about such fantasies. Some have feared that indulgence in them somehow represents an inadequacy, or an inability to gain complete pleasure with a partner, male or female. Others have been concerned that the very fact of fantasizing might threaten the partner. Some women, too, have worried that their fantasies, particularly if they are woven around a situation that a woman might never act out in the "real" world, represent serious emotional disturbance.

But sexual or erotic fantasies are in fact a natural part of a woman's sexual and emotional life. All women fantasize at some time or another. A sexual or erotic fantasy may be a fleeting image, or it may be an elaborately worked out story or stories that a woman returns to again and again. Until recently, we knew very little about women's sexual erotic fantasy life, mainly because women have been scared to speak out, and because sexual behavior and information about sexuality has predominantly been defined and produced by men: the secret world of women remained largely unknown. However, with the publication of books such as *My Secret Garden* by American writer Nancy Friday, and the work of American researcher Shere Hite, women themselves have been speaking out and breaking the silence surrounding female sexuality.

As a result of such work, we now know that women's sexual fantasies cover a rich and wide-ranging area. They may include sex with a stranger, fantasies of pain and torture, voyeurism, exhibitionism, and a whole range of likely and unlikely encounters with men and women. Research also shows that fantasies can occur at any age, and with any woman whether she is in an unsatisfactory or satisfactory relationship. For all women, fantasies are an expression of need, desires, and dreams. They may be used to compensate for an unsatisfactory sexual relationship, or to enhance a good sexual experience. Either way, they are an addition to a woman's sexual and emotional life; and they enable women to imagine situations that they may not want to put into practice. They may be a closely-guarded secret, or shared with an understanding partner. Either way, they can be a rich and healthy addition to a woman's life.

Sexual fantasies

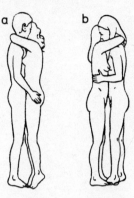

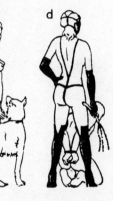

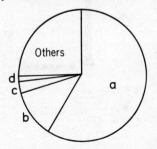

Fantasies during masturbation
Most women fantasize while masturbating, so surveys have revealed. In the diagram below, the bars show the percentages of masturbating females who fantasize in many ways.
a Heterosexual fantasies 60%
b Lesbian fantasies 10%
c Animal fantasies 4%
d Sado-masochistic fantasies 1%

©DIAGRAM

The older woman

Although sexual topics are now much more openly discussed, the sexual needs and behavior of older people are often subject to considerable misunderstanding and even embarrassment. In society's eyes, and particularly among the young, it is still not considered "correct" for older people, who are probably parents and grandparents, to have the same sexual yearnings and desires as younger people. Such an attitude is ill-founded, and stems largely from society's current emphasis on youth and youthful attractiveness.

There is no doubt that the sex drive does decline with age. In men, this starts in the twenties and then proceeds gradually through life

Psychological problems
An older couple (**1**) with a previously enjoyable sex life (**2**) may find this threatened (**3**) by problems such as the following:
a Disharmony about non-sexual matters may disrupt the couple's physical relationship
b Attitude of mind may make the couple think they are too old for sex
c The couple may still enjoy sex, but feel embarrassed about what others might think
d Unimaginative lovemaking may lead to boredom with sex
e Worry about declining sexual prowess may lead one partner to seek reassurance elsewhere, often with someone younger
f Another response to fears of sexual decline is to reject sex completely
g Worries about non-sexual matters – such as retirement or money – may interfere with sexual performance

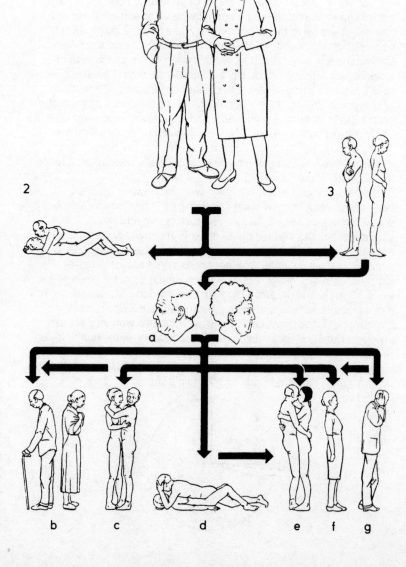

until about age sixty, when the rate of decline decreases. In women, there is usually no appreciable decline at all until about age sixty, after which the rate of decline is very gradual. Clearly, this is in no way consistent with the erroneous idea that old people should have no sex lives. People who enjoy sex earlier in life generally continue to do so as they get older; and although the aging process may make it necessary to adapt their lovemaking to some extent, most older people remain capable of intercourse for as long as their general health will permit.

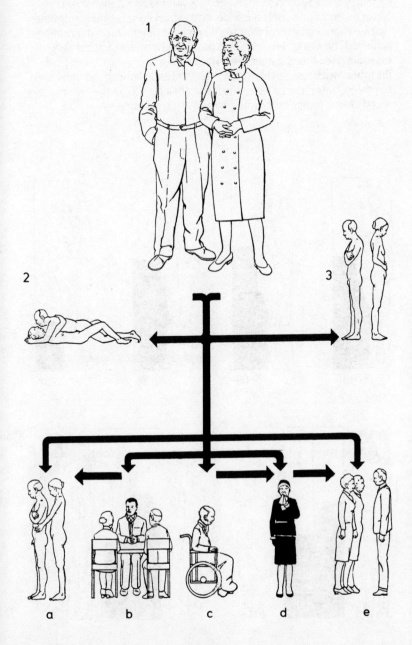

Practical problems
Here we look at some of the practical problems that older people (**1**) may have to overcome if enjoyment of sex (**2**) is not to come to an end (**3**)
a One partner may still be interested in sex but the other may not be
b Physical problems associated with aging of the reproductive system may make intercourse uncomfortable unless they are treated
c Illness or infirmity may make intercourse difficult: but trying special positions may help
d Death of one partner often ends the sex life of the other since many older people are not interested in finding a new mate
e People who would like a new partner cannot always find one: women outnumber men in older age groups, and some are naturally shy about meeting new people

©DIAGRAM

The ability to enjoy lovemaking can continue well into old age, particularly if a couple makes the effort to understand and respond to the various changes that age brings to the natural pattern of sexual response. All too often, older couples give up intercourse because they mistakenly interpret these changes as signs of forthcoming impotence. Lovemaking may have to become a more leisurely affair as a couple gets older, but the benefits of maintaining the physical side of a relationship into old age can be great. Older men generally need a longer period of sexual excitement before an erection occurs. One survey found that men aged 48–65 took an average five times as long to achieve an erection as men aged 19–30. Indeed, a man who could attain an erection in only a few seconds when he was young may find that he requires several minutes when he is older. Once an erection is achieved, however, an older man has the advantage of being able to maintain it for much longer. Feelings of ejaculatory inevitability tend to disappear with age, giving greater control and allowing the older man to prolong intercourse almost indefinitely if he adopts the technique of withdrawing temporarily whenever orgasm is imminent.

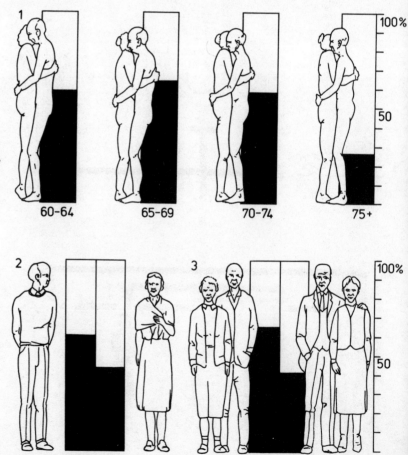

Comparisions of sexual activity
These diagrams are based on a Duke University study of older people living in and around Durham, North Carolina. People taking part were volunteers and none was institutionalized. All still having intercourse either regularly or intermittently were classed as "sexually active."
1 Sexual activity by age
The study showed comparatively little variation in those who were sexually active in the first three age groups. But over 75, there was a big drop – usually attributed to illness.
2 Men compared with women
The level of sexual activity was higher among men (61%) than women (44%), but more women were widowed or had ailing partners.
3 By socio-economic status
Those of low status had a higher level of sexual activity.

60-64   65-69   70-74   75+

100%

50

Although orgasm is reached more slowly by older men, orgasm itself is completed more quickly and orgasmic contractions are no longer as strong. The force of ejaculation is reduced, and the seminal fluid is thinner and reduced in quantity. Even so, orgasm remains a pleasurable experience. After ejaculation the older man tends to lose his erection very quickly and it may be some time – hours or even days – before he is capable of another. If a couple wants intercourse more often than the man's capacity for erection allows, he can use his greater ejaculatory control to avoid orgasm – further erections will then be no problem. Older women will probably find that their cycle of sexual response is much less affected by age than is that of their partner, although in women, too, sexual arousal does tend to take rather longer as they get older, and orgasm is typically more rapidly completed. The menopause does not usually reduce a woman's sex drive; and even if it does, this effect is usually only temporary. Intercourse may, however, be made painful by vaginal dryness, thinning vaginal walls, and strong uterine contractions during orgasm. All these problems are directly caused by estrogen deficiency and can be alleviated with hormone treatment.

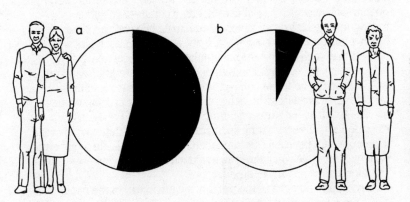

Sex and marital status
Of persons taking part in the North Carolina survey, sexual activity was reported by 54% of those who were married (**a**) and by 7% of those who were single, divorced or widowed (**b**). Although the sex drive often remains strong enough for sex to continue within marriage, it is not often strong enough to lead to extramarital sex.

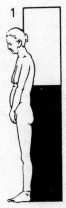
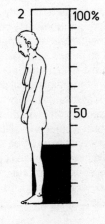

Masturbation
These diagrams show the importance of masturbation as a sexual outlet among older women.
1 Among unmarried women aged 50–70, about 60% probably masturbate, so surveys have revealed.
2 About 30% of older women are believed to masturbate to supplement coitus.

©DIAGRAM

281

5.02 Sexual violence

Male images of women

Images of women derive from a multiplicity of sources – cultural, familial, and media – and are, of course, confirmed or moderated by personal experience. Historically, both the well-being of women and the function of childbearing required the support of men, and so women were traditionally regarded as dependents. Submissiveness and chastity therefore came to be the qualities most valued because they enabled men to retain a woman's effective control of fertility. Women were even regarded as little more than part of the family's wealth and had few or no rights.

Today, too, stereotypical images of women – their nature and their proper functions – sometimes circumscribe and limit women's freedom to do as they wish; and women who act "inappropriately" are open to public censure or abuse. In some cultures, religious restrictions also place strict limits on female behavior and impose heavy penalties upon those who do not stay within set limits with the excuse that such control is for a woman's own protection.

But even in more permissive societies, certain traditional images of women and the codes of conduct thought appropriate to them are still prevalent. Accordingly, breaches of such behavior are sometimes used as excuses for harassment and assault, and have even been regarded as actively inviting such crimes. The fact that a woman is a lesbian, wears revealing clothing, is hitch-hiking or is out alone after dark may even be considered as evidence that she is not "respectable" and therefore a justifiable target.

Stereotypical images of the place of a woman within the family – the self-sacrificing mother, the faithful but sexually available wife, and the loyal, loving daughter – are familiar in classical literature; but these images are in many respects just as potent today, and refusal or inability of a woman to comply with her partner's or other family members' expectations may result in punitive violence. Abuse suffered or witnessed in childhood will also in turn produce distorted images and so perpetuate patterns of abuse.

Pornography, which promotes the idea that a woman's body is merely a tool for male sexual gratification, is merely one end of a spectrum of fantasies about women promulgated by the media. Violence against women in movies and on television is also frequently eroticized, and women are all too often portrayed either as helpless victims whose virtue must be saved by the hero, or as jealous and vengeful villainesses whose rejection of conventional meekness and obedience is seen as particularly threatening. There remains a great deal still to be done in order to correct such extremes.

The term sexual abuse generally covers forms of sexual assault other than that of rape. But because legal definitions of rape may vary from place to place, sexual abuse may include penetration of the vagina by foreign objects, intercourse with a minor, and incest, as well as forced oral sex, mutilation, anal penetration, and other forms of molestation such as touching or stroking of the genitals or breasts. Although abuse of females frequently takes the form of sexual abuse, the motivation of the offender is not always attributable to sexual impulses. As with rape, sexual abuse is often used to humiliate, insult, or maintain control over a woman. In many countries, sexual abuse of a woman by her husband may not even be a criminal offence and is therefore unlikely to be reported by the victim, making estimates of its occurrence hard to obtain.

Despite much-publicized cases of rape and other forms of sexual abuse committed by strangers, statistics show that a woman or girl is more likely to suffer abuse in her own home and at the hands of someone she knows – partner, relative or family friend. Assault by a stranger is more likely to be forcible and to take place out of doors or in an automobile, whereas a known and trusted person – striking in the home or workplace – is often able to use threats, cajoling, or bribery to ensure the victim's silence. Men are the abusers in up to 95% of cases and are usually aged between 18 and 44 years, though older men are more heavily represented in cases of child molestation. Women have been implicated in cases of systematic or ritual abuse of children, and have been blamed for enabling or even encouraging the abuser to continue his activities by not speaking out.

Available statistics tend to be misleading because particular groups are likely to be under-represented. Abuse among poorer families may be brought to light by a social worker, whereas wealthy families are better able to keep it a secret.

INCEST AND CHILD ABUSE

Incest legally consists of intercourse between close relatives, although it is sometimes extended to homosexual relationships and child abuse within the family. Child abuse is most often committed by a single adult against one particular child, but instances of a parent abusing all the children are not unknown, and considerable public attention has been focused on cases of organized abuse of many children for supposed occult purposes or commercial gain. Proving abuse may be very difficult: doctors vary in their reliance on diagnostic methods, and courts have been reluctant to accept wholeheartedly evidence obtained by encouraging the child to describe the abuse using anatomically accurate dolls. Childhood abuse frequently results in disturbed behavior, which may be the main or only indicator of its occurrence, and can cause lifelong emotional problems. Despite widespread public abhorrence and media attention, there is increasing evidence that sexual abuse of children is widespread throughout all social strata.

Domestic violence

Every year, millions of women of all classes, races and ages suffer violence and battering in their homes. They may be beaten by sons or brothers, but most usually it is husbands or male partners who inflict both mental and physical violence on women. It is difficult to find exact statistics because, like rape, domestic violence is seriously under-reported. Nevertheless, what evidence exists suggests that the problem of domestic violence is enormous. In Peru, for instance, 70% of all reported crimes are of women being beaten by their partners; in Japan, wife-beating is the second-most frequent reason given for divorce initiated by women; and in the UK, it is estimated that in one in every hundred marriages women suffer severe physical violence every year. Brutality itself may range from repeated punching, kicking, attempted strangulation, use of weapons, burning and scalding through to humiliation, degradation, and severe mental torture. It may also include sexual abuse.

Domestic violence, or so-called "wife-battering," is not new. The reasons for it are complex, and closely linked to the oppression of women in general and prevailing male views of women as objects and possessions. It has also been argued that violent men are those who feel powerless outside the home, and that domestic violence against women is their one means of achieving feelings of power.

The law, too, often compounds the situation. While to some extent it protects children, it has been slow to recognize violence against women. In many countries, women have very little actual or legal protection against abusive husbands and partners; and in some parts of the world, male violence toward "their" women is either accepted as part of the prevailing culture or ignored. Even where wife-battering is a recognized evil, police and others may be slow to intervene on the grounds that domestic violence is a family affair.

Violence within the home can continue for many years; and the battered woman may find it difficult to leave, particularly if there are young children, or if her partner is the breadwinner. If she does leave, there may be difficulties in finding a new home, childcare facilities, and a job. Many battered women, too, suffer considerable feelings of guilt, embarrassment, and low esteem – feelings that may make it even harder for them to leave a violent situation, and which may even force them back after leaving. Some women are also terrified of further violence toward themselves or their children if they do leave.

Any woman who is being battered needs help, and to get away from a violent situation. For most battered women, a shelter or refuge provides an immediate and safe place to stay for both themselves and their children. It provides advice, support, and the opportunity for a battered woman to regain strength and confidence. There is a desperate need for more such refuges, but women's shelters do exist in most major cities, and addresses can be found through women's centers and the telephone directory. In the long term, a sympathetic lawyer, evidence of mental or physical cruelty from doctors and social workers, and support from family and friends will enable a battered woman to establish her own independence.

MENTAL CRUELTY

Mental cruelty toward a woman can take many forms within a marriage or cohabitation: sometimes it consists of systematic denigration of a woman to undermine her independence and self-respect; it may result from distorted or unrealistic attitudes toward women which lead to unreasonable behavior; or it may be a consequence of unwillingness to adapt one's own life style to the needs or wishes of others.

The distinction between unreasonable behavior and mental cruelty can be hard to clarify. Mental cruelty, however, generally implies a conscious desire to hurt another person, whereas unreasonable behavior is usually a consequence of lack of appreciation for the other person's point of view. Both are capable of causing great distress; and the degree to which either can be overcome depends upon how committed each partner is to the relationship and how willing each is to change.

Well-publicized divorce cases of "golf widows" and parsimonious spouses illustrate extreme forms of unreasonable behavior which often seem to stem from a basic lack of interest in the sharing aspects of marriage on the part of the husband. On the other hand, mental cruelty is usually an indication of a man's determination to make a relationship work, but on his terms alone. Typically, the relationship begins extremely well – both partners are swept off their feet and may think that they have found the ideal mate. However, once the initial euphoria subsides, each partner becomes aware of the other's unsympathetic character traits. In a normal relationship, adjustment takes place on the part of both partners; but in cases of mental cruelty, a man's desire to exert absolute control over his partner may show itself in constant criticism, unprovoked rages, and financial manipulation to destroy her independence. A woman's sense of self-esteem might lead her to abandon the relationship at the earliest sign of such behavior; but if she already suffers from feelings of low self-worth and has already invested much emotional energy in the relationship, she may be reluctant to give it up – particularly if unpleasant episodes are followed by attempts at reconciliation. Women who have been discouraged from assertiveness in childhood may be more vulnerable to these techniques of emotional subjugation.

WHERE TO GO FOR HELP

The hardest part of escaping from a bad relationship is regaining enough self-respect to say "no more." Acquiring or relearning assertiveness skills can be an important step in this process, and a changed response to bullying tactics may assist in allowing a healthier dialog to develop. If the man can be persuaded that a problem exists, a marriage counselor or family therapist can be brought into the situation. But more often the woman has to seek help alone; and psychotherapy may be of particular assistance in providing clarification of how and why control of the relationship is sought by one partner and surrendered by the other.

©DIAGRAM

Rape

The forcing of sexual intercourse upon an unwilling woman is one of the most serious of all sex crimes. Violent and hostile, its total violation of personal and physical privacy can have a devastating effect on the victim.

Amazing as it may seem, babies only a few months old have been raped, as have women over the age of 80. In some countries, the legal definition of rape also includes indecent assault, and the penalty varies considerably throughout the world. Punishment for a convicted rapist for instance, can range in different countries from a short prison term to a life sentence or even death. (Statutory rape applies to those crimes of intercourse where the victim is judged incapable of consenting – perhaps because she is under age or mentally subnormal).

Even today, rape remains one of the most unreported of all crimes: and there is no way of knowing whether the apparent increase in the incidence of rape actually results from a greater willingness among victims to report that they have been raped. (One UK survey showed that over a ten year period, the number of rapes reported rose by about 30 percent. In another study in which 400 women were interviewed, around 25 percent stated that they had been raped.)

Young girls and women under the age of 25 are the most likely rape victims. Rapists, too, tend to be young. They are also generally otherwise perfectly ordinary members of society, leading normal lives, with families and holding down a job. More often than not, too, the rapist is someone who is known to or at least recognized by the unfortunate victim.

Many rapes occur in or near the victim's home, often during the daytime; and despite another common myth that women who are raped must in some way have "asked for it," research suggests that only in fewer than 5 percent of cases can women be said to have encouraged the attack by either their appearance or behavior.

Although the courts today are more sympathetic to rape victims than they once were, it is still often difficult for a woman to win a rape case. Victims are therefore strongly recommended to seek the help of a rape victim support group.

Common rape scenarios
a A woman of 20, living on her own in a rented apartment, is attacked by a man who breaks in one Sunday afternoon. She recognizes him as a local window cleaner.
b A young student accepts a lift from her former teacher when waiting for a late-night bus and is raped in the car after she has been driven to a remote country lane.
c An elderly widow forgets to use the safety chain and is raped by an intruder who forces his way into the home at 10 o'clock one morning.
d A teenage girl of 15 walks across a park on her own in broad daylight in order to take a short cut, and is raped by a man who first approaches her to ask if she knows the time.

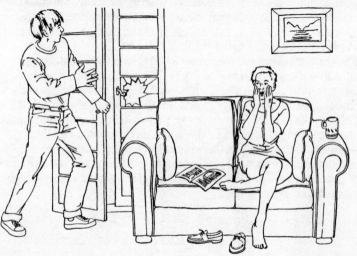

EFFECTS OF RAPE

Rape is traumatic and can be both physically and emotionally damaging. It has been noticed, however, that women who talk out the experience with others do recover more quickly. Anger, disbelief, hostility toward men, fear of sexual relationships, guilt, self-disgust, intense humiliation and severest depression – all are common emotional responses to the experience of rape. But supportive counseling is almost always helpful. It should be remembered, too, that a boyfriend, husband or father may well also benefit from counseling in such circumstances. A young child, meanwhile, will of course require very careful treatment and indeed may not even understand at all what has happened to her. Some feel tremendously ashamed and may feel they have to keep the rape secret, even though the memory of the event remains vivid: and some may not even have the words to describe what happened.

IF RAPE OCCURS

A woman who has been raped and who wants to bring charges must stay in the same clothes and not wash away evidence of rape; call the police as soon as possible; go directly to a hospital or doctor, whether prosecuting or not; get support from a friend, rape center, or women's group; and prepare herself for possible skepticism and humiliation both from the police and, later, the courts if she decides to prosecute her attacker. Doing so could protect others, remember. Rape centers have been set up by women in several countries in order to provide advice, support and emergency facilities. Likewise, some police departments are beginning to set up specially-staffed 24-hour rape units. The police will probably involve you in lengthy questioning, and will arrange a medical examination to establish whether intercourse did indeed occur. You will usually be able to request a woman doctor if you would prefer this. But even if you do not report an incidence of rape, you should certainly see your own doctor or attend an STD clinic for checks for infection as well as injury. It is also possible that you will be offered a morning-after pill which should be effective as contraception if taken within a day or so.

Changes in the law that have been suggested are that the need for medical evidence be removed and that questions about a woman's sexual life be prohibited. In some parts of the world, too, the penalties for rape probably also need changing because "life" or "death" minimum penalties often make conviction harder to obtain.

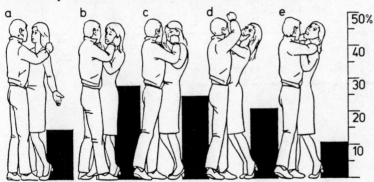

Use of violence
Beating was involved in nearly half the rapes in one U.S. study: other victims suffered choking and "roughness." In nonviolent cases, victims had been shown weapons or were threatened verbally.
a No physical force 15%
b Roughness 28%
c Beaten 25%
d Beaten brutally 21%
e Choked 11%

©DIAGRAM

MYTHS OF RAPE
"Rape is mainly interracial"
The attitudes of the police, the courts, and of society in general toward rape have been formed more by myth than by reality to try to excuse rapists' behavior, and to lay the blame for rape onto women.

It is commonly, but incorrectly assumed that black men frequently rape white women. In fact, usually rapist and victim are of the same racial background.

Time and time again, women are also blamed for provoking rape, and for leading men on, either by their appearance or their behavior. Again, studies show this to be incorrect.

"Women create dangerous situations"
It is often said that women invite rape by putting themselves into dangerous situations – by walking home alone, by hitch-hiking, by going alone to a bar. But many rapes could happen to a woman who never left home unless accompanied by someone she knew.

Sexual aggressiveness in men is also often excused by the myth of a spontaneous "uncontrollable" sex drive. In fact, most rapes are premeditated, whether they involve one attacker, two or several. It is often argued, too, that many women use the accusation of rape simply for revenge purposes. But only a small percentage of rape charges are dismissed by police as "unfounded" – a technical term, often just meaning "unsuitable for prosecution."

Age of victims and rapists
This diagram, based on a US rape study (M. Amir, *Patterns of Forcible Rape*), shows percentages of rape victims (**A**) and rapists (**B**) in different age groups. Among rape victims, 28% were aged 14 years or under, and 38% were aged 15-24 years. Of rapists in the study, 66% were aged 15-24 years, and 24% were aged 25-34.

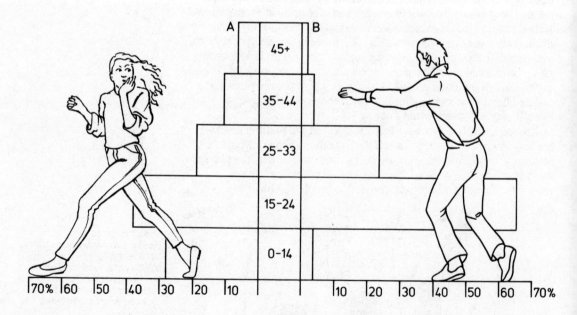

EVIDENCE REQUIRED

In a rape case, the judge will instruct the jury to weigh the victim's testimony very carefully on the grounds that sexual charges are "easy to make but difficult to prove." The evidence required to prove rape varies. In some countries or states, the victim's testimony only is sufficient; in others, corroboration is needed either as a matter of course or whenever the victim's testimony is not considered credible. Corroboration is generally medical – signs of intercourse, or physical injury, for instance.

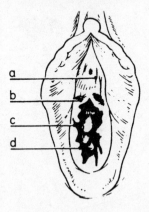

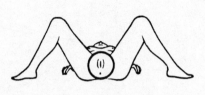

Possible physical signs of rape
a Scratches
b Bruises
c Tears
d Seminal fluid

RAPE AND THE COURTS

Strangely, the victim in a rape case often seems to receive harsher treatment than the suspect. The reasons are complex. They include the rules of evidence and society's attitudes to women and to sex.

The main issues in a rape case are to prove that the defendant is the rapist, to prove the victim's lack of consent, and to prove resistance by the victim.

In a rape case, as in all criminal cases, "the defendant is innocent until proved guilty." Burden of proof falls on the prosecution. But because of its nature, there are rarely any witnesses to rape and so the outcome may well depend on who is the more credible – rapist or victim.

Defense tactics usually rely largely on the idea that rape is a woman's fault: that is, an unaccompanied woman, an unmarried woman, or one with some sexual experience (for example, on the Pill) is either asking for rape or has not been raped at all. In effect, a woman has her character and personal life put on trial to such an extent that she may well begin to doubt or blame herself.

In order to cope with such defense, a woman who brings charges should get advice and support from a women's group and rape center; memorize details of the rape; stress the force or duress used; and emphasize beyond all possibility or doubt her lack of consent.

Self-defense

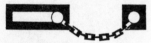

Preventing attack

At home
Windows should be kept locked and hallways and entrances kept well-lit. Outside doors should be fitted with bolt locks and chains. A woman living on her own should use initials rather than full name in the telephone directory and on any mailbox. Half of all rapes happen in the home.

While out
Women should keep to well-lit and peopled areas. Non-restrictive clothing should be worn for ease of movement in case of pursuit. As she approaches her home, a woman should have her door key ready to avoid delay in entering.

When hitch-hiking
A woman should know the license number of the car, check for inside door handles, and know how to get out quickly. Lifts with more than one man in a car should be refused, and a woman should avoid getting into the back of a 2-door car. Better still, she should never hitch-hike alone.

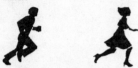

If trouble threatens
Panic must be avoided. No woman should fight if she can escape – but if she cannot, she should not be afraid to cause hurt. Loud yells – "fire" not "help" – may bring people. If overcome, talking – though unlikely to stop rape – may prevent extra violence.

It has been estimated that one reported rape takes place every 7 minutes in the USA. Rape is increasing rapidly; and to cope with this growing threat, it is becoming vital for women to learn how to defend themselves.

The diagrams on these two pages show some of the defense tactics that a woman can use if she is attacked from either the front or from behind.

Points to aim for

Eyes

Nose

Neck

Groin

Knee

Shin

Instep

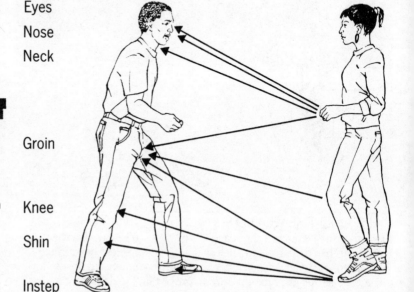

Weapons
No woman should carry weapons that can be used against her. But she can carry some articles which, if used fast, are effective.

a Pepper-shaker
b Artificial lemon full of vinegar
c Hairspray
d Personal alarm

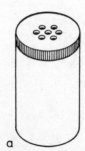
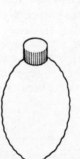
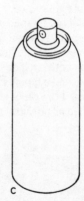
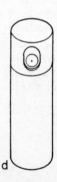

a   b   c   d

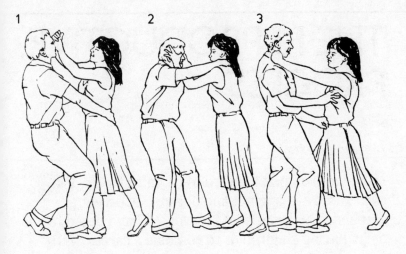

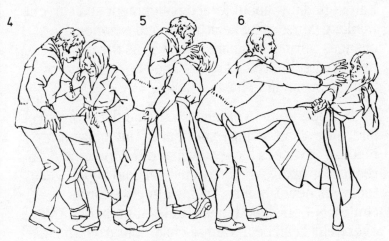

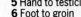

Defense tactics if approached from the front
1 Double fist to bridge of nose
2 Thumbs into eyes
3 Fist to the side of neck
4 Knee to groin
5 Hand to testicles
6 Foot to groin

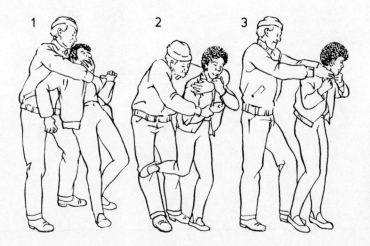

Defense tactics if approached from the rear
1 Hand to testicles
2 Foot to knee
3 Bend little finger outwards

©DIAGRAM

THE REPRODUCTIVE PROCESS

Most women look forward to having a family. But patterns are changing: and because of career demands particularly, many women have opted to delay having children or to combine a career with parenting.

Latest findings about fetal development and current thinking concerning health care and emotional changes during pregnancy, as well as the birth process itself, are clearly outlined here for every woman planning to have a child.

In the past, some women have found the problem of infertility a shattering experience. But amazing medical advances have now made childbearing a reality for many who previously had no hope; while today, as never before, highly effective forms of contraception should mean, at least in theory, that every child can be a wanted child right from the start.

Chapter six

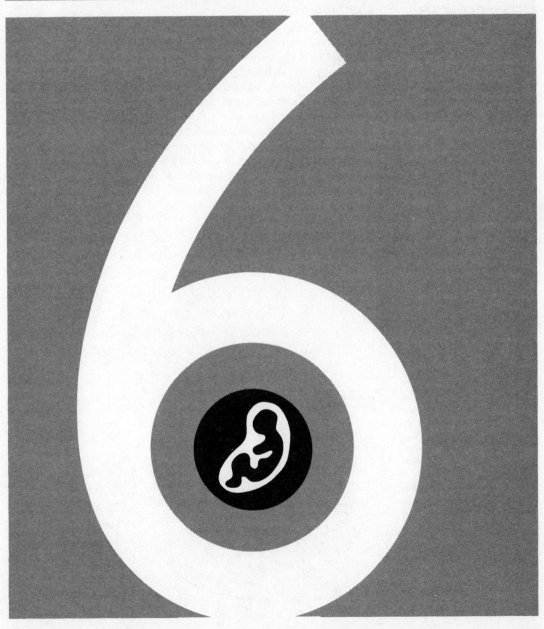

6.01 Reproduction

Intercourse

EJACULATION

Sperm have more than 1ft (0.3m) to travel before reaching the female vagina. As shown in the diagram *below*, at ejaculation, muscular contractions in the testes (**a**), epididymis (**b**) and along the vas deferens (**c**) propel the sperm toward the penis. On their way, they mix with the seminal fluid secreted from the seminal vesicles (**d**) and prostate (**e**). The resulting semen is propelled through the urethra (**f**) into the woman's vagina (**g**).

Sperm production occurs inside the testes at a rate of millions a day. While developing, they are stored in the epididymis. Each sperm is miniscule, visible only under a powerful microscope, and takes 60–72 days to mature. By contrast, in a woman just one mature egg is normally produced each month.

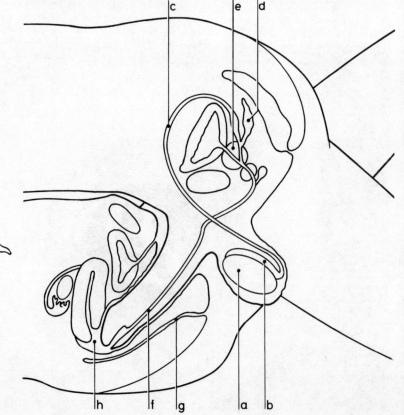

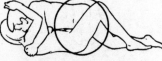

Expulsion of semen from the male sex organs at ejaculation during intercourse

a Testes
b Epididymis
c Vas deferens
d Seminal vesicle
e Prostate gland
f Urethra
g Vagina
h Seminal pool

CONCEPTION

The diagram *below* shows the eight stages on the route of the male sperm from ejaculation to fertilization of the female egg or ovum.

1 During the two weeks before ovulation, a number of egg follicles have been maturing in the ovary. A week before ovulation, one suddenly accelerates its growth.

2 Ovulation occurs as the mature egg bursts from its folicle. Muscular contractions propel it along a Fallopian tube. If not fertilized within 24–48 hours, the egg will degenerate.

3 During intercourse, about 400 million sperm may be ejaculated by the man into the woman's vagina. Of these, only one will fertilize the ovum. The sperm travel fast, aided by muscular spasms, and possibly cover 1in (2.5cm) in 8 minutes.

4 The sperm arrive at the cervix. The seminal fluid has liquified, and about half the original sperm have died in the acidic conditions of the vagina. The remainder pass through the cervical mucus. Normally a barrier to sperm, vaginal mucus can be easily penetrated at the time of ovulation.

5 Sperm reach the top of the uterus. There are possibly only thousands of the original number left, and it has taken them under an hour to arrive. About half now turn into the wrong Fallopian tube.

6 The remaining sperm swim into the top of the Fallopian tube that contains the matured female ovum. If conditions are favorable, sperm may survive here for up to 72 hours. Should ovulation not have taken place, sperm can therefore wait for a newly-developed ovum to arrive.

7 A few hundred sperm complete their journey along the Fallopian tube to the female ovum. Enzymes released by the sperm heads now break down the ovum's outer wall.

8 One male sperm penetrates the ovum and fertilization occurs. The cell wall immediately hardens, preventing other sperm from entering. The nuclei of the two cells fuse together and a new human life is conceived.

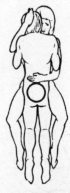

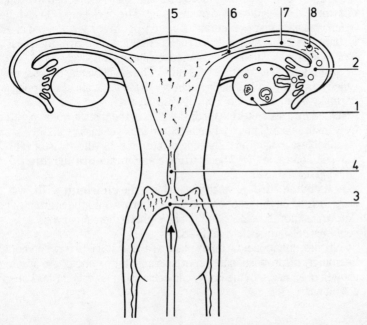

The route of the sperm from ejaculation to conception
1 Egg follicles mature in the ovary
2 Ovulation
3 Ejaculation of sperm into vagina
4 Arrival of sperm at the cervix
5 Sperm reach the uterus
6 Sperm enter the Fallopian tube
7 Sperm journey to the ovum
8 Fertilization occurs

© DIAGRAM

Fertilization

Fertilization, implantation and early development

1 Fertilization
2 First cell division (day 1)
3 Morula stage (day 4)
4 Blastocyst stage (day 7) when implantation occurs
5 Internal cells differentiate (day 10). At this stage nourishment is drawn by diffusion from the uterus by the chorionic villi
6 Embryo form yolk sac (day 15)
7 Umbilical cord develops (day 20)
8 25-day stage

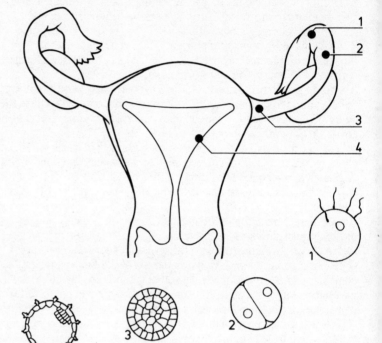

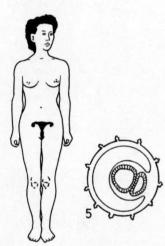

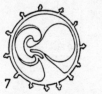

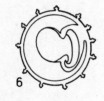

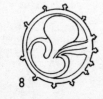

Fertilization occurs in one of the Fallopian tubes within a day of ovulation. There may be as many as 100,000 sperm in the Fallopian tube, or as few as 100. But more than one sperm is needed to produce enzymes to break down the ovum's wall. The nuclei fuse (**1**) and the ovum wall hardens, preventing the entry of other sperm. Soon after fertilization, the ovum begins to divide (**2**), first into two, then into four, and so on. The first division takes about 24 hours.

Subsequent divisions take less time. The small bundle of cells, now called a **morula**, looks like a mulberry (**3**). The ovum at this point will normally be about to enter the uterine cavity.

Helped by a little uterine fluid, the cells of the morula are separated by a small space. The outer cells flatten into a cellular wall (the "trophoblast"), and the remaining cluster of cells (the "blastocyst") moves to one side (**4**). The **amniotic sac**, **placenta** and **fetus** develop from these.

By about the 7th day, small projections, the **chorionic villi**, will have formed on the trophoblast. These burrow into the uterus wall (known as the "endometrium"). The embryo then undergoes continual cell differentiation (**5–8**).

Cell differentiation now takes place at a vital stage of development. Seemingly disproportionate repercussions (for example, the stunted growth of an organ of the body) can occur from damage or loss of one cell alone.

Implantation in the uterus also establishes a basis of embryonic nutrition. After about 18 days, the nervous system begins to form and continues to develop until a few weeks after birth.

By the end of the first month, the embryo is about the size of a tapioca grain, with millions of cells intricately organized to carry out specific functions. A primitive heart is now formed. It is already 10,000 times bigger than the original ovum.

Implantation
The enlarged sections of the blastocyst (*below*) show how it burrows into the uterus wall (the endometrium).

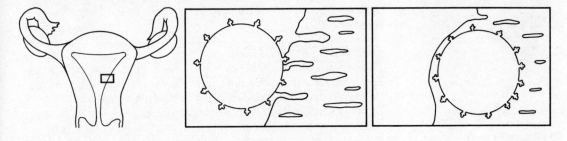

MULTIPLE FERTILIZATION

Since the advent of fertility drugs, multiple births have become increasingly common. A drug, stimulating the growth of follicles, may cause the release of more than one ovum from the ovary. Triplets, quads, and quins may develop from 3, 4 and 5 ova, with 3, 4 and 5 placentae, and 3, 4 and 5 amniotic sacs respectively. A single ovum may also split, as in the case of identical twins or triplets.

Quads may be the result of two split ova, or of two single ova plus one split one. The sharing of the placenta is dependent upon whether or not the ovum has split. On rare occasions when the uterus is stretched to its ultimate capacity, the same amniotic sac may be shared.

Identical twins are the result of one ovum splitting soon after fertilization. (Siamese twins are the product of a splitting which for some reason has been arrested before completion.) The twins lie within separate sacs of amniotic fluid, though they share the same placenta and so will be of the same blood group. The splitting of the ovum also means that they will share the same genetic structure: that is, they will be of the same sex with very similar features.

Non-identical twins are the result of two ova being fertilized by two sperm. Thus they may or may not be of the same sex or blood group and will only share the general resemblances of any two children born of the same parents. Multiple births tend to be a trait inherited and carried by women rather than men.

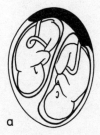
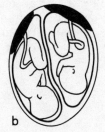

Twins
a Identical twins, sharing the same placenta
b Non-identical twins with separate placentae

■ Placenta

a   b

Aiding conception

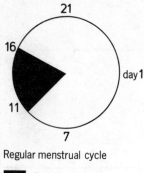

Regular menstrual cycle

■ Fertile phase

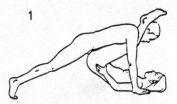

1

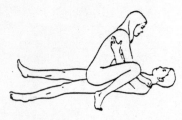

2

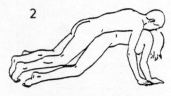

Techniques of intercourse
1 Full penetration positions
2 Recommended position for retroverted uterus

TIMING OF INTERCOURSE

Chances of conception may be improved by concentrating intercourse on the woman's fertile phase of each month. If the charts that she keeps show that she has regular 28-day periods, her fertile phase will usually lie between days 11 and 16. With irregular cycles of between 27 and 35 days, chances of pregnancy improve if intercourse occurs on five alternate days, starting with the 13th day of the cycle. (Intercourse on all the fertile days would exhaust the man's sperm output.)

TREATING INFECTION

The cervix is often affected by a discharge. The cause is sometimes unknown, but may be due to venereal disease or other diagnosable infection, or to foreign bodies such as forgotten tampons or contraceptive devices. Treatment usually involves a course of pessaries, or sometimes antibiotics. (Occasionally, the cervix is cauterized under anesthetic, to burn away chronically infected tissue.) Infection may impair fertility. Risk of spreading infection may also prevent investigatory techniques.

TECHNIQUES OF INTERCOURSE
Full penetration

Sometimes infertility is due to poor coital connection. When obesity is the cause, if the woman hooks her knees over the man's shoulders during intercourse, this flexes the hips and allows deeper penetration. (Care must be taken in case pain occurs.) When the cause is vaginal tightness, then (perhaps after treatment by dilation) the woman should squat over the man, as he lies on his back, and slowly lower herself onto his penis.
Retroverted uterus

In about 10% of women, the uterus is tilted back, and the cervix forward. The typical position of intercourse may then not bring the semen into contact with the cervix. Most women have no difficulty in becoming pregnant despite this. Conception can be aided in such cases if the woman uses a face-down position (lying or kneeling), with the man entering her from behind. The lying position should make the pool of semen bathe the cervix but may cause cystitis if the penis bruises the woman. Alternatively, the woman can change from a kneeling position to a lying one after intercourse ends.

Fertility in any woman is usually improved if the woman remains fairly still for at least half an hour after intercourse ends. It also seems that the second half of a man's ejaculate – the fluid from the seminal vesicles – is actually likely to harm the sperm, while that of the prostate, in the first half, protects it. So a couple can sometimes increase their chances of parenthood if the man withdraws from the vagina halfway through his ejaculation. (The couple should also abstain from further intercourse for 48 hours afterwards.)

IMPROVING RECEPTIVITY

Mechanical devices and ointments may be useful for improving the sperm receptivity of various parts of the woman's genitals.

Dilation of the vagina with glass dilators or with the fingers helps in many cases where vaginal tightness prevents successful penetration.

Douching to make the cervical mucus more alkaline may improve the chances of the cervix taking up viable sperm. The woman sits in a bath and douches the upper part of the vagina with warm water containing bicarbonate of soda. For this purpose, she uses a douche equipped with tube and nozzle. This method should only be used when a post-coital test has shown that it is appropriate.

Vaginal acidity seems to make sperm move up toward the cervix. Most vaginas have natural acidity, but occasionally an ointment is prescribed to enhance this. The ointment is inserted on the day before intercourse since use on the actual day of intercourse may produce acid conditions strong enough to kill the sperm.

Synthetic hormones are sometimes prescribed. The receptivity of the cervix to sperm depends largely on the hormonal balance. Lack of estrogen may make it unreceptive. Synthetic estrogen given for 4 or 5 days around ovulation may improve receptivity.

Infertility

A practical indicator of infertility is a couple's failure to achieve conception in a year or more of intercourse, without contraception. It is estimated that out of every 100 couples, 10 cannot have children, and 15 have fewer than they wish. So a quarter may be below normal fertility. The causes can involve either or both partners; the woman in 50–55% of cases, the man in 30–35%, and both in about 15%. The most common is failure to ovulate, due to hormonal failure. This may result from actual disorders of the hormone mechanism, or from emotional stress and other psychological factors. Hormonal imbalance can also prevent a fertilized egg attaching itself to the wall of the uterus, while emotional stress may operate directly by setting up spasms in the Fallopian tubes that prevent them transporting the egg.

A second group of causes concerns the vaginal and cervical fluids. These may be inadequate for sperm transport, or even actively hostile to sperm movement or survival. (Again, hormonal imbalance may be involved.)

A third group are congenital, including a hymen or vagina too tight for penetration, and common malformations such as fusion of the small vulval lips; a vagina divided in two or totally absent; a uterus divided in two; or uterus and cervix absent.

Another possible cause in this group is tilting (retroversion) of the uterus, so that the sperm do not normally find their way in.

Finally, there is infertility that is linked with other disorders in the sex organs, including infection with venereal disease, cystitis, growth of fibroids, polyps, cysts, or cancer; and effects of exposure to high doses of radiation. These may affect the ovaries or block the Fallopian tubes.

Infertility tests

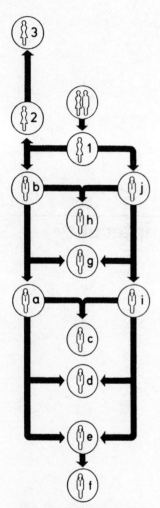

Working relationships within the medical team investigating infertility

1 Clinic secretary
2 Clinic nurse
3 Clinic social worker

INVESTIGATIONS

Diagnosis may prove simple. But, if necessary, a woman's doctor may refer her to a team of specialists using advance techniques of investigation and treatment.

A **post-coital test** is usually made 6–18 hours after intercourse, and as near as possible to the day of ovulation. A mucus specimen is taken from the cervix. Microscopic study of this shows the quantity and quality of the sperm present. Both depend on the material originally ejaculated by the male and the condition of the woman's cervical mucus. The mucus should be most receptive to sperm at ovulation, but hormonal imbalance may distort this. Infertility sometimes also results from incompatibility between mucus and sperm.

The health of and hormonal influence upon the uterus lining can be tested by **dilatation and curettage** (or **scraping**). The resulting stretching of the cervix helps sperm penetration, and so may itself aid fertility.

Salpingography is X raying of the uterus and Fallopian tubes, to reveal their internal condition, by introducing into them an X ray-opaque, oily or water-soluble dye. It is done before ovulation to avoid possible ovum damage. Sometimes the procedure itself helps: the dye unsticks adhering tube walls, and pregnancy follows.

In a **gas test** (**insufflation**), carbon dioxide is blown through the Fallopian tubes, revealing and sometimes even clearing blockage. But it gives no detailed information, and some consider it outmoded.

Uteroscopy includes use of a periscope instrument to give an internal view of the uterus via the vagina.

Laparoscopy gives a good external view of uterus, tubes, and ovaries, without a large abdominal incision. Carbon dioxide gas is blown through a hollow needle into the abdominal cavity. This distends the abdominal wall, and allows a clear view of the reproductive organs through a laparoscope introduced through a tiny abdominal slit.

Various specialists may be involved, as shown in the diagram *left*.

a Surgical gynecologist, specializing in investigating and operating on the female reproductive organs

b Medical gynecologist, advising on non-surgical treatments

c Histologist, analyzing tissue samples taken by the surgical gynecologist from the ovaries or uterus lining

d Radiologist, interpreting X rays of, for example, the Fallopian tubes

e Endocrinologist, looking for disturbances in the hormones of the endocrine system

f Biochemist, providing the endocrinologist with precise measurements of hormone levels

g Psychiatrist, to help overcome psychological barriers to pregnancy

h Geneticist, assessing risks of inherited abnormality, and advising termination if necessary

i Urologist, specializing in disorders involving the urinary tract

j Andrologist, specializing in investigating the male reproductive system

INFERTILITY IN MEN

Male infertility is of two kinds: cases where there is no ejaculation (that is, impotence): and cases where the quality of the ejaculate is poor, as shown by sperm concentration, shape, and mobility.

Sperm concentration depends not only on sperm production, but also on the amount of seminal fluid. Both very small and very large amounts are unfavorable to fertility. A small amount will fail to buffer the sperm against the acidity of the vaginal fluids. A large amount dilutes the semen too much, and makes it more likely to spill out of the vagina. The higher the number of abnormal sperm forms, the less the likelihood of fertility, too.

Sperm movement indicates the length of life of the sperm and is significant because they may need time before encountering an egg to fertilize. For some reason not yet understood, sperm also need to survive for some time in the female reproductive tract before they are capable of fertilizing an egg.

Causes of poor sperm production can include such factors as heat around the testicles due, for example, to tight underclothing, obesity, or working conditions; poor health, inadequate nutrition, lack of exercise and excessive smoking or drinking; emotional stress; and prolonged abstinence which can increase the number of abnormal sperm.

More specialized factors (some of which can cause sterility) include certain birth defects; failure of the testes to descend before puberty; and some childhood diseases and other illnesses (for example, mumps if it occurs in adulthood rather than childhood).

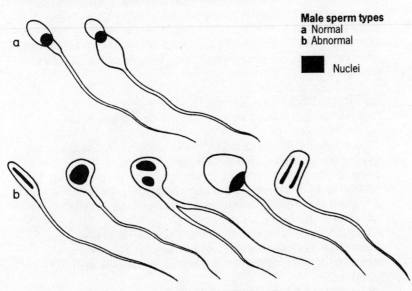

Male sperm types
a Normal
b Abnormal

◼ Nuclei

Treating infertility

FERTILITY DRUGS

These have given remarkable results in recent years.

Clomiphene is usually the first drug tried when failure to ovulate is suspected. Just how it works is unclear (in fact, it was originally tested as a contraceptive, and found to have the reverse effect.) The woman may need no more than a single 5-tablet course taken during one menstrual cycle: with luck, ovulation follows less than a fortnight afterwards. If no pregnancy occurs after a month, a second course may be tried, and so on up to 6 courses, with intervals. About 30% of those given the drug conceive. Only one ovum is released at a time, so multiple pregnancies are unlikely. (Twins occur in about 7% of cases.) Ovarian cysts are a possible side-effect; otherwise the drug seems harmless.

Pergonal is more controversial. It is an extract of FSH and LH hormones obtained from menopausal women. (FSH and LH stimulate the ovaries to produce estrogen and progesterone, the hormones that prepare the uterus for pregnancy.) Patients receive the drug by injection under closely controlled hospital conditions. Good supervision should yield no more than one or two ova; miscalculation may produce either none or a large number. Most unwanted multiple births due to fertility drugs stem from Pergonal, and such births carry increased risks to mother and babies alike.

Hypothalamic releasing factors are substances produced by the hypothalamus at the base of the brain. They stimulate the pituitary to produce FSH and LH. Such hypothalamic releasing factors are now made synthetically, and have cured infertility which was due to poor pituitary action. A hormone pump may be worn for this purpose.

Anti-spasmodics do not promote ovulation: they are used simply to get existing ova to their destination by preventing the Fallopian tubes going into spasm. (In some women, such temporary spasms block ova transport.)

OPERATIONS TO AID FERTILITY

A number of operations may be performed to improve fertility in appropriate cases.

Operations on the **vulva** include opening cysts and abscesses, and dividing the small lips of the vulva if these have fused. Where the **hymen** is too thick and rigid to be stretched, it may be cut and stitched back. A narrow **vagina** may also be widened and lined with a skin graft; and the longitudinal division that sometimes separates the two sides of the vagina can be removed.

A badly torn **cervix** can be treated by plastic surgery. Repeated miscarriages between the 14th and 28th weeks are sometimes prevented by stitching the cervix. Dilation may also aid sperm penetration.

A **backward-tilting (retroverted) urterus** can be brought forward by inserting a special plastic pessary into the vagina, or by shortening the ligaments between uterus and groin. **Fibroids** can be cut away from the uterus wall. The wall that sometimes divides a uterus can also be removed.

Fallopian tubes cannot be cleared when totally blocked, as a result of old infection. But the "petals" at the ovarian ends of the tubes may need teasing out; and if the uterus end of a tube is blocked, this can be cut away and the shortened tube rejoined to the uterus.

Sometimes tubes are intact but hampered by bands of tissue that prevent them moving to collect the ovum from the ovary. These bands can be cut away.

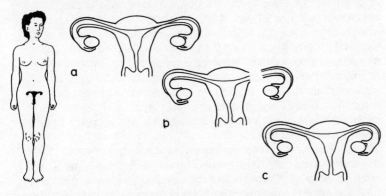

Clearing a Fallopian tube
a Fallopian tube blocked
b Blocked section removed
c Shortened tube rejoined

Cutting a wedge from the **ovaries** allows egg release, when this is blocked by certain ovarian cysts. Removal of other cysts may also aid pregnancy. Probably a third of all gynecological operations are for ovarian cysts.

ARTIFICIAL INSEMINATION
This involves the artificial transference of semen onto the cervix – usually by syringing through a tube on 3 or 4 successive days around ovulation. After insemination, the woman remains lying down for about half an hour. Artificial insemination with the partner's sperm may be used when physical or psychological causes prevent normal intercourse or ejaculation; or when the man's sperm count is low, or the woman's cervical mucus is hostile to his sperm. It can be carried out in a clinic or surgery, or (using special equipment) by the couple at home. Use of the sperm of an anonymous donor is called for when the partner is totally infertile, or when his chromosomes are known to carry hereditary disorders. The donor is carefully chosen to match the partner in appearance and to be free from disease. Babies conceived by artificial insemination develop no differently from those conceived in the ordinary way.

PSYCHOTHERAPY
There are women in whom long-term failure to ovulate derives ultimately from psychological stress. These cases include those showing clear mental symptoms, such as severe depression. However, there may be no surface symptoms but still some underlying unhappiness or insecurity. In some men and women, long-term trauma may also interfere with the actual sexual act. For other couples, the desire and struggle for fertility will itself give rise to mental tension, with emotional or physical consequences such as male impotence. Psychotherapy or some other form of counseling may prove very effective.

New fertility techniques

Several new methods of achieving fertility, many of them still largely experimental, have been developed in recent years. Those which involve donation and freezing of sperm, ova or embryos, with theoretical possibilities for genetic engineering, have raised complex social and moral issues; and certain research is now subject to legal restrictions. Most of the new techniques rely on the use of ultrasound scanning for detecting when ovulation will occur and allowing the removal of ova. Fertility drugs may also be used to encourage the ovaries to produce several ova at a time. But the success rate of these methods is currently low; and the expense and complexity of the procedures involved may deter some couples. The long-term effects of fertility drugs, freezing and of "test-tube" fertilization are also as yet uncertain. Risk of multiple pregnancy needs to be assessed very carefully; and at all stages, women should be given accurate information and consulted over such matters as how many ova or embryos will be implanted.

In some cases where the man has a low viable sperm count, it is possible to use a centrifuge to concentrate the active sperm. These can then be injected straight into the woman's abdominal cavity at the time of ovulation, circumventing "hostile" cervical mucus, in a technique known as **Direct Intraperitoneal Insemination (DIPI)**. Alternatively, ovum and sperm may be mixed and injected into a Fallopian tube by **Gamete Intrafallopian Transfer (GIFT)** or the space behind the uterus (**Peritoneal Oocyte and Sperm Transfer or POST**). These methods will work only for women whose Fallopian tubes are undamaged.

In vitro fertilization (IVF) is performed mainly for women whose Fallopian tubes are not functioning normally, but who are otherwise healthy. It can also be used to get round the "hostile mucus" problem or a low viable sperm count. But IVF may be difficult to obtain as part of a public health program because it is very expensive. The procedure basically involves inducing ovulation (usually with Pergonal); collecting the resulting ova by laparoscopy; mixing the ova with sperm in a nutrient solution in the laboratory; and finally transferring one or more multi-celled embryos into the uterus. Superfluous embryos may be frozen for later transfer attempts. Problems with timing ovulation, fertilizing the ovum and getting it to grow under laboratory conditions, as well as inducing the correct uterine conditions for successful implantation, account for the low success rate of IVF.

Donor sperm, ova, or embryos are also sometimes used in the procedures described above so that in theory a woman may become a surrogate mother and actually bear a child for another woman who is infertile; or a woman may bear a child conceived as a result of fertilization by her partner's sperm of another woman's ovum.

Pregnancy

The **HCG (Human Chronic Gonadotrophin)** test for pregnancy is made on a sample of woman's urine which should be taken to the clinic or doctor's office. It takes about 2 minutes to carry out and is 95% accurate after the 40th day of pregnancy.

For the test, a drop of a substance which neutralizes HCG (anti-HCG) is combined on a glass slide with a drop of the woman's urine. A minute later, another substance is added (latex rubber particles with HCG). If there is no HCG in the urine, the anti-HCG will fix onto the HCG in the latex rubber particles, forming milky lumps or "curds." This is a negative result. But if the woman is pregnant, the HCG in her urine will be fixed by the anti-HCG in the first mixture, and when the rubber and HCG is added, there will be no anti-HCG left to combine with the added HCG. The particles will not form lumps but remain smooth. Subsequent physical diagnosis is essential, however.

Home pregnancy tests can be carried out 5–7 days after a missed period; but to be certain, the test should be repeated a few days later. Pregnancy testing kits can be bought from a pharmacist.

Clinical diagnosis can be made between the 6th and 10th weeks: The two stages of the examination are quite painless; they cause mild discomfort only if the woman is not relaxed. A speculum is inserted into the vagina in order to look at the cervix, which is a bluish color in pregnancy. Then, after removal of the speculum, the doctor gently inserts two fingers into the vagina, while pressing on the abdomen with the other hand, in order to feel whether the uterus has enlarged. The test will also show up any swellings in the uterus, while a Pap or smear test is often taken at the same time to check for cancer.

Pregnancy tests

Home pregnancy testing kit
These take a variety of forms. It is therefore important to follow instructions carefully. The test shown here is the Predictor test. It is described in outline only. Full details are in each pack. Having collected some early morning urine:
1 Liquid from the dropper tube is squeezed into the test tube, and turns purple.
2 The dropper tube is then used to draw up urine. Five drops of urine are place in the test tube, and its stopper replaced. Shake the tube, remove the stopper, and replace on the stand.
3 Remove the indicator strip, holding it by the end nearest the sachet opening. Place in the test tube. Wait.
4 Rinse the tip for a few seconds. If the top of the indicator strip is pink, this indicates pregnancy.

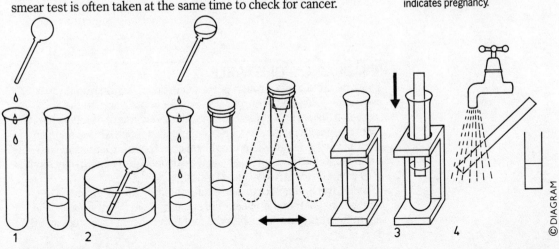

1   2   3   4

© DIAGRAM

The course of pregnancy

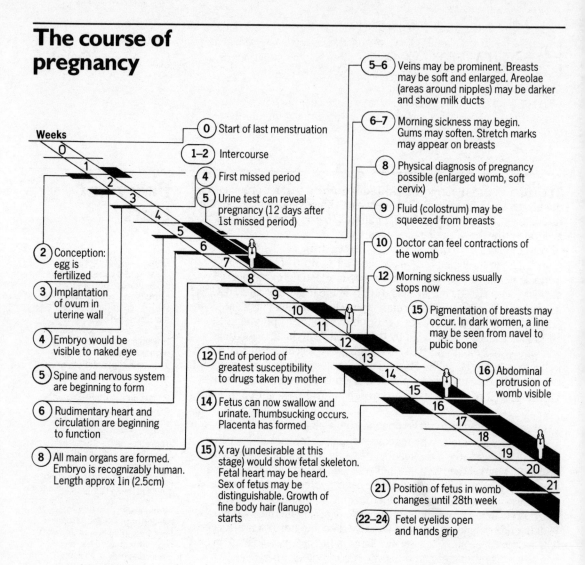

Weeks

0 Start of last menstruation

1–2 Intercourse

4 First missed period

5 Urine test can reveal pregnancy (12 days after 1st missed period)

5–6 Veins may be prominent. Breasts may be soft and enlarged. Areolae (areas around nipples) may be darker and show milk ducts

6–7 Morning sickness may begin. Gums may soften. Stretch marks may appear on breasts

8 Physical diagnosis of pregnancy possible (enlarged womb, soft cervix)

9 Fluid (colostrum) may be squeezed from breasts

10 Doctor can feel contractions of the womb

12 Morning sickness usually stops now

15 Pigmentation of breasts may occur. In dark women, a line may be seen from navel to pubic bone

16 Abdominal protrusion of womb visible

2 Conception: egg is fertilized

3 Implantation of ovum in uterine wall

4 Embryo would be visible to naked eye

5 Spine and nervous system are beginning to form

6 Rudimentary heart and circulation are beginning to function

8 All main organs are formed. Embryo is recognizably human. Length approx 1in (2.5cm)

12 End of period of greatest susceptibility to drugs taken by mother

14 Fetus can now swallow and urinate. Thumbsucking occurs. Placenta has formed

15 X ray (undesirable at this stage) would show fetal skeleton. Fetal heart may be heard. Sex of fetus may be distinguishable. Growth of fine body hair (lanugo) starts

21 Position of fetus in womb changes until 28th week

22–24 Fetel eyelids open and hands grip

PREGNANCY TIMETABLE

This timetable gives a rough guide to certain milestones and occasional problems in pregnancy. Some events relate to the mother-to-be, while others involve the development of the fetus.

Most people think of pregnancy lasting nine months. But calendar months vary in length. Our chart irons out these variations by showing a timespan of 40 weeks. These can be divided into nine 31-day months (279 days) or ten 28-day (lunar) months.

Traditionally, most doctors use lunar months for pregnancy calculations, dating the onset of pregnancy from the first day of the last menstrual period, despite the fact that conception occurs about 14 days later.

Some dates shown are only approximate. There are large variations in the timing and even appearance or non-appearance of certain signs or symptoms. One factor that especially affects some variations is whether the mother-to-be is expecting her first second or a subsequent child.

On page 402, you will find a chart that you can use to work out the expected date of delivery from the date of the first day of your last period.

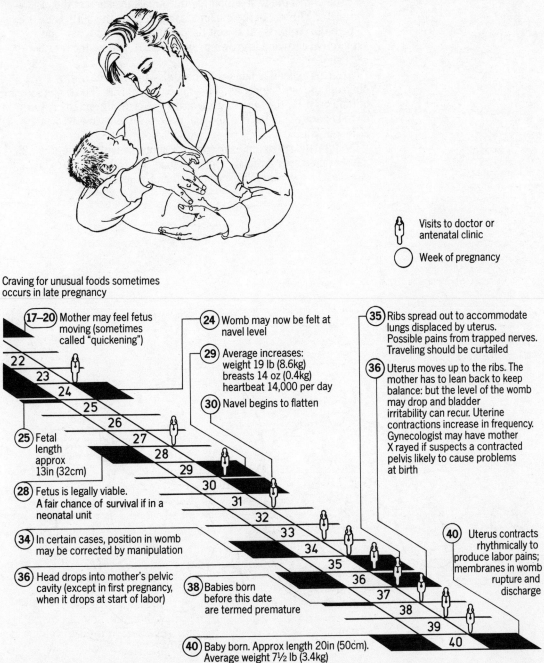

Visits to doctor or antenatal clinic

Week of pregnancy

Craving for unusual foods sometimes occurs in late pregnancy

(17–20) Mother may feel fetus moving (sometimes called "quickening")

22
23
24
25
26

(25) Fetal length approx 13in (32cm)

27
28
29

(28) Fetus is legally viable. A fair chance of survival if in a neonatal unit

30
31
32

(34) In certain cases, position in womb may be corrected by manipulation

33
34
35

(36) Head drops into mother's pelvic cavity (except in first pregnancy, when it drops at start of labor)

36
37

(38) Babies born before this date are termed premature

38
39

(40) Baby born. Approx length 20in (50cm). Average weight 7½ lb (3.4kg)

40

(24) Womb may now be felt at navel level

(29) Average increases: weight 19 lb (8.6kg) breasts 14 oz (0.4kg) heartbeat 14,000 per day

(30) Navel begins to flatten

(35) Ribs spread out to accommodate lungs displaced by uterus. Possible pains from trapped nerves. Traveling should be curtailed

(36) Uterus moves up to the ribs. The mother has to lean back to keep balance: but the level of the womb may drop and bladder irritability can recur. Uterine contractions increase in frequency. Gynecologist may have mother X rayed if suspects a contracted pelvis likely to cause problems at birth

(40) Uterus contracts rhythmically to produce labor pains; membranes in womb rupture and discharge

Development of the embryo

The tiny embryo has embedded itself in the wall of the uterus; and up to the 8th week of pregnancy, the uterus contains the growth without enlarging in size.

Between the 4th and 8th weeks of life, the embryo develops from a small limbless object resembling a white kidney bean only ⅛in (4mm) long into a miniscule but complete human being, all of 1⅝in (40mm) from head to toe.

By the end of the first 2 months, the initial formation of the organs is complete. The sex of the embryo is apparent by the 50th day.

The embryo starts off as soft tissue. But by the 40th day, the skeleton of cartilage is growing; and by the 45th day, the first bone cells appear.

The arms appear as buds at 30 days. By the 40th day, they differentiate into hands, and lower and upper arms. The fingers are in outline only. By the 50th day, the arms are growing and the fingers have separated. (The legs and feet develop in the same way as the arms but later.)

The fetal heart continues to form for about 2 months; but at 30–35 days it takes over circulation of the blood, which has hitherto been circulated via the umbilical cord and the placenta.

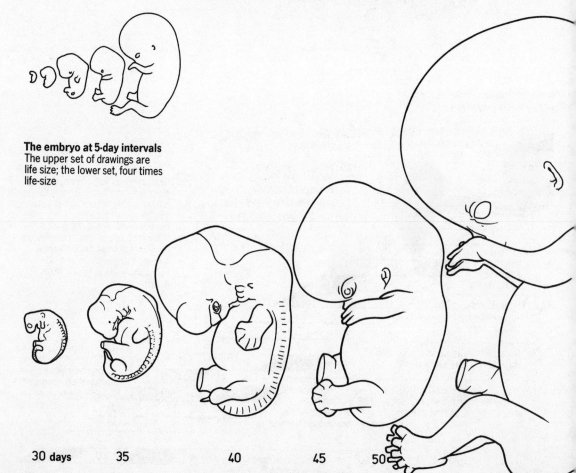

The embryo at 5-day intervals
The upper set of drawings are life size; the lower set, four times life-size

30 **days**   35   40   45   50

THE SUPPORT SYSTEM

The **placenta** develops during the first 10 weeks of life from the spot where the chorionic villi first burrowed into the uterine wall. The placenta, which looks like a bath cap roughly 8in (20cm) in diameter, and about 1lb (0.45kg) in weight when fully developed, has a maternal (outer) and embryonic (inner) surface. The outer surface is divided into roughly 20 lobes of chorionic villi and tiny blood vessels. The flow of blood to and from these vessels is supplied from the mother's uterine artery and vein. The inner surface, covered by a layer of amnion, has tiny vessels radiating out from the umbilical cord at the center. The **umbilical cord**, which links the embryo to the placenta, supports and protects two arteries and a vein which carry blood to and from the embryo.

The placenta acts as both a pool and a filter. The cells of the maternal surface fill with blood from which the blood vessels on the embryonic surface draw not only oxygen but also, by diffusion, proteins and vitamins which are essential to fetal growth. Waste products will be drawn from the embryo's blood vessels in the same way. But though there is this free exchange, the blood systems of the mother and embryo are quite separate. The placenta is largely protective in function, but there are some drugs and viruses against which it has no defense. The placenta also produces the hormone progesterone, upon which the pregnancy depends. The placenta, or afterbirth, is expelled after the birth of the baby.

The amniotic sac (or bag of waters) is a sac of tough membrane, the amnion, within which a fluid (largely water with some protein) is contained. The sac forms around the embryo soon after it has become attached to the uterus wall. In it, the embryo has complete freedom of movement until about the 30th week. It is the growth and gentle pressure of the amniotic sac which slowly enlarges the uterus, and so the abdomen, giving the overt sign of pregnancy.

The fluid cushions the embryo from knocks. It maintains a constant temperature and so also insulates the embryo, providing a level of water-conditioned central heating. It absorbs the waste excreted by the embryo, and is the medium with which the fetus first learns to swallow.

In cases of multiple birth, each fetus normally develops in its own sac. On average, at the 36th week of pregnancy, the sac contains about 2.4 pints (1.1 liters). By the 40th week, however, roughly one-third of this will have been lost.

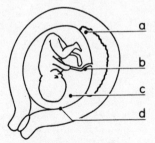

Cross-section through the uterus
a Placenta
b Umbilical cord
c Amniotic fluid
d Amnion

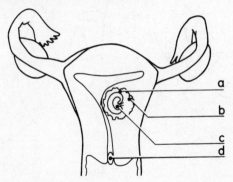

Vertical section through the uterus 35 days after fertilization

a Chorionic villi
b Placenta
c Embryo
d Mucus plug

Fetal development

After the stage at which the sex of the embryo can be determined (approximately the 8th week), it is referred to as a fetus.

During the next 7 months the organs of the fetus grow rapidly, so that by the time the baby is born, all the organs have increased their weight 120 times. Weight increases from about 1oz (28.3gm) at 8 weeks to 7¼lb (3.4kg) on average at birth. This means the fertilized egg will have increased 5000 million times. (Over the next 20 years, weight increases only 20 times.)

Length increases from 1⅝in (4.1cm) at 8 weeks to 20in (50.8cm), from crown to heel, at birth (that is, 12½ times).

Growth gradually slows down just before birth, but rapidly speeds up after the first few days of birth. Besides general fetal growth, head and body hair, and nails, are growing by the 18th week. By the 30th week, fat is deposited under the skin, making it smoother and more rounded, and less red and wrinkled.

Eyelids, which have been growing, close over the eyes in the 9th week, to open again in the 22nd week.

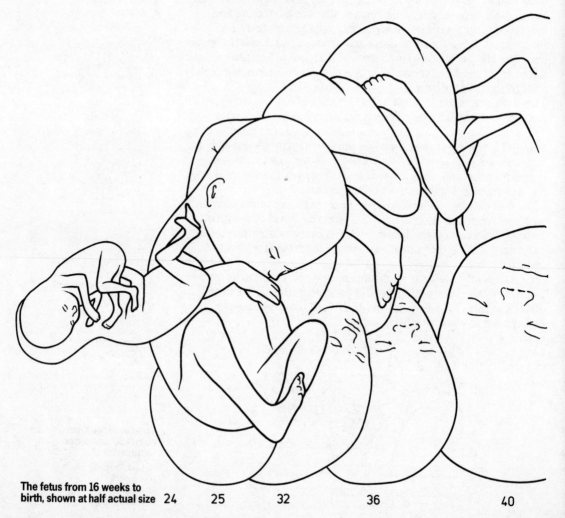

The fetus from 16 weeks to birth, shown at half actual size 24   25   32   36   40

On the internal front, at 14 weeks the heart pumps about 6 pints (2.8 liters) a day. By the 18th week, it can be heard externally by placing an ear on the mother's abdomen. At around 38 weeks, the heart pumps around 720 pints (340 liters) per day. Muscular reflexes develop on eyelids, palms, and feet, and the swallowing reflex starts at the 14th week. Thumbsucking also takes place around this time.

Fetal movements, or "quickening," can be felt at the 18th week. Urination into the amniotic fluid begins around the 14th week. Premature live birth is possible at 22 weeks, but survival prospects are poor. Babies born at 24 weeks, though, can often be kept alive in intensive care units, and with the use of special respirators.

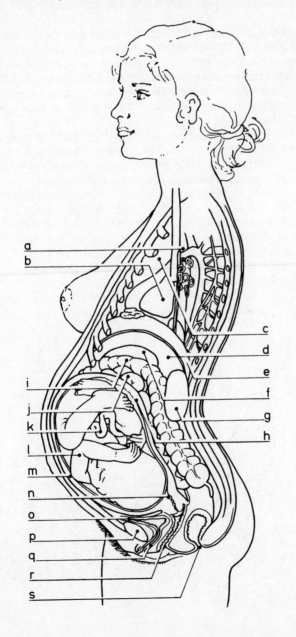

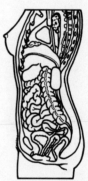

The baby in the uterus (*left*) showing position of surrounding organs as compared with the non-pregnant state (above)

a Trachea
b Heart
c Lung
d Liver
e Diaphragm
f Stomach
g Kidney
h Placenta
i Large intestine
j Small intestine
k Umbilical cord
l Fetus
m Uterus
n Cervix
o Bladder
p Pubic bone
q Urethra
r Vagina
s Anus

©DIAGRAM

311

Physical changes in pregnancy

Usually the first sign of pregnancy is a missed period. But if periods are normally irregular, the time of ovulation is uncertain and so amenorrhea is not a definite diagnosis of pregnancy.

The most obvious physical manifestation of pregnancy after the 3rd month is the swelling of the abdomen as the uterus expands beyond the pelvis. (The swelling causes stretchmarks which may remain after birth.)

Between the 4th and 5th months, the mother feels the **fetal movements** ("quickening") for the first time. The sensations are faint at first but get stronger. From the 5th month, the fetal heart can be heard with a stethoscope and fetal movements seen from the outside.

The mother's **weight** gradually increases (on average by between 25 and 30lb – or about 11½–13½kg). She will begin to feel tired because of her shape and size, increasingly so toward the end of pregnancy. Her **posture** changes, as she has to lean back to balance the baby's weight. Because of this, backache is often experienced. Eventually she may have to walk with a waddling movement, with her legs slightly apart.

Most symptoms of pregnancy, some of which bring about discomfort (in turn causing insomnia) result from changed **hormone levels** and the increased pressure of the growing fetus. The altered hormone levels of pregnancy also cause changes in emotional states, and there seems to be a general pattern common to most women (though not all). In the first 3 months, there are often extreme swings in mood, with an ambivalent response to pregnancy. But by the second trimester, the woman has generally accepted the fetus and prepared for it, and will be adjusting to hormonal changes.

About two-thirds of women experience **morning sickness** usually from the date of the first missed period until the second or third month, when it often ceases abruptly. It varies in severity, from

The changing female shape throughout pregnancy

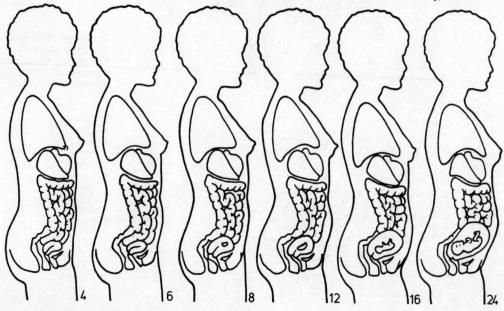

4   6   8   12   16   24

nausea in the morning only, to vomiting during the day. The exact cause of morning sickness is not known, though it is thought that the increase in estrogen is responsible. The body eventually adjusts but while nausea continues, it is a good idea to eat small frequent meals rather than large ones. Dry toast in the morning may help, and greasy or spiced foods should be avoided.

The **breasts** soon start to enlarge in preparation for feeding. They may itch, tingle or feel heavy, and are sometimes painful. Their veins become prominent. By the 16th week, they start to secrete a thin fluid from the nipples ("colostrum"). The areolae also become mottled due to increased pigmentation. (Increased pigmentation may also appear on the face and external genitals, and a dark line may run from the navel to the genitals.)

As the fetus grows, so does the mother's appetite. But pressure and reduced mobility of the stomach induced by hormones reduce the capacity for large meals. There may be **cravings** for certain foods, however. With some women, this extends to the truly unusual – coal, for example – and is then known as "pica." By contrast, certain foods and substances may become repulsive for some women. Coffee, meat, alcohol, wine and fatty foods are examples.

Reduced mobility of the large intestine increases the possibility of **constipation**, and therefore **hemorrhoids**. Dried fruit or bran will ease constipation. Laxatives should be avoided.

Relaxation of the esophagus sphincter can cause regurgitation and heartburn during pregnancy, but a good diet should ease this situation.

The pressure of the uterus on the bladder makes **urination** more frequent. This happens in the 2nd and 3rd months and also near term, when the fetus settles down into the pelvis.

Fetal pressure on the main leg veins in the groin may also cause **varicose veins**. The veins in the legs dilate as a result of the pressure of blood trying to return to the heart.

Cravings
Quite often in pregnancy, a woman has cravings (known as "pica") for certain foods. This can sometimes be an indication of a particular nutritional requirement; but quite why pica sometimes takes such unusual and extremely varied forms – such as the desire for coal, chocolate or strawberries – remains very much a mystery.

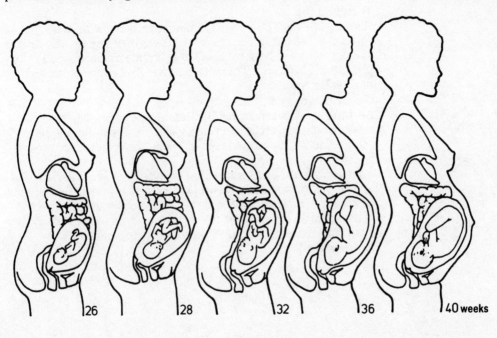

26 | 28 | 32 | 36 | 40 **weeks**

© DIAGRAM

Health care during pregnancy

It is essential that every pregnant woman maintains good health, learns about infant care, and bears healthy children. Essentially, she (and her partner) should also learn what is happening to her and what to expect. Good antenatal care has substantially reduced maternal and infant mortality.

The woman will usually first go to her doctor or antenatal clinic to have her pregnancy confirmed. The approximate date of the birth will be determined, and the doctor will carry out a full consultation entailing discussion of past illnesses and operations, present health, and current complaints. A general and then obstetric examination will reveal any conditions which may affect the pregnancy, for which treatment will be given. This enables the doctor to anticipate possible complications. Any previous pregnancies, miscarriages, or abortions will also be considered, and questions answered.

The physical examination entails a general medical check, a urine test, blood test, blood pressure test, and obstetric investigation.

The mother-to-be continues her visits to the antenatal clinic every month until she is 7 months pregnant, and then every 2 weeks until she is 9 months, with a weekly check thereafter until the birth. Visits will be more frequent if any previous illnesses (diabetes, heart disease, or hypertension, for instance) are likely to cause complications. At each visit, the baby's position in the uterus will be checked. When the fetal head settles down into the pelvic cavity, this suggests that the mother's pelvic shape and size are normal. An examination will also be made to ascertain the position of the fetal head, and a cervical check made at the same time.

Illness

Any fever, chill, heavy cold, or other illness during pregnancy should be reported immediately to the doctor. **German measles (rubella)**, contracted up to the 12th week of pregnancy, may interrupt the development of the fetus and lead to deafness and heart defect.

Weight gain

A gain of 25–30lb (11.3–13.6kg) from conception to birth is normal. Any more than this is unnecessary and even undesirable. At term, the average fetus weighs about 7lb (3.2kg) and the amniotic sac and placenta 2½lb (1.1kg). The mother carries the balance as fats and fluids in her tissues.

General care

Bathing is safe and relaxing. But water in the vagina is best avoided, although only dangerous if forced in under pressure. Douching is unnecessary, as the vagina is self-cleaning, and in pregnancy may not be safe.

The genitals and breasts should be kept clean, as secretions become heavier during pregnancy. **Dental care** is also important, as the gums become softer and so more easily injured by food and toothbrushes. Injured gums are susceptible to infection which can cause loss of teeth, and regular dental inspections during pregnancy are recommended.

Unless there is a history of miscarriage, or possibility of complications, **intercourse** during pregnancy will not harm the fetus. Near term, intercourse in some positions may be uncomfortable for the woman, disturbing for the fetus, and difficult to achieve other than in a new position, however.

ROUTINE TESTS

A **blood sample** taken early in pregnancy may be tested for any or all of the following: syphilis, AIDS, toxoplasmosis, immunity to rubella, presence of anemia, levels of hormones (such as HCG and estriol) and a protein (known as "alpha-fetoprotein" or AFP). High levels of AFP may indicate the presence of a neural tube defect, and ultrasound or amniocentesis can then be used to check for this. Abnormally high levels of HCG may be caused by hydatidiform mole (see p. 328). Measurements of AFP, HCG and estriol can be used, together with the mother's age, to assess the risk of Down's syndrome. **Urine samples** will be tested throughout pregnancy for the presence of infections, and excess glucose or protein in the urine (a warning sign of **pre-eclampsia**). Ultra-sound tests (see p. 324) may also be routine.

Blood pressure measurements are routine at antenatal clinics to give warning of the development of **toxemia**. Its cause is unknown but its effects can be severe. The arteries supplying the uterus go into spasm, reducing the blood supply to the placenta, with possibly fatal results to the fetus.

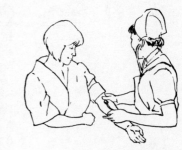

EXAMINATIONS

Abdominal examinations are made to test for muscle tone and possible enlargement of liver and spleen, and after the 12th and 28th week to check on growth and the position of the fetus.

Pelvic examinations for structure and dimensions are made as part of pregnancy confirmation. Breasts and nipples will also be examined, and legs for signs of varicose veins.

©DIAGRAM

315

EXERCISE AND RELAXATION

Relaxation helps to relieve tension during pregnancy and pain during labor. A comfortable position is important for practicing it. The floor, a bed or chair are all suitable. In the later stages of pregnancy, lying on your side may be more comfortable than on the back. Concentration on each part of the body is required. After practice, a sensation of "floating" can often be felt.

Breathing exercises will help you to gain control over the various muscles which will be used in labor. Slow, deep breathing is used to aid relaxation during contractions. Later on, rapid shallow panting is used, speeding up as each contraction intensifies.

The posture of a pregnant woman is altered as the abdomen enlarges. Strain on the back and abdomen can be avoided by standing correctly. The whole spine length can be pressed against a wall, while tucking in the buttocks and abdomen, keeping the head up and shoulders back, and maintaining this posture. Humping and hollowing the back mobilizes it and prevents it aching.

Labor positions can also be practiced to strengthen the inner thigh muscles and control of breathing.

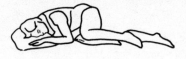

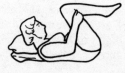

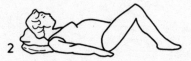

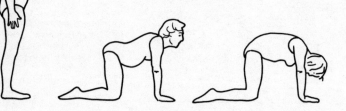

Keeping fit during pregnancy
1 Relaxation practice
2 Breathing exercises
3 Posture exercises
4 Labor exercises

DIETARY NEEDS

Eating for two is definitely out! A woman's average calorie requirement is about 2300; and the fetus requires only an extra 300. So intake should only increase slightly. It is important that extra emphasis is put on proteins, vitamins, and minerals. (Your doctor may prescribe supplements in some instances, perhaps of iron or folic acid, which is a form of Vitamin B aiding development of the fetal nervous system.) Wholefoods are preferable to refined. But vitamin and mineral supplements should only be taken on the doctor's advice. A woman who is breastfeeding her child should allow 500 calories per day above her usual requirements when she starts feeding.

Malnutrition during pregnancy can seriously affect the fetus. It may even die from undernourishment, a factor revealed in autopsy not only by low weight, but also by stunting of each individual organ and low cytoplasm content of the body cells. More usually, the baby is born alive but underweight. Low birthweight also carries with it increased risk of cerebral palsy, epilepsy, autism, blindness, deafness, mental subnormality, and neonatal death. Some sources estimate that a third of all long-term childhood handicaps are associated with low birthweight.

Low birthweight is not always totally due to malnutrition, but it is a major factor. In Guatemala, a nutritional program reduced low birthweight from 20% to 5.1% of births. This is below that of many industrialized countries, so it is not just in "developing" countries that there is room for nutritional improvement. But careful nutrition must begin before the 20th week of pregnancy. Any later improvement in diet has only limited effect.

Ideally, a pregnant woman should follow a normal healthy diet, increasing calorie intake marginally. But many women find that their appetite in pregnancy is small or unpredictable; and poverty may be a factor. At the very least, wholewheat bread and milk are preferable to tea or coffee and biscuits. The minimum diet, shown *below*, should be followed each day. Interestingly, some pregnant women find that they can face cold food more easily.

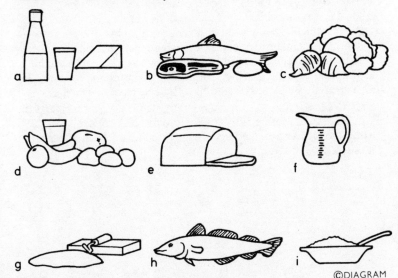

©DIAGRAM

Minimum recommended diet during pregnancy
a 1 pint (½ liter) milk, or ½ pint (¼ liter) and 2oz (57g) of cheese daily
b Portion of meat or fish, or an egg daily
c Portion of root or raw green vegetable daily
d Fruit, orange juice, and/or potato daily
e Wholewheat bread daily
f 1 pint (½ liter) of water daily
g Liver or oily fish once a week
h White fish once a week
i Bran, if needed, to avoid constipation

Risks in pregnancy

Factors within a woman's control
Drugs
Alcohol
Smoking
Diet
Weight

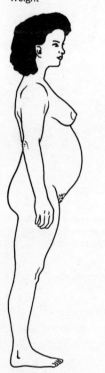

Factors outside a woman's control
Viral infections
Rhesus incompatibility
Sexual infections

Abnormalities at birth can be caused by various factors and every expectant mother worries about them. On this page, we list some of the chief dangers in pregnancy. As far as **accidents** are concerned, a fetus can only be damaged by a blow directly into the uterus. Falls are more likely to damage the mother than the fetus. But although the fetus is well protected, its development can be seriously affected by many of the risks mentioned.

Some **genetic disorders**, of course, can be inherited by an infant. Examples are hemophilia and sickle-cell anemia. Congenital abnormalities are also more likely to occur in babies born to women under 16 and over 40.

There are many factors in the environment, too, that can put an unborn infant at risk – air and water **pollution** for example. A woman can lessen the risk from **radiation** by avoiding X rays, although today these are generally only given in order to detect and prevent a greater risk. Always advise your dentist that you are pregnant.

INFECTIONS

The amniotic sac protects the fetus against most bacteria. But virus infections in the mother's bloodstream may cross the placenta and sometimes cause damage.

Rubella (German measles) in a woman in early pregnancy can cause fetal death or deformities such as deafness, blindness, brain damage, and retarded growth. Rubella in the first 3 months of pregnancy causes defects in up to 50% of babies, and is often considered grounds for abortion. There is also slight risk in the 4th and 5th months. But if the mother has previously had the illness, or a vaccine against it, she is unlikely to contract an infection strong enough to spread to the fetus. (Vaccination cannot be given during pregnancy.) See p.329, too.

Other vaccinations should also be avoided during pregnancy, smallpox among them; but some can be given after the first 14 weeks. Your doctor will be able to advise about this.

CMV (cytomegalo virus) is spread between adults by close personal or sexual contact. It is found on the cervixes of a number of pregnant women, usually without obvious symptoms. It can cause low birthweight, prematurity, deafness, and mental retardation if it infects the fetus. No vaccine is available. But only when it is contracted for the first time during pregnancy is it usually strong enough to infect the fetus; and only 1 infected baby in 10 suffers permanent damage.

Syphilis in the mother can cause death, deformity, or disease in the fetus, unless the mother is treated before the 16th week of pregnancy.

Mumps, chickenpox, and **fevers** (as in influenza) are sometimes also suspected of causing deformities.

SMOKING

As well as affecting a woman's own health, smoking may affect the health of her unborn baby. It is widely accepted that there is a connection between smoking and pregnancy complications, and studies have shown that smoking while pregnant results in a lighter baby and an increase in perinatal mortality. Effects of smoking in pregnancy have also been found to persist into childhood. Probably the dangers are most severe if smoking continues after the first 3 months, and not all effects have been totally proven. Fetal breathing movements are, however, a direct measure of fetal health and well-being; and smoking has been shown to reduce the incidence of fetal breathing movements and must therefore be considered damaging to fetal health. A study of 18 normal pregnant women has shown that just two cigarettes smoked consecutively produce a dramatic reduction in these breathing movements.

Statistics also suggest that women who smoke when pregnant tend to produce lighter babies than non-smoking mothers. One British study showed that only 4% of the live babies born to non-smoking mothers weighed less than 5lb 8oz (2.5kg) compared with over twice that percentage born to mothers smoking at least 20 cigarettes a day when pregnant.

A study made in California included the smoking habits of *both* parents. It showed that babies weighing less than 5lb 8oz (2.5kg) at birth were most common when both parents were smokers.

The diagrams shown are based on a survey taken in the UK of 17,000 children whose progress had been followed from birth. They compare the mental abilities of 11-year-old children of mothers who smoked during pregnancy with those of non-smoking mothers. Children of mothers who smoked up to 9 cigarettes daily were some 5–5½ months behind in school progress, and those of mothers who smoked over 10 cigarettes daily were 5½–7 months behind, compared with children of the same age of non-smoking mothers. In addition, the survey noticed that children of smoking mothers tend to be 2in (5.1cm) shorter than the children of non-smokers.

Comparative mental abilities of children of smoking and non-smoking mothers

a Reading ability
b Mathematical ability
c General ability

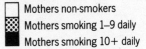

☐ Mothers non-smokers
▨ Mothers smoking 1–9 daily
■ Mothers smoking 10+ daily

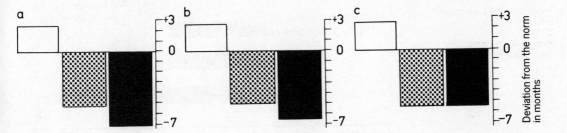

Deviation from the norm in months

ALCOHOL

An occasional drink does no harm during pregnancy. But recent studies suggest that an increasing number of babies are being born seriously deformed or mentally retarded because their mothers have been drinking heavily during pregnancy. It has even been claimed that 1 in 3 women who drink heavily must expect their child to be mentally or physically defective. But so far evidence is mainly from actual alcoholics. The diagrams below are based on a US study of 23 children born to chronically alcoholic mothers. They were compared with children of non-alcoholic mothers and matched for socioeconomic group, race and maternal age, as well as other factors.

Diagram (**a**) shows mortality rates among the newborn babies. 17% of those born to alcoholic mothers died within 1 week, as opposed to 2% of those born to non-alcoholic mothers.

Diagram (**b**) compares birthweight, length and head circumference of two sets of infants. Comparisons were based on a measurement of normality that generally only 3% of babies fail to achieve. In the survey, 13%–32% of the children of alcoholic mothers failed to reach the measurement. Diagram (**c**) shows that at the age of 7, 44% of the children born to alcoholic mothers had a very low IQ.

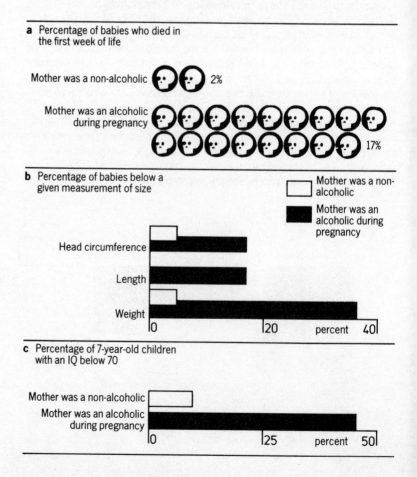

a Percentage of babies who died in the first week of life

Mother was a non-alcoholic — 2%

Mother was an alcoholic during pregnancy — 17%

b Percentage of babies below a given measurement of size

☐ Mother was a non-alcoholic

■ Mother was an alcoholic during pregnancy

Head circumference

Length

Weight

0   20   percent   40

c Percentage of 7-year-old children with an IQ below 70

Mother was a non-alcoholic

Mother was an alcoholic during pregnancy

0   25   percent   50

DRUGS

Doctors today recommend that women avoid all drugs during pregnancy unless they are absolutely essential for the mother's well-being. The fetus maintains its hold on life through the umbilical cord and the work of the placenta. Oxygen and nutrients pass from the mother's circulation into that of the fetus via the placenta and umbilicus, and carbon dioxide and other waste products pass back the same way. As a result, most substances in the mother's bloodstream will reach the fetus. In the case of drugs, recent studies show that, as with thalidomide, effects on the fetus can be disastrous, particularly during the first 3 months when the fetal organs are forming.

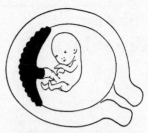

Some of the drugs that cross the placenta and what the effects on the fetus might be

Drugs	Placenta	Effects on fetus
Caffeine (in coffee and tea) Tannic acid (in tea)		Stimulate fetal nervous system
Sleeping pills		Depressant
Tranquilizers		Possible malformations; but some now designed specifically for safe use by pregnant women
LSD and other psychedelic drugs		Increased risk of miscarriage; possible chromosome damage
Cocaine; amphetamines		Acts as stimulant on fetus
Heroin; morphine		Possible fetal addiction; and dreadful withdrawal symptoms
Aspirin		Large amounts can cause miscarriage or hemorrhage in newborn
Phenacetin		Possible damage to fetal kidneys
Antibiotics a Streptomycin, gentamycin b Sulphonamides (long-term) c Tetracycline		Associated with deafness in infants Can cause jaundice Possible deformities; stains teeth
Antihistamines		Possible malformations: some now designed specifically for safe use by pregnant women
Cortisone		Fetal and placental abnormalities – possibly stillbirth; cleft lip
Progesterone (for hormone deficiency and possible miscarriage)		Genital abnormalities in female infants
Antithyroid		Possible goiter
Nicotine (in cigarettes)		Low birthweight

©DIAGRAM

Inherited disorders

Sadly, the birth of a stillborn baby or affected child is often the first time that parents become aware that they carry a genetically inherited condition. There is a large number of these disorders, most of which are extremely rare; others – such as cystic fibrosis, sickle-cell anemia and hemophilia – are more common. Because these conditions are inherited in different patterns, the chances of other children being affected vary in statistical probability and according to sex, and one or both parents may be a carrier. Some disorders are not apparent at birth and develop in childhood or even later in life. A genetic counselor is therefore the most appropriate source of information. She or he will also be able to advise on the possibility of screening future pregnancies.

Metabolic disorders are characterized by a defect in the body's biochemistry. In some instances, the results of these defects can be partially rectified: in **phenylketonuria**, for instance, adherence to a diet lacking in one amino acid that cannot be metabolized can prevent severe mental subnormality. **Hemophiliacs**, who cannot make a blood-clotting substance, can be given it by injection to control bleeding; and replacement pancreatic enzymes and antibiotics help in the treatment of **cystic fibrosis**. Drugs and dialysis may also be used to try to rid the body of harmful substances.

Among some of the most common inherited disorders are the following: **Duchenne muscular dystrophy** (a sex-linked inheritance that affects young boys, causing muscular swelling and weakness, and then wasting); **cystic fibrosis** (a recessive inheritance whereby a couple who are both carriers have a 1 in 4 risk of a child who produces abnormally thick mucus that causes lung infections and digestive problems); **sickle-cell anemia** (a recessive inheritance in which abnormal hemoglobin causes misshapen red blood cells which break up and disrupt circulation); **hemophilia** (a sex-linked inheritance in which boys have an inability to produce the blood-clotting factor); **phenylketonuria** (an inability to metabolize phenylalanine resulting in brain damage unless a strict diet is followed); **galactosemia** (an inability to metabolize galactose resulting in cataracts and mental deficiency); and **Tay-Sachs disease** (affecting the nervous system, fatal within the first few years of life, and for which the gene is carried by 1 in 27 of Jews originally from Eastern Europe, and 1 in 300 of the rest of the population, but both parents must be carriers for there to be a 1 in 4 chance of the child being affected).

CHROMOSOME DISORDERS

Some congenital conditions are not inherited from affected parents but arise at fertilization and occur because more than the usual number of chromosomes are present in each of the body's cells. An extra sex chromosome results in abnormalities of the genitals, and possibly other malformations and sterility. **Down's syndrome** (mongolism), caused by the presence of an extra chromosome 21, is an hereditary condition in a few families but more usually occurs as a non-inherited form in older mothers. Affected children have varying degrees of handicap; and there may be congenital heart defects and mental retardation.

Congenital defects
Disruption of the embryo's early development (by illness of the mother, drugs, environmental or genetic factors) may also cause malformations. Most of these are relatively minor and either pass undetected or require only minor surgery (such as hernia repair). Those which are very severe usually result in miscarriage. A large number of defects at birth come into the category of "**neural tube defects**," varying from absence of the brain (**anencephaly**) at one end of the spectrum to minor hidden protrusion of the spinal cord membranes at the other. **Spina bifida** is a condition caused by the spinal canal having failed to close around and protect the spinal cord. Affected children need surgery to prevent infection and further damage to the nerves. There may be **hydrocephalus** (excess fluid around the brain), paralysis of the legs and incontinence.

Not all the tests listed *below* will be used in every pregnancy. Blood and urine samples, blood pressure measurements and ultrasound scans are, however, likely to be performed at some stage of pregnancy in clinics in developed countries; but amniocentesis, chorionic villus sampling and fetoscopy are only used if abnormality of the fetus is suspected. The fact that a test is available does not mean that it will automatically be performed: for example, a woman offered amniocentesis for the detection of Down's syndrome may decide that the risk outweighs the advantage in her case, particularly if she would not seek abortion if the fetus were to be found abnormal. Consultation with the specialist concerned should be offered before invasive procedures, and the implications of possible findings discussed before deciding to go ahead.

AMNIOCENTESIS

This is the method by which amniotic fluid is extracted from the uterus, and analyzed for possible fetal abnormalities. A growing number of fetal abnormalities can now be detected, including **Down's syndrome** and **spina bifida**. Those who might want the test are women who have already given birth to a defective child; women carrying a serious disorder; and women aged over 40, since they have approximately a 1-in-50 chance of delivering a child with congenital abnormalities.

Amniocentesis is best carried out between the 12th and 16th weeks of pregnancy. A local anesthetic is given and a needle inserted into the uterine cavity. Amniotic fluid is withdrawn and the cells in it studied for defects.

Amniocentesis is quickly performed and usually causes little discomfort, but it results in miscarriage in around 1% of pregnancies and the results take up to 3 weeks, which may mean that if an abnormality is found, the mother must make a decision about abortion at a relatively late stage. The test is also used to detect neural tube defects if ultrasound is unavailable.

CHORIONIC VILLUS SAMPLING (CVS)

This technique is still under development and may be performed either by inserting a narrow tube through the cervix or by inserting a needle through the skin of the mother's abdomen under ultrasound guidance. Cells from the developing placenta are obtained and analyzed in the laboratory for inherited or chromosome disorders. The level of risk and efficiency depends on the experience of the operator; and miscarriage may occur spontaneously at the stage of pregnancy at which this test is performed. The test can be performed earlier in pregnancy than amniocentesis – from 8 until 11 weeks – and results are available in 2–3 weeks, enabling an earlier decision about termination where a disorder is found.

Testing for risks

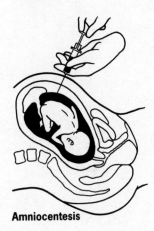

Amniocentesis

ULTRASOUND

This technique is quite often used for routine screening in pregnancy, with scans performed at around 16 weeks and, in some centers, late on in pregnancy. The first scan is performed to measure the fetus, and so check its age against expected date of delivery, and to screen for a multiple pregnancy and obvious physical malformations. Later scans can check on the position and progress of twins and small babies, and also ensure that the placenta is functioning properly and not covering the entrance to the birth canal ("placenta previa"). It is also sometimes possible to determine the sex of the baby. Ultrasound is also used as a guidance technique in amniocentesis, chorionic villus sampling, fetal blood sampling and fetoscopy, and is able to give warning of poor oxygen supply to the baby and may be used if a mother has previously lost a baby because of placental insufficiency. Ultrasound is generally considered to be a safe technique because it is non-invasive and no adverse effects have yet been discovered. However, its efficiency relies heavily on the skill of the operator; standards vary, and suspected abnormalities should be confirmed by another operator or by further tests. The main preparation involves making sure you have a full bladder, so you should drink plenty of water and not go to the bathroom for at least two hours beforehand. In the examination room, you will lie comfortably on your back, and your exposed abdomen will be swabbed with oily fluid to ensure good contact with the transducer. This instrument is passed over the abdomen until the area being investigated appears cloudy on the screen. Watching the viewer, many mothers "see" their babies for the first time during an ultrasound scan. The procedure only takes 5–45 minutes; and afterwards you should be able to go straight home. The obstetrician will discuss any findings with you at a later date, and you may be asked if you would like to know the sex of your child if this has been determined during the scan.

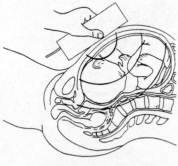

Position during ultrasound procedure
A transducer is passed over the abdomen until the area to be investigated appears on the viewing screen

FETAL BLOOD SAMPLING

Direct sampling of the baby's blood can be achieved from about 18 weeks onward. A needle is inserted under ultrasound guidance to the point where the umbilical cord joins the placenta, and a small amount of blood is withdrawn. The blood can be tested for a variety of conditions and results take only 7 days. The risk of miscarriage is around 1%. The technique is also used to transfuse the fetus in cases of rhesus incompatibility (see p.327).

FETOSCOPY

This method of testing involves the insertion of a tiny telescope through the mother's abdominal wall into the uterus under ultrasound guidance. The operator can then examine the fetus under direct vision and take samples with a needle. The procedure cannot be performed until about 18 weeks and, because of the need for sedation and hospitalization and higher risk of infection and miscarriage, it is only likely to be done if other tests have proved inconclusive. It will also reveal the sex of a baby and possibly such visible defects as a cleft palate.

Complications of pregnancy

The majority of pregnancies are completely normal, but there are some in which complications may develop. If left unattended, these conditions can become serious, but the main purpose of antenatal care is to detect potential dangers and, where possible, to prevent them from happening.

The chart *below* shows which unusual symptoms should be reported immediately to a doctor and the possible causes of such symptoms.

Danger signs	Possible causes
Severe abdominal pain, possibly with slight bleeding, in first few weeks of pregnancy	Ectopic pregnancy
Vaginal bleeding with or without abdominal pain the first 28 weeks of pregnancy	Threatened miscarriage
Vaginal bleeding with or without abdominal pain after the 28th week of pregnancy	Premature separation of placenta (abrupto placenta, if pain; placenta previa, if painless)
Severe swelling of fingers and face, with blurred vision and headaches, after the 20th week of pregnancy	Toxemia of pregnancy
Gush of water from the vagina at 28–36th week	Rupture of membranes (bursting of amniotic sac)

ECTOPIC PREGNANCY

Bleeding and pain in early pregnancy (6th–12th week) may be caused by an ectopic pregnancy. In this condition, the fertilized egg has failed to reach the uterus and has implanted within a Fallopian tube.

If the fertilized egg does not reach the uterus within seven days, the tiny arm-like protrusions ("chorionic villi") which will have formed by then will burrow into the wall of the Fallopian tube. This will then become sorely distended as it can only stretch to a limited extent.

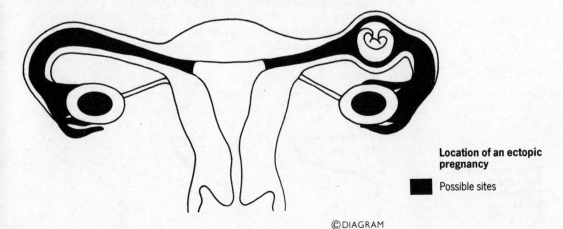

Location of an ectopic pregnancy

■ Possible sites

©DIAGRAM

The chorionic villi will continue to burrow into the wall in search of nourishment – which is obviously restricted. Eventually they will break through the muscular wall or into an artery causing bleeding and pain. Loss of the embryo is inevitable unless it escapes into the cavity of the abdomen and the chorionic villi burrow into the wall where eventually a placenta will develop. Healthy babies which have developed within the abdomen have occasionally been delivered (by Cesarian section).

Ectopic pregnancies are not common, and since the same hormones are secreted as in a normal pregnancy, they are not always detected until discomfort is felt. One in every ten women who has had an ectopic pregnancy is liable to have another. They are often due to prior inflammation of the Fallopian tube.

MISCARRIAGE

About 1 in 6 woman miscarry, and a threatened miscarriage is the usual cause of bleeding in the first half of pregnancy. Known more correctly as a "spontaneous abortion," miscarriage occurs most often at the 6th or 10th week. The fetus detaches itself from the uterus and is expelled. The most common causes include a major abnormality in the fetus (about 50% of aborted fetuses are found to be abnormal); death of the fetus; faulty hormone production; anatomical defect or functional abnormality; illness or infection; a defective sperm or ovum; or psychological conditions.

There are different kinds of miscarriage at different stages of pregnancy: threatened, inevitable, complete, incomplete, and missed are the most usual.

The symptoms of a **threatened miscarriage** will generally appear during the first few weeks. Bleeding (red or brown), without pain, occurs. At this stage, it is uncertain whether the miscarriage is inevitable, and in 80% of cases the threat passes and pregnancy continues. But if the cervix opens, then miscarriage will transpire.

In a **complete miscarriage**, the uterus empties itself of the entire pregnancy. **Incomplete miscarriage** leaves varying amounts of tissue in the uterus and a D&C (dilatation and curettage) is required. In a **missed abortion** the fetus has died but remains in the uterus. It is eventually aborted and a D&C is usually given. A miscarriage can be a tense and despairing time, and many women still feel expectant of the birth even though they are no longer pregnant. It can be a shattering experience, but there are support associations (see useful addresses, p.408). After a first miscarriage, the chance that the next pregnancy will be successful is high.

Three main types of miscarriage
a Threatened
b Inevitable
c Incomplete

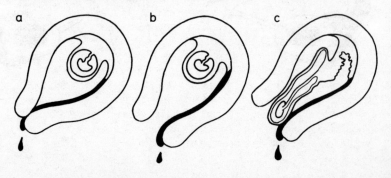

REPEATED MISCARRIAGE

Miscarriages occur more frequently in older mothers (over 35), in those who have had difficulty in conceiving and where there have been two previous miscarriages. Sometimes they can be due to an **incompetent cervix**, in which case an obstetrician may suggest inserting a stitch so that the cervix is closed throughout the pregnancy. The procedure is carried out under anesthesia, and the stitch is removed late in the pregnancy. In any event, your obstetrician will monitor your pregnancy particularly carefully if you have a history of miscarriage.

DISPLACED PLACENTA

Hemorrhage after the 28th week of pregnancy may be caused by two fairly rare conditions: **placenta previa**, in which the placenta lies in the lower part of the uterus; and **abruptio placenta**, in which the placenta separates prematurely from the uterus.

A woman with placenta previa will be hospitalized after the 28th week. A Cesarian may be necessary, but in 20% of cases delivery is normal. Most cases of abruptio placenta continue normally, and in only 25% is separation too great for the infant to survive.

RUPTURE OF THE AMNIOTIC SAC

A sudden gush of water from the vagina after the 28th week generally means that the amnoitic sac in which the baby grows has burst and amniotic fluid is escaping. If this occurs before the 28th–36th week, it may often precede premature labor. The woman is hospitalized and drugs or sedatives may be given to discourage labor. After the 36th week, labor will either be allowed to continue or will be induced as the baby is sufficiently mature to survive.

RHESUS INCOMPATIBILITY

Blood is denoted **rhesus positive** if it contains the rhesus factor. If it does not contain the factor, it is **rhesus negative**. (85% of people are rhesus positive). Normally, being rhesus negative is of no consequence; however, problems can arise in pregnancy when a rhesus negative woman is carrying a rhesus positive child. (If the father is rhesus positive, this is likely in three out of four pregnancies.)

In the course of labor or birth, it is quite likely that the child's blood will get into the mother's system. If this happens, antibodies will be produced in the mother to protect her against the rhesus positive blood of the baby. But these antibodies are small enough to pass through the placenta in a subsequent pregnancy, and so inactivate the blood of the fetus, if it is again rhesus positive.

The dangers increase with each subsequent pregnancy. In a severe case, the fetus may suffer from anemia, jaundice, or a weak heart. One in 200 pregnancies is complicated in this way. If the child is likely to be moderately affected, it is usually given a complete transfusion of rhesus negative blood shortly after birth. As there is no rhesus factor in negative blood, no antibodies are formed, and within 40 days the baby's own rhesus positive blood will have replaced the transfused blood, which is broken down in the liver. In serious cases, the fetus can be transfused while still in the uterus.

How rhesus incompatibility works
a A small amount of fetal rhesus positive blood enters the blood system of the mother, whose own blood is rhesus negative
b This causes the mother to produce antibodies to inactivate the rhesus positive blood
c During a subsequent pregnancy the mother's antibodies pass through the placenta and inactivate the fetal rhesus positive blood. But an injection of anti-rhesus globulin protein will destroy any of the cells left in the mother's blood after a first pregnancy or termination, and also following each future pregnancy.

+ Rhesus positive blood of fetus
O Antibodies

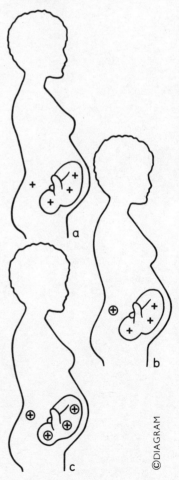

Maternal disorders

A wide range of disorders may affect the mother (and the baby she is carrying), most of which are rare. Some arise as complications of the woman's body adjusting to the state of pregnancy; others are of infectious origin. Blood and urine samples from pregnant women are tested to pick up most of the most dangerous complications. However, routine testing for certain conditions such as AIDS and toxoplasmosis (a disease spread by cat feces which can cause blindness in the baby), is not universal.

Edema (swelling of the face, fingers, and legs) is normal in pregnancy and is not usually of any significance. However, sudden swelling – particularly of the face – should be reported as it may be a sign of pre-eclampsia (see *below*). **Carpal tunnel syndrome** – tingling, numbness and pain in the wrist and hand – sometimes occurs for the first time in pregnancy. Diuretic (water-reducing) drugs are usually effective in relieving the condition.

Pre-eclampsia (also known as **toxemia**) is a serious complication of late pregnancy and occurs in about 10% of women who are pregnant for the first time, less frequently in subsequent pregnancies. Warning signs include high blood pressure, protein in the urine and sudden edema. There may also be headache, vomiting and blurred vision. If two high blood pressure readings are taken and there are also other signs, the mother will be admitted to hospital as **eclampsia** (a highly dangerous condition with fits and coma) may occur unpredictably and put both mother and baby at risk. Early delivery of the baby is likely to be necessary.

Women who are already known to have **diabetes** will be advised by their physician to exercise tight control over blood glucose levels even before they become pregnant. This lessens the risk of miscarriage and fetal abnormalities in the early stages. Insulin requirements gradually increase during pregnancy; and those who have previously been using tablets will probably be switched to insulin treatment until after the birth. Mothers who can achieve stringent control of blood glucose through home blood-testing have no more complications of pregnancy than non-diabetic women and should be able to carry the baby to term and avoid intervention in labor. Once labor starts, the diabetic mother should not eat and will probably be placed on an insulin and glucose drip. Babies born to mothers with high blood glucose levels tend to be large and puffy, requiring early (possibly Cesarian) delivery, and may have breathing problems and low blood sugar, needing special care. **Gestational diabetes** is the name given to diabetes arising for the first time during pregnancy. Affected women are often overweight, and alterations in diet may be sufficient to prevent complications; however, insulin injections may be needed until after the birth.

Hydatidiform mole affects a higher proportion of Asian women and those aged under 20 or over 40. It is a condition in which faulty fertilization of the egg takes place. The result is overgrowth of the trophoblast as a collection of fluid-filled cysts without development of a fetus. The woman has typical symptoms of pregnancy, including severe morning sickness. Treatment consists of removal of the abnormal material by vacuum curettage. Women who have had hydatidiform mole will subsequently be advised not to become pregnant for 2 years and will be followed up with regular tests because there is a chance (up to 10%) that a malignant condition may ensue. If caught early by this form of screening, it responds very well to treatment with anticancer drugs; and pregnancy may later be possible.

SEXUAL INFECTIONS

AIDS testing is not routine in pregnancy: but if a mother suggests she is a carrier of the HIV virus, she may want to have the AIDS test. If it is positive, she may then decide whether to continue with the pregnancy. If so, the baby can be carefully monitored during its early years. Research has yet to show for sure to what extent the virus can pass from mother to child in the womb.

Syphilis If a pregnant woman has syphilis, her baby is also likely to be infected as the organism can cross the placenta. However, antibiotic treatment early in pregnancy cures the disease and the baby will then be born healthy.

Gonorrhea and **chlamydia** do not cross the placenta but the baby may be infected as it passes through the birth canal. Treatment during pregnancy is therefore desirable. Both diseases cause eye infections in the newborn which need treatment with antibiotics, and chlamydia can also cause a respiratory tract infection in young babies.

If a woman suffers from **genital herpes**, she should inform the obstetrician or midwife who will be looking after her. Herpes is thought not to cross the placenta; but if sores are present at the time of delivery the baby may be infected and be extremely ill. Cesarian section is used during active infection to prevent the baby coming into contact with the virus.

OTHER INFECTIONS

Any infection which causes a high temperature and general illness should be reported in pregnancy. While most viruses are unlikely to do harm, high fever may result in miscarriage.

Pregnant women who have not had **rubella** (German measles) and have not been immunized should avoid contact with anyone who has the disease or has a rash. If contracted in the first 4 months of pregnancy, the virus may cause the baby to be handicapped by blindness, deafness or mental retardation. A blood sample can be tested to confirm immunity, and many countries have immunization programs; but women who are already pregnant cannot be immunized as this would harm the fetus.

The effects of **polio** can be severe in pregnancy. Most developed countries have immunization programs. **Cytomegalovirus** is a common virus which usually causes only a mild illness. However, if contracted for the first time in pregnancy, it may cause brain damage and other malformations.

Toxoplasmosis is caused by a parasite found in animal and bird feces. An infected woman may not feel unwell but the disease can cause severe malformations and even death of the fetus. Some countries screen blood samples for the disease; and pregnant women are probably best advised to avoid handling pet feces if possible.

6.03 Childbirth

Methods and choices

Labor and delivery are, for many women, the most alarming aspects of pregnancy. As with the physical changes of pregnancy itself, an understanding of the processes involved helps to relieve anxiety. A woman has 9 months to prepare for birth, and in order to participate fully in the experience she should become acquainted with all the available possibilities. But each woman's experience is essentially personal and individual: whether she delivers at home or in a hospital, with or without drugs, and with or without the presence of a partner or friend should in the final analysis be for her to decide.

NATURAL CHILDBIRTH

Natural childbirth is the process of giving birth without the automatic use of drugs or obstetric techniques. The idea was popularized in the 1930s by the English doctor, Grantly Dick-Read. It is based on the assumption that much of the pain of childbirth is caused by tension, itself due to the woman's anxieties and fears about labor. If these are eliminated, tension is relieved and pain will be lessened.

Psychoprophylaxis

The psychoprophylactic method of childbirth was introduced by a French doctor, Fernand Lamaze. He felt that relaxation was not enough, and introduced pre-learned muscular and breathing exercises to be used by the woman during labor. With these, a woman is no longer helplessly passive but can actively participate in the process of birth.

Although this is the basis of childbirth preparation today, a woman should not feel she has failed if she opts for artificial pain relief during labor.

HOME OR HOSPITAL?

Fifty years ago, it was normal for a woman to have her child at home. In Holland over half of all deliveries are still carried out in the home, with absolute safety. In the US and Britain, however, home births are rare. Most doctors prefer to deliver in hospital, where the facilities for any possible complications are immediately available. However, given an absence of complications, there is no reason why a woman who wishes to do so should not deliver her child at home. The advantages are obvious – your own room, a familiar atmosphere and possibly the presence of friends can greatly ease the doubts and tensions of labor.

Some women feel safer delivering in a hospital, though; and it is generally recommended that a woman have her first child there. After the first birth, it is often possible to predict whether the next will be normal. The risks of pregnancy and labor rise for the third and subsequent births, and for mothers under 17 and over 35 – so these are usually delivered in a hospital. A pregnant woman will also be admitted for a hospital birth if there is any evidence or suspicion of possible difficulty or danger – toxemia, diabetes, rhesus incompatibility, prematurity, multiple birth, difficult fetal position, or a small pelvis. Unfortunately, the choice of a home or a hospital delivery today largely depends on the facilities available. The main aim of doctors has been to lower risks, and even though hospital birth is not essential for many women, it has become part of a routine for greater safety.

ALTERNATIVE BIRTH STYLES

The possibly damaging effects on a woman of a prolonged, painful, and distressing childbirth are now well recognized. But it is argued that some of the methods of delivery commonly used can have a lasting and detrimental effect on a child. There have been three main advocates of a new approach to birth: R. D. Laing, the Scottish psychologist; Frederick Leboyer, the French obstetrician; and the American psychoanalyst, Elizabeth Fehr. All have concerned themselves primarily with the well-being of the child and consider that not only is it aware of its time in the womb but also of its arrival into the world. Its initial impressions are said to be critical to its future development. R. D. Laing argued that cutting the umbilical cord too soon is a major cause of birth traumas. The cord linking mother and newborn child still carries on its functions of providing blood, oxygen, and nutrients even after the actual birth. Immediate severance causes unnecessary shock to the baby, which can be avoided by leaving the cord uncut until it has naturally ceased to function. According to Laing, if the cord is left for 4 or 5 minutes until the baby's own circulation has taken over, the process is more natural and non-traumatic.

Frederick Leboyer, in his book *Birth Without Violence*, also advocates not cutting the cord until it has ceased to function. In addition, he believes that the newborn child's eyes, ears, and skin are hypersensitive, and should be treated gently and with respect. Struggling out of the womb into bright lights and noise, being put on hard scales and hung upside down (which immediately forces the spine into an unaccustomed angle) are all alien to a being who has been 9 months in the womb. Leboyer suggests that lights and noise in the delivery room should be at a minimum, that the baby should be placed on the mother's stomach before the cord is cut, and that the child should then be placed in a bath of water at body temperature and allowed to move and "open-up" in a calm, unhurried way. Certainly Leboyer has noted that a baby born in this way opens its eyes and will usually give just one cry (as opposed to a torrent of tears and red-faced rage) having satisfied everyone of its ability to breathe.

Elizabeth Fehr believed that a traumatic birth left a permanent impression. She introduced into psychoanalysis the process of "rebirthing," by which a person retraces his or her life backward toward birth. As a result of her investigations, she concluded that auditory hallucinations suffered by schizophrenics might well be related to sounds heard by the child as it struggled from the womb. Her work has given impetus to the movement for gentler birth styles.

INDUCED LABOR

Labor may be induced artificially if the health of the mother or fetus is in danger, or if the birth is overdue. Labor will normally begin within 24 hours of induction, and if it is also accelerated (see *below*), tends to be shorter than a spontaneous labor. The contractions follow the same pattern as spontaneous labor, even though each stage may take much less time.

The frequency of induction varies greatly from place to place. The following are the main conditions in which induction is justified.
Pre-eclampsia (also known as **toxemia**) is a major medical cause of induction. It is characterized by high blood pressure, edema and proteinuria (protein in the urine) in the woman. Although the danger to the mother is slight, danger to the fetus increases with severity. Should **eclampsia** (in which fits occur) develop, the mortality rate is very high for both the mother and the fetus.
Post-maturity also accounts for many inductions. If the fetus remains in the uterus after term, it will continue to grow, making for a difficult birth. Placental function begins to fall off after the 40th week, and it is usual to induce by the 42nd week because of risk to the baby.
Hemorrhage, which is caused by the placenta separating from the uterus before birth, accounts for a number of inductions, too. In difficult cases, a Cesarian section may be required. **Rhesus incompatibility** also necessitates induction in some cases.

METHODS OF INDUCTION

Induction of labor can involve use of prostaglandin pessaries which are inserted into the vagina in order to ripen the cervix. If necessary, this can be followed by artificial rupture of the membranes. Fluid is drained off and labor usually begins within 24 hours. The rupturing of the amniotic sac does not itself make for any difficulty in delivery. If labor does not proceed at a satisfactory rate, however, it can be accelerated with use of an intravenous infusion of oxytocin to stimulate uterine contractions. The oxytocin is given throughout labor, though not for more than 10 hours.

Amniotomy
Artificial rupture of the amniotic sac or bag of waters is termed "amniotomy."
a The baby is protected by the cushioning of the amniotic sac.
b Once it has been ruptured, however, and the waters escape through the vagina, labor can proceed.

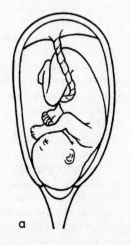

a

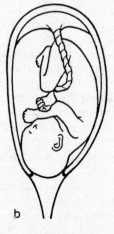

b

BREATHING EXERCISES

At the beginning of labor, deep abdominal breathing helps to relieve pressure. Once contractions increase so that they harden the abdominal wall, deep chest breathing is more helpful. The mother should then continue to change as labor progresses, each time alternating her normal breathing (between contractions) with the learned form (used during the contractions). Once delivery begins, expulsion breathing is used.

Preparing for birth

The four types of breathing used during labor
- **a** Deep chest breathing for early first stage
- **b** Shallow chest breathing used in the middle stage
- **c** Shallow rapid breathing (panting) for transition
- **d** Expulsion, in which the breath is slowly exhaled while the woman bears down to push against the baby

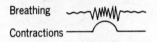

Breathing

Contractions

COPING WITH PAIN

A woman who delivers in a hospital can use a variety of pain-relieving or pain-killing drugs, if she feels she needs them. There are two kinds: analgesics and anesthetics.

Analgesics relieve pain and may either be inhaled or injected. During early labor, painkillers are rarely necessary, but narcotics such as Demeral (Pethidine) may be given.

Barbiturates, also used in the past, are now not generally given, as they can cause breathing to stop in some cases.

Inhalant analgesics can be self-administered and the intake controlled as needed.

Regional anesthetics are injected into the woman's body at a specific point, the anesthetic completely blocking off pain. The **epidural block** is probably the most efficient. Anesthetic is injected into the epidural cavity which lies between the spinal cord and its covering, the dura. It numbs the entire region from the lower abdomen to the feet, and can be readministered during labor. Although an effective pain-reliever, it can lessen the mother's ability to push and may result in a forceps delivery. Other regional anesthetics include the **pudendal nerve block**, given immediately before a forceps delivery, and the **caudal block**. Both anesthetize the pelvis. A **parcervical block** (not widely used everywhere) can be injected into the plexus, making the cervix and upper vagina completely insensitive. A regional anesthetic is also given before an **episiotomy** (surgical opening of the perineum to prevent tearing, often criticized for being performed unnecessarily.

Possible sites for drug administration
- **a** Intravenous infusion
- **b** Injections
- **c** Inhalation
- **d** Injections

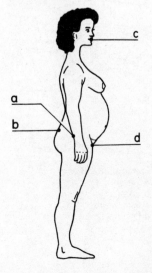

© DIAGRAM

Drugs used in labor are carefully supervised but most do cross the placenta and can make the newborn infant drowsy and slow to suck. These effects, although undesirable, are temporary and should be weighed against the possible long-term effects on a woman of a painful and distressing labor.

Hypnosis is another method of pain relief sometimes taught to pregnant women. Not everyone, however, is able to master self-hypnosis: and those who try it may find they need additional relief. **Acupuncture** is also sometimes used.

RISKS AND BENEFITS

Narcotics used in labor may depress the vital functions of both mother and baby. However, unwanted effects can be reversed within seconds by a powerful narcotic antagonist. The sedative-tranquilizer substances used in modern obstetrics pose no threat. Systemic medication is a valuable method of procuring pain relief in labor.

There is no discernible risk to mother or baby from a few deep inhalations of **anesthetic gases**. The technique is considered safer than the use of narcotics, although not as effective as epidural anesthesia.

Paracervical blocks are not widely used and carry some risk of constriction of the uterine artery which may cause fetal distress. They are not used if there is any hint of abnormality on the fetal monitor. The mother may suffer a reaction to the local anesthetic and there may be concealed bleeding due to damage to the uterine artery.

Pudendal blocks should permit trouble-free use of forceps and the repair of an episiotomy (incision to widen the opening of the vagina) or perineal tear. But the anesthetic cover may be patchy, requiring use of a local anesthetic as well. This technique does not relieve the pain of uterine contractions. There is rarely any risk to the baby but the mother's complications may include toxic reaction to the anesthetic.

The prominent risk with **epidural blocks** is of puncturing the dura matter so that some of the anesthetic solution enters the spinal canal. This results in temporary loss of sensation in the legs. A slight drop in blood pressure follows these injections so they are not used if there has been any prior bleeding. Epidurals are not used either if there are neurologic problems in the mother or if there are indications of fetal distress.

Caudal analgesia is like an epidural but blocks a smaller area. It is used for a shorter period and rarely brings serious complications.

In **spinal anethesia** the drop in blood pressure is usually greater. This can be counteracted with intravenous fluids. Apart from backache, the commonest complication is headache, occurring within a day or so of delivery and sometimes lasting several days. Postspinal headache is due to leakage of cerebrospinal fluid through the dura mater. It recedes with treatment or when the dura reseals itself by natural means. But this form of anesthesia is rarely used.

General anesthesia carries its usual risks, plus the fact that the unconscious mother may inhale regurgitated stomach contents. Even for a Cesarian section, local anesthesia may therefore be preferable, except in a life-threatening emergency.

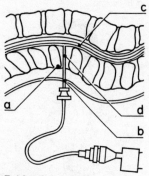

Paracervical block
The diagram shows the nerve supply for the uterus, cervix, and vagina. Most of the nerves for this area collect together at the paracervical ganglion or plexus (**a**). When local anesthetic is injected here, the cervix and upper vagina are desensitized, without impairing the ability of the uterus to proceed with labor.

Epidural anesthesia
a Vertebra
b Syringe
c Spinal cord
d Epidural space

Labor

BIRTH POSITIONS

The diagrams show some of the positions currently used for delivery. The **dorsal**, in which the woman lies flat on her back with her knees up and separated, and the **left lateral** in which she lies on her left side, knees toward her chest, are still the most typical in many western countries. But the **lithotomy** position is one still used sometimes in the USA, although there has been a movement in recent years toward use of a birthing stool and birth in a supported upright position.

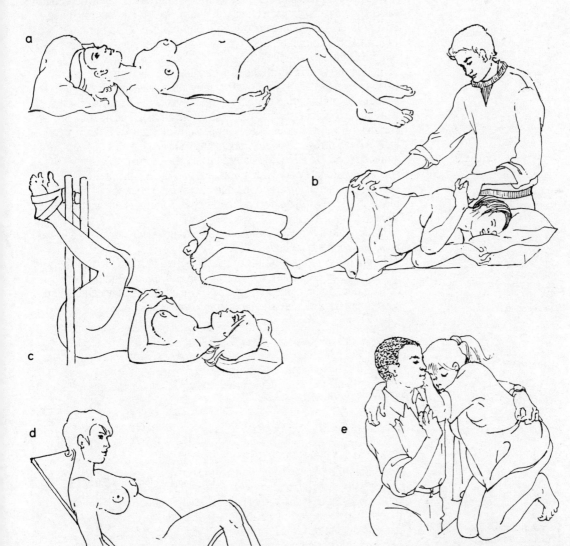

Positions during labor
a Dorsal
b Left lateral
c Lithotomy
d Semi-upright
e Upright or squatting

© DIAGRAM

DURATION OF LABOR

Labor itself has three distinct stages. In the first stage, the cervix is "effaced" and "dilated," to allow the fetus to pass without damaging it. The second stage is the actual delivery of the baby; the third, delivery of the placenta or afterbirth.

First stage

Before delivery can begin, the uterus must undergo a change in shape to permit the fetus to pass through the cervix. The upper uterus pulls the lower uterus and cervix up around the head of the fetus.

This process takes about 8 hours for women having their first child (also known as "primigravidae"), and may take 4–5 hours for those having their subsequent children ("multigravidae"). By the time effacement is completed, contractions are occurring about every 3–5 minutes, and lasting 40–90 seconds. The mucous plug which was lodged in the cervix throughout pregnancy is now displaced, as the cervix begins to dilate to allow the baby a free passage through. The process, a continuation of effacement, reveals the **amnion** (or bag of water) surrounding the baby's head. If the amnion has not been ruptured already, it is usually ruptured during dilation, either by the baby's head or by the doctor delivering. This releases a quantity of amniotic fluid. To allow the baby to pass, the cervix must dilate to accommodate its head, which is about 4in (10cm) in diameter. As dilation proceeds, contractions become more frequent and intense; by full dilation they will be occurring every 2–3 minutes and lasting 60–90 seconds.

Dilation takes from 3–5 hours for a woman having her first child, and less for subsequent children.

During the early stages, there is little active participation on the part of the woman. Generally she remains up and about, waiting for contractions to increase in frequency. Once labor is fully established, she should then choose the most comfortable position.

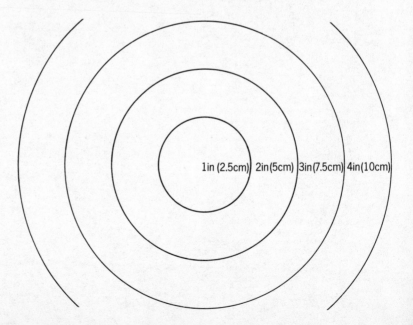

1in (2.5cm) 2in (5cm) 3in (7.5cm) 4in (10cm)

Cervix dilation
The full dilation (widening) that allows the baby to pass – 4in (10cm) – shown at its actual diameter. The time taken to achieve full dilation depends on whether it is a first birth, and also varies with the individual mother.

THE FIRST STAGE OF LABOR

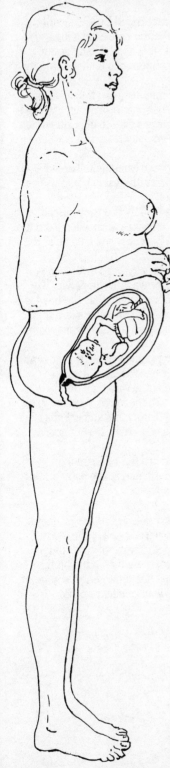

First stage
During this stage, the mother should take up any position she finds most comfortable

a Partial effacement
Contraction and retraction of the uterus shorten the neck of the cervix.
Contractions now every 10 minutes

b Full effacement
Contractions every 5 minutes

c Partial dilation
Continued contraction and retraction dilate the cervix.
Contractions every 2–5 minutes

d Full dilation
The fetus is able to pass through the cervix without damaging it.
Contractions every 2–3 minutes

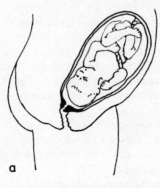

a

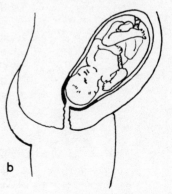

b

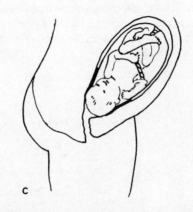

c

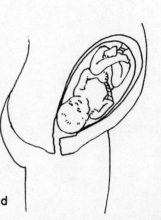

d

©DIAGRAM

TRANSITION

Transition to second stage

The transition to the second stage is characterized by feelings of
pressure in the low pelvis, backache, and often nausea and leg
cramps. At this point, when tension rises, it is helpful and comforting
for the woman's partner or a friend to prompt her to do her antenatal
breathing exercises.

Contractions continue, once every few minutes, and there is an
increasingly uncontrollable desire to push or bear down – like trying to
relieve severe constipation. However, it is not safe to bear down until
full dilation has been achieved, as the cervix may tear.

Second stage

When the cervix is fully dilated, bearing down can begin. The baby is
now being pushed out of the uterus and down the vagina, and will be
delivered in anything from 5–50 minutes.

If there is danger of the perineum being torn by the baby's head, an
episiotomy may be performed. The doctor makes an incision from the
vagina obliquely down toward the anus. This cut is sewn up after the
delivery is completed.

The fetus begins its journey on its side, usually head first.
Contractions of the uterus force the fetus down into the pelvis. The
head is rotated downward beneath the pubic arch and, as the head is
born, it rotates back to its original position. The shoulders and then
the body follow the same pattern of rotation as they are delivered, and
the baby is born.

The second stage is now completed – in primigravidae or first-time
mothers it takes up to one hour, in multigravidae less. Mucus is
extracted from the mouth and nose of the baby, who may be
suspended upside down to drain mucus from the lungs. The umbilical
cord is clamped and cut, sometimes immediately and sometimes after
some minutes. In a week, the stump of the cord will dry out and
fall off.

The baby on delivery is wet and covered in a fatty substance,
"vernix." As oxygen begins to circulate in the lungs, the baby's color
will change gradually from a bluish tone to pink.

Third stage

The dorsal position is generally adopted for delivery of the placenta,
expelled within 30 minutes of the baby. As birth occurs, the uterus
retracts quite markedly. The placenta is not capable of contraction or
retraction, and shears away from the uterus. Light traction on the
cord aids its delivery. The placenta is then checked to ensure none of
it is left inside the uterus, since this could lead to infection and
hemorrhage.

SECOND AND THIRD STAGES OF LABOR

Second and third stages
a A full dilation of the cervix signifies the beginning of delivery.
The woman bears down to help expel the baby. Contractions every 2–5 minutes
b The baby's head passes through the cervix and rotates to squeeze beneath the pubic arch
c The head is born, and rotates back to its previous position. The baby's shoulders rotate to pass through the pelvis
d The right shoulder, then the left, is born
e The baby breathes spontaneously. Mucus is cleaned from the face and air passages. The umbilical cord is clamped
f The placenta is delivered within 30 minutes of the birth

©DIAGRAM

Problem births

PREMATURE BIRTH

A premature baby was once defined by weight: under 5½lb (2.5kg). But low birthweight, full-term babies have totally different problems from the true premature baby, who is better defined as one born before the 36th week of pregnancy. Often the cause of premature labor is unknown, but possibilities include lack of antenatal care, poor health, multiple pregnancy, and a small placenta.

After the birth, the premature baby is placed in an incubator. Its skin is red and wrinkled, lacking fat deposits, and body heat is hard to maintain. Problems can also arise with breathing, as the respiratory system is possibly underdeveloped. It cannot suck well, and has a feeble cry. But if adequately cared for, it will become as healthy as a full-term baby.

BREECH BIRTH

Normally the fetus moves from breech to vertex position between the 24th and 28th week. However, some fail to do so, and 3.5% remain in the breech position till birth.

A normal-sized baby in the breech position will usually be delivered with no problems for mother or child. But a small maternal pelvis or a large fetal head may lead to difficulty.

The duration of delivery can be critical: a long delivery may even result in oxygen starvation if the head squeezes the umbilical cord, and a short delivery may cause damage to the fetus and mother. Breech delivery is in three stages: the breech and legs are born first, then the shoulders, and finally the head. Forceps are usually used to help ease out the head gently and to avoid injury.

Breech birth
1 Breech presentation with baby's head at the top
2 The bottom passes through the cervix and rotates to squeeze under the pubic arch
3 The legs are born first, then the shoulders, and finally the head

MULTIPLE BIRTHS

Twins are born on average once every 85 births; triplets once every 7,500 births; quadruplets once every 650,000; and quintuplets once every 57,000,000 births.

Difficulties may arise in multiple births. They tend to be premature, and so must be delivered in a hospital. Labor, however, is usually straightforward as each baby is small. The birth canal is dilated after the birth of the first baby so that subsequent ones are born easily. **Toxemia** of pregnancy and **anemia** occur more frequently in a multiple pregnancy. The maternal death rate in twin pregnancies is also greater. In larger multiple births, the likelihood of fetal death also rises steeply.

CESARIAN BIRTH

Cesarian section is an operation carried out on a pregnant woman to deliver her baby, if this is not possible through the vagina. Reasons for it include fetal distress, a low-lying placenta, a very small pelvis, obstructive fibroids, a transverse fetal position; and previous uterine injury.

An anesthetic (often an epidural rather than a general) is given before the operation. A cut is made below the navel into the abdomen and uterus, and the baby is delivered through this incision.

It is possible for a woman to have several Cesarian sections, but 4 is thought to be enough. Only in the last 25 years has the Cesarian section become a routinely safe operation. Now it accounts for over 10% of all deliveries in the USA, and is often used in preference to a difficult forceps delivery.

VACUUM EXTRACTION

Vacuum extraction is used as an alternative to simple forceps delivery. It can be started before the cervix is fully dilated. A metal cup is inserted into the vagina and placed against the fetal head. It is connected to suction equipment, the vacuum formed being strong enough to allow the fetus to be pulled gently out of the uterus. Scalp tissues are sucked into the cup, but within a few hours of delivery any swelling subsides.

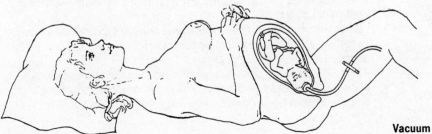

Vacuum extraction

©DIAGRAM

FORCEPS DELIVERY

Frequency of a forceps delivery varies greatly from country to country. In the USA an average of 50% of births involve forceps, and about 13% of births in the UK are forceps deliveries, for instance.

Forceps are used in the second stage of labor to aid the progress of the fetus in the following circumstances: slow or no fetal progress; maternal distress, as in pre-eclampsia exacerbated by the effort required during labor; and fetal distress.

They consist of two curved blades that interlock and fit closely around the fetal head. One blade is inserted into the uterus and located in position around the head. The other blade is then inserted and, when positioned, locked into the first blade. Gentle traction draws the fetus down through the vagina. Local anesthetic and an episiotomy may be needed.

The cervix must be fully dilated to allow insertion of the forceps blades and damage will be caused to the cervix and vagina if the fetus is pulled through before dilation. The amniotic membranes must be ruptured, if they are not already, and bladder and rectum should be empty. The forceps can only be applied to the fetal head.

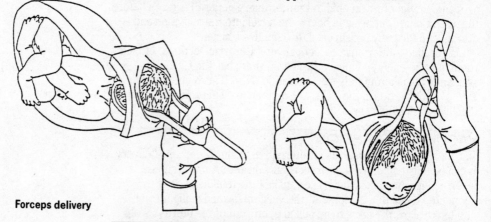

Forceps delivery

EMERGENCY BIRTH

In 80% of cases, a woman can deliver without any problems; but if a birth begins unexpectedly, the help of a doctor or hospital should always be sought. If no help is available, then it is best simply to give encouragement to the mother, and to allow nature to take its course without interference. Let the mother bear down (push against the baby) as soon as she wants to do so and do not worry whether full dilation has occurred, for any damage to the cervix can be repaired later in hospital. Pain is not normally a problem, if the atmosphere is kept calm and quiet.

After the birth, clean the mucus from the baby's mouth and nose. Breathing should begin within 30 seconds. Do not cut the cord. Keep mother and baby warm.

More than about ½pt (.25 liter) of blood from the uterus (not the placenta) signifies hemorrhage. In this case only, the abdomen should be massaged to try to ease the bleeding after the delivery.

Stillbirth

In an age of high-tech medicine and newspaper stories of the survival of tiny premature babies, it is particularly distressing when a baby is born dead or dies soon after birth: we somehow expect every life to be savable, every defect repairable.

There are many possible causes of stillbirth or death at around the time of birth: genetic or accidental defects in development, prematurity in cases of late miscarriage, and illness in the mother are all common reasons. Alternatively, a birth which was expected to be straightforward may be complicated by factors which could not have been foreseen. Whatever the cause, the effect upon the mother and father is likely to be the same. A stillbirth is a bereavement and should be treated as such, both by medical staff and members of the family. In the past, it was often the practice to avoid letting the mother see her baby. It is now realized that such attitudes did little to help parents cope with their grief and even caused further distress by encouraging the suppression of grief.

It is entirely natural for parents to feel guilt, however misplaced, and this may surface in anger at each other or at medical personnel: these emotions should not be repressed but dealt with as they occur. The mother's body has been changed by pregnancy and the process of childbirth, but there is no baby to suckle or hold, resulting in a deep physical as well as emotional sense of loss.

The death of a baby who would have been severely handicapped can be especially hard to cope with: on the one hand, parents are worried about how they came to have an abnormal baby, but they may also feel some relief that they do not have to face the problems of bringing up the child, which in turn may lead to a sense of guilt. If a genetic defect is involved, counseling from a geneticist is important regarding future pregnancies and the prospects of having an unaffected baby. The obstetrician may also be able to offer an explanation for premature delivery or birth problems.

The time of coming home from hospital without a baby is distressing for parents and difficult for family and friends who may not know how best to help, but talking about the baby is unlikely to offend the parents and may be actively welcomed. Crying is not something to be embarrassed about – it is a normal part of the grieving process, and grandparents and children should feel that they too have an opportunity to mourn. A self-help organization can sometimes offer the opportunity to speak to a befriender, someone who has also experienced the loss of a child and knows what the parents are going through. Grief proceeds through stages: the mother and father will probably feel very lonely and unable to offer each other much support at first, particularly if they have to work or attend to other children. There may also be sexual difficulties if couples are anxious to start another pregnancy too soon – lovemaking may become mechanical and be a source of distress rather than comfort. For this reason, and to avoid the emotional conflicts that birth of a new baby near the anniversary of the stillbirth may bring, parents are usually advised to give themselves time to recover fully before they contemplate having another baby.

Health checks for the baby

Immediately following birth, a mother should be allowed to have direct skin contact with her baby, so that **bonding** can begin as early as possible. Indeed, this can even take place prior to the cutting of the cord. The midwife or obstetrician will then want to examine the baby, and record its weight and length, as well as confirming that it is breathing well and appears healthy.

Only five minutes old possibly, the baby is given certain ratings against a test known as the **Agpar scale** which assess **heart rate, breathing, skin color, muscle tone** and certain **reflex responses**.

The baby's **head** size is also checked, as are the **genitals**, the upper mouth for any sign of a **palate defect**, and the legs for any indication of a **dislocated hip**.

The newborn baby will also be watched for signs of **jaundice**. Around half of all babies develop this. It usually disppears after about a week, however, with frequent feeding and exposure to sunlight. A more serious type of jaundice can be due to incompatibility of the mother's and the baby's blood, and this will require careful treatment.

The newborn's reflexes
- **a** Stepping reflex, soon lost
- **b** The grasping reflex
- **c** The rooting reflex for the nipple
- **d** The Moro or startle reflex

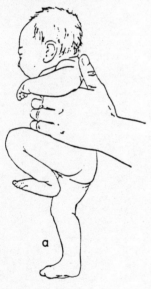

a

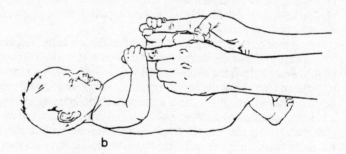

b

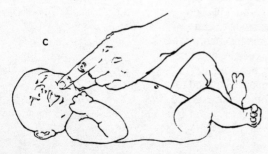

c

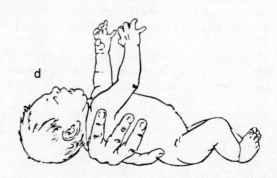

d

BIRTH DEFECTS

Thirty live births in every thousand have some kind of congenital malformation. Some may be so severe that life is not possible; others may be so trivial that life is not affected. Many, but not all defects are obvious at birth. Some, such as defects in the heart or kidneys, may be discovered within a few days, while others are only detected after many years or by chance during surgery or autopsy.

Malformations are either of genetic origin or due to external factors such as infection, drugs, or high-energy radiation which affect the pregnant woman. Congenital defects are one of the most important causes of death in the first and later weeks after birth.

Embryo development is a continuous process following a strict sequence. Any interruption or disorganization of these processes at any time may result in a malformation. Usually the earlier the interruption occurs, the more severe the defect.

THE MOST COMMON DEFECTS IN THE NEW-BORN

Defect	Rate*	Description
Double ureter	300	Two ureters from one kidney. Usually without symptoms or significance. Very occasionally obstructs urine flow, causing infection. Genetic. Surgery if necessary.
Male inguinal hernia	80	Hernia in the groin, between the muscles of abdomen and thigh. Developmental. Surgery needed.
Mental subnormality (except Down's syndrome)	17	Varying degrees of defect from a variety of different causes.
Spina bifida (often with hydrocephalus)	10	Spina bifida – defect leaving spinal cord exposed; hydrocephalus – obstruction in skull causing collection of cerebrospinal fluid under pressure. Genetic, or result of antenatal injury or infection. Surgery to prevent paralysis or death.
Anencephaly	6	Absence of brain and top part of skull. Replaced by fibrous tissue. Invariably fatal. More common where baby has very young or old mother.
Cleft lip and palate	5	Lip and palate not fused. Difficult breathing, feeding, and speaking. Partly genetic. Associated with thalidomide and rubella. Plastic surgery required.
Down's syndrome	3.5	Rate rises to 200 if mother is over 40. Caused by extra chromosome. Characterized by mental retardation, heart defects, Mongoloid features, protruding tongue.
Celiac disease	2.5	Disorder producing a sensitivity to gluten, part of the protein found in some cereals. Chronic diarrhea and malnutrition. Treatment dietary, recovery usual, but slow.

*Rate per 10,000 live babies

©DIAGRAM

After the birth

For about 10 days after birth, there is a steady loss of a bloody substance (**lochia**) from the vagina, as the placental site and uterine lining break down. The breasts produce colostrum for the first few days. This is then replaced by milk. Sometimes the breasts are overfull and painful. For a day or two after the birth, the mother may also experience some constipation, and difficulty in urinating; or she may urinate involuntarily, especially when coughing or laughing. This is caused by muscle slackness in the pelvic area and is best treated by early mobilization and reassurance. Changes in hormone balance often cause the mother to be depressed and weepy for a short while after giving birth. This is called the "3rd or 4th day blues."

Menstruation normally returns after about 24 weeks (if the mother is breastfeeding) or 6–10 weeks if not. Ovulation starts in the first case after about the 20th week. Women who do not breastfeed can therefore become pregnant much sooner; while the longer women breastfeed, the lower the likelihood of pregnancy, although this is not always the case.

POSTNATAL TIMETABLE

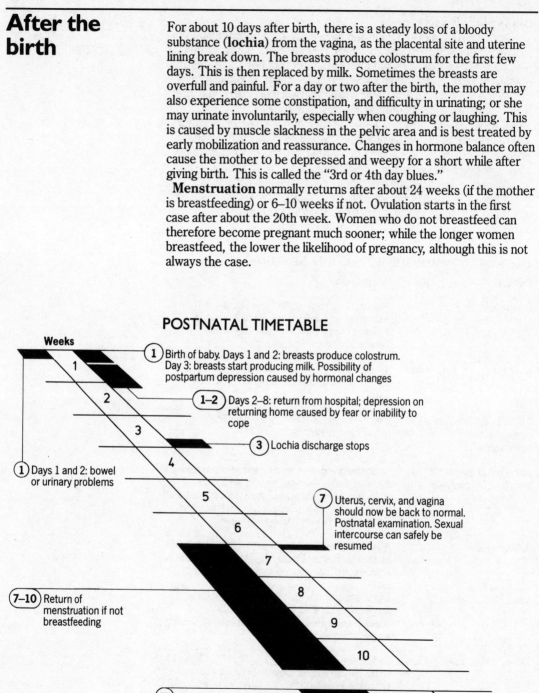

Weeks

(**1**) Birth of baby. Days 1 and 2: breasts produce colostrum. Day 3: breasts start producing milk. Possibility of postpartum depression caused by hormonal changes

(**1–2**) Days 2–8: return from hospital; depression on returning home caused by fear or inability to cope

(**3**) Lochia discharge stops

(**1**) Days 1 and 2: bowel or urinary problems

(**7**) Uterus, cervix, and vagina should now be back to normal. Postnatal examination. Sexual intercourse can safely be resumed

(**7–10**) Return of menstruation if not breastfeeding

(**25**) If breastfeeding, probable return of menstruation by now, if not earlier

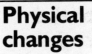

Physical changes

THE UTERUS

The **puerperium** or "postpartum" period is the name given to the weeks during which the uterus and other organs return to their normal size. The uterus, cervix, and vagina undergo immense stretching during pregnancy and labor; but within 6 weeks of the birth, evidence of the pregnancy is difficult to find. The uterus weighs, after birth, about 2½lb (1kg); and after 2 weeks, about 11oz (350g). In rare cases, the uterus retroverts following pregnancy.

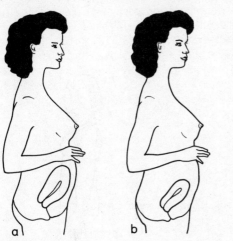

a   b   c

The uterus
a After birth
b 1 week after birth
c 6 weeks after birth

INTERCOURSE

Medical opinion generally favors delaying the resumption of intercourse until after the postnatal examination. Some people, however, argue that problems are unlikely provided that there is no vaginal discomfort and the discharge of lochia has ceased.

In any case, it is wise to wait until you feel ready. Reduced interest may be due to emotional upheaval, sleepless nights, or a lowered estrogen level. Other problems may include muscular cramps during intercourse or pain from stitches after an episiotomy. Pregnancy is possible before menstruation resumes or during lactation. A diaphragm used before the birth will no longer fit, and the Pill should not be used if breastfeeding, unless the progesterone-only "minipill" is prescribed. Condoms with spermicides are otherwise recommended.

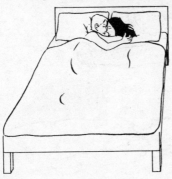

Postnatal exercises

These are important for most women, as they retone muscles (especially those of the pelvic floor), stimulate blood circulation, and promote good posture.

They should be done as many times as possible each day as soon as the mother is up and about. Some abdominal exercises can be performed while feeding the baby (see exercise 1) or around the home (see exercise 2).

Exercise 1
Tighten abdominal muscles while sitting in correct posture position

Exercise 2
Stand straight, pull in abdomen and buttocks. Tighten up inside

Exercise 3
Lie flat on floor, back straight (**a**). Feet must be held by another person or a heavy item of furniture. Cross arms on chest, raise body to forward position (**b**), then lie back (**c**). Arms can be stretched forward above head before lying back

1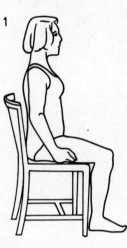

2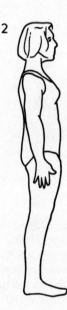

3a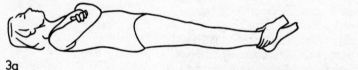

b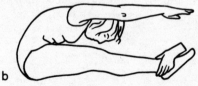

c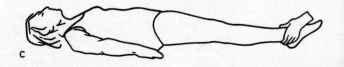

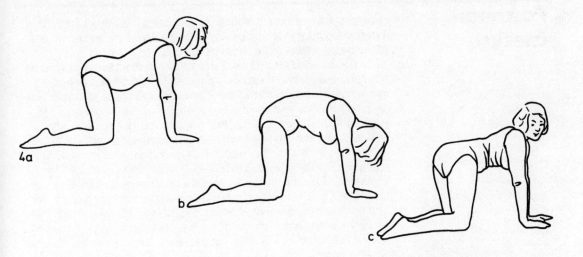

4a

b

c

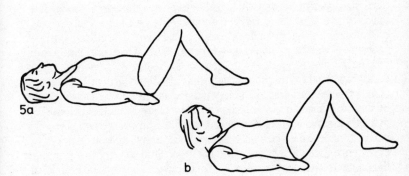

5a

b

Exercise 4
Alternately hollow (**a**) and hump
(**b**) back, abdominal muscles
held tightly
Hollowing back, move head and
hip first to right, then to left (**c**)
Exercise 5
Lie relaxed on floor, with knees
bent, feet flat (**a**). Draw in
abdomen tightly, then raise head
(**b**) Hold for few seconds, then
lower head slowly. Repeat 10
times
Exercise 6
Lie on back with legs straight.
Move feet up and down, and
round in circles (**a**).
Tighten kneecaps, tense leg
muscles (**b**).
Ankles crossed, press thighs
together, and tighten up inside
(**c**)

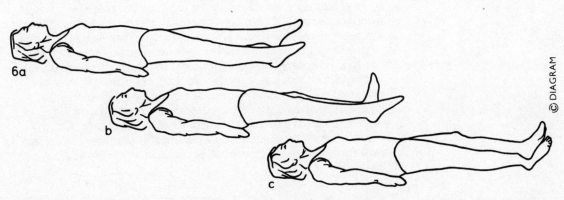

6a

b

c

© DIAGRAM

349

Postnatal checks

Around 4–6 weeks after the birth of your baby, it is important to have a postnatal check which will be carried out either by your doctor or at the hospital where you had your baby.

The doctor or obstetrician will check that the uterus is once again its normal size and that any stitches you may have had are now healed. You will also be weighed to check that you are fairly close to your pre-pregnancy weight; your blood pressure will be checked, as will your urine; and you will be given the opportunity to talk over any anxieties you may have, as well as receiving advice about contraception. It could be, too, that if you had not previously been immunized against German measles (rubella), the injection will be given now. This will protect against certain possible deformities in a future child if you caught rubella during a subsequent pregnancy: but it is important that, if you are immunized at this stage, you do not conceive for the next three months. You will, of course, also have been given details of when the baby should attend a postnatal clinic for developmental checks.

Emotional changes

The delivery of a baby instantly turns the pregnant woman into a "mother." From now on, the responsibility of meeting her infant's needs, of nurturing and educating that child, falls on her shoulders – a burden which can be shared to a variable extent with a partner or other family members. The sudden materialization of the silent floating fetus, the repository of so many hopes and dreams, as a bawling, irascible creature who never sleeps is as likely to provoke the reaction "What have I done?" as "Isn't motherhood wonderful?" With the birth of a first baby comes the realization of lost independence and freedom – life can never be the same again; and alongside emotions of joy and achievement there may be sensations of panic at the apparent fragility of the newborn and lack of confidence in the ability to care for it. Some women do not experience these fears, and some babies do little but feed and sleep; but the postpartum period is still a time of immense physical and emotional adjustment. Hormonal changes can produce violent alterations in mood and feelings about the baby which have no rational explanation.

The baby is, at first, an unknown quantity, and lack of a routine or pattern in the first few weeks can be very tiring and stressful, particularly for women who like to feel in control of their lives. Lack of sleep makes it difficult to think properly and produces irritability. A sense of insecurity about handling the baby may be sensed by it, leading to further tension and lack of confidence. Motherhood is not an instinct that lies dormant in women and surfaces miraculously at childbirth: it has to be learnt. However, as a mother finds out more about her baby and how to treat it, anxiety usually subsides. Child care experts can offer helpful advice about purely practical matters, but ultimately most would agree that each mother knows best about her own child, even if that knowledge is arrived at by the unscientific process of trial and error.

Stress produced by a difficult birth or the abrupt changes in life style after birth may contribute to the development of postpartum depression, particularly if there are other sources of tension or anxiety in the home and family.

POSTNATAL DEPRESSION

The baby blues are rapidly being acknowledged as a significant after-effect of childbirth. Though the intensity ranges from mere anxiety to severe psychosis, most women experience depression of some kind during the postnatal period.

This is not confined to first-time mothers: some women experience depression after the birth of each of their children.

Almost every mother goes through a "low" period about 3 days after the birth, roughly coinciding with the time the breasts begin to produce milk rather than colostrum. Many more women, however (about 10%), experience severe depression on return from hospital. These feelings may last only a matter of days but, particularly in a woman who is physically run down, may persist for a few months. It has been estimated that about 1 in 600 women are affected in this way.

Among the feelings most commonly experienced during depression are confusion, shock, insecurity, inadequacy, fear of inability to cope with the baby, and even disappointment about its sex or appearance. Many women are frightened because they cannot rationalize their anxieties, and many fear a deterioration of their relationship with their partner. Postpartum depression is often attributed to hormonal imbalance (high levels of estrogen and low levels of progesterone) following childbirth or a difficult birth, but evidence is as yet inconclusive since depression has been noted in adoptive as well as natural mothers. Some women react by becoming hyperactive, while others are temporarily unable to cope with the most simple of tasks and may appear confused.

Probably the single most important cause of postpartum depression is society's glorification of motherhood which sets up uncertainty and guilt in women who doubt their ability to be loving, caring mothers.

Treatment for the depression can involve drugs, but it is usually preferable to treat the cause rather than the symptoms. If the mother receives help, support, and constant reassurances from her family, friends and other mothers, the chances of a quick recovery are high.

Postnatal support groups can be of enormous benefit to those mothers suffering from severe depression.

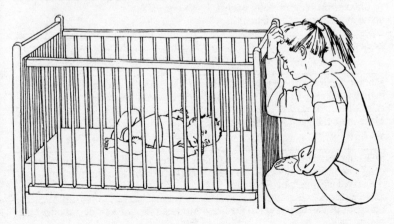

© DIAGRAM

Feeding

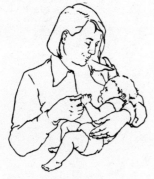

More and more women in western countries are choosing to breastfeed their babies. Most doctors welcome this, for they regard breastfeeding as the safest and most natural method of infant feeding, and many mothers agree that it is an enjoyable and rewarding experience. Some women, however, are uncertain about breastfeeding. Perhaps they have commitments that would make it impossible; or they may find the whole idea distasteful. Even those who had planned to breastfeed may experience problems that force them to turn to bottle feeding.

Current breastfeeding propaganda may make mothers who are bottle feeding their babies feel inadequate and uncaring. This should be ignored. Although breastfeeding is preferable for most babies, the vital physical contact between mother and child can be as intimate, warm, and loving whether the baby is fed by breast or bottle.

Mothers who do decide to breastfeed should ensure that they take sufficient rest as tension and the inability to relax can reduce the milk supply. Diet is another important factor. The lactating mother should ensure that she eats a high calorie diet with particular emphasis on foods rich in protein, vitamins, and calcium.

If the breasts become engorged, use of a cold compress or breast pump to draw up some milk may help. A breast pump can also be used to enable a mother to feed her baby with breast milk if for some reason the baby cannot take milk from the breast. Some pumps convert to a bottle. Sore nipples do not necessarily imply failure with breastfeeding, and can be treated on advice from your doctor, nurse or midwife. Special creams, exposure to warm air and avoiding use of soap often help.

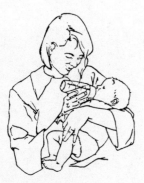

A SUMMARY OF ADVANTAGES AND DISADVANTAGES

Breastfeeding	Bottle feeding
Milk instantly available, at the correct temperature, and sterile	Milk needs mixing and (usually) heating. Equipment must be sterilized
Antibodies protect the baby against some infections for first 6 months	No equivalent
Breast milk is free	Bottles, milk, sterilizing equipment and teats must be purchased
Mother cannot tell how much milk the baby has taken	Mother can see at a glance how much milk the baby has taken
Mother's health and well-being affect the milk supply	Milk supply is independent of the mother
Milk supply usually adjusts itself to the baby's needs but cannot always meet the occasional need for extra milk	Extra feeds present no problem but there can be risk of overfeeding
Some drugs can be passed to the baby via the milk	Mother's medications do not affect the baby

Cot death

Tragically, about 1 baby in 500 dies suddenly, usually between the ages of 8 and 20 weeks. The reasons for this are often unclear, and there may be more than one factor involved. (The term "sudden infant death syndrome" is used if no cause can be found at autopsy.) Autopsy, which is carried out in most countries, may reveal a previously undetected abnormality or unsuspected disease to which the death can be attributed. More often a combination of several otherwise survivable factors, such as a mild respiratory infection, is to blame. Most deaths occur in winter, in cities, and are more common in boys and in families of lower socio-economic status. Children of heavy-smoking mothers are also at increased risk.

In around 7% of cot deaths, an inherited enzyme deficiency is found. The abnormal gene responsible comes from both parents, and each of the couple's children will have a 1 in 4 chance of inheriting the deficiency. If another child (such as an identical twin of a victim) is diagnosed as being affected, special measures can then be taken to try to prevent cot death.

Some babies have a tendency just to stop breathing. Special monitors are available which sound an alarm if breathing stops for a set period of time, but even these cannot be completely effective as sadly it is not always possible to revive the baby.

Babies react unpredictably to infections such as the common cold which are widespread in the winter months. Rarely, too, a child that appeared perfectly well when put into its cot or pram may later be found dead.

Recent research suggests that babies laid down to sleep on their backs are statistically less likely to be victims of SIDS (sudden infant death syndrome) than those who lie prone. This may be because a baby lying on its back is more able to a kick off the covers if it is hot. Hyperthermia (too high a body temperature) has been put forward as a possible factor in some cases.

To have a baby die unexpectedly is a deeply distressing event for the parents and family, and this distress may be added to by the legal necessity for autopsy and, possibly, an inquest. Because the causes of cot death are often obscure, other people sometimes make uninformed comments or judgments. Parents may feel that they are in some way to blame, that they have failed to look after the baby properly, and will need reassuring that there was nothing they could have done differently to prevent their baby's death. Subsequent babies are very unlikely to suffer cot death, but the mother will be encouraged to participate fully in antenatal care, and tests may be performed after the birth if an inherited condition was responsible for an earlier death. A support society can provide information about cot death and may be able to offer the services of a befriender, someone who has personally lost a child and can help bereaved parents deal with their grief.

Pregnancy and after

During pregnancy, a woman's body changes dramatically. Most obvious is its increase in size and weight. As the breasts swell and the belly juts out farther and farther, many women become convinced that their bodies will never return to their former shape, but the body need not alter permanently. Eating correctly ensures that a woman does not put on excess weight, and correct posture and gentle controlled exercise ensure that after the baby is born, the body returns easily and quickly to its previous shape, if not an even better one.

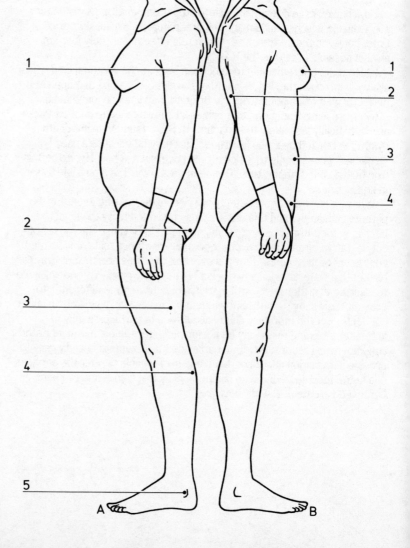

Possible problems
A Pregnancy
1 Backache caused by extra abdominal weight throwing greater strain on the back
2 Hemorrhoids (piles), stretched veins that occur around the back passage (anus), aggravated by constipation
3 Varicose veins
4 Cramp
5 Swollen ankles
B Post-pregnancy
1 Sagging breasts if a good supporting bra is not worn during pregnancy and after
2 Backache from failure to readjust posture after the baby's birth
3 Sagging stomach from lack of exercise
4 Poor bladder control and prolapse of the womb if pelvic floor muscles not strengthened by exercise

CONCEPTION AND CONTRACEPTION

For pregnancy to occur, several conditions must be fulfilled: semen from the man must enter the woman's vagina; the semen must contain healthy male sperm; the sperm must find conditions in the vagina in which they can live; the living sperm must make their way into the woman's uterus and (possibly) the Fallopian tubes; they must find an egg there ready for fertilization; and the egg, once fertilized, must be able to implant itself in the uterus.

By preventing any one of these, contraception is achieved. But it is important to note three things. Firstly, sperm may reach the vagina even if the penis does not enter it. (Sperm ejaculated onto the vulva or surrounding skin can still swim into the vagina.) Secondly, although conditions in the vagina are hostile to sperm, they can live there for 6 hours or more. Any barrier to prevent sperm moving up into the uterus must therefore last at least this long after intercourse. Thirdly, once sperm have reached the uterus, they can live 4 – 5 days or more. So, to avoid conception, there must be at least this time gap between the arrival of sperm in the uterus and the arrival of the egg.

A normal fertile woman experiencing regular intercourse with a normally fertile man stands about a 60% chance of becoming pregnant in any one month. For the woman who intends to have intercourse but not babies, some form of safe, effective contraception is essential.

CONTRACEPTIVE ADVICE

Availability of contraceptive advice is restricted in some countries by legal factors. The range of methods available may also vary, and not all may be subsidized by a public health program. In developing countries, women are more likely to be offered injectable progestogens or sterilization as part of a population control program. But in developed countries, most family doctors will provide advice about contraception. Alternatively, you can visit a family planning clinic whatever your marital status; and you can either go alone or with your partner. You will be asked certain questions about your health, a vaginal examination may be given, and blood pressure and weight will be checked in order to recommend the most suitable methods. Pharmacies, of course, display certain contraceptives (such as condoms, contraceptive sponges and spermicides) for general sale, and dispense others (such as the Pill) on prescription. Routine family planning services are all confidential: but young women may want to check first with an advice center about the likelihood of their parents being informed before contraception is prescribed.

Birth control

©DIAGRAM

Sites of contraceptive
methods
1   Condom
2   Diaphragm (cap)
3   Spermicides
4   IUD
5a Female sterilization
5b Male sterlization

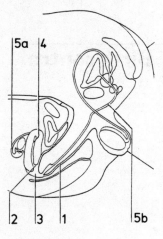

TECHNIQUES OF CONTRACEPTION

There is a wide variety of contraceptives in use today, none of which is ideal. Many concentrate on keeping sperm out of the uterus. Caps and condoms aim to provide a physical barrier; spermicides, a chemical barrier. Withdrawal modifies the sex act, by an attempt at keeping sperm out of the female tract completely. Other techniques – generally more effective – concentrate on interfering with the ovum. Oral contraceptive pills usually affect its development and release. Intrauterine devices (IUDs) are thought to prevent the ovum implanting in the uterus.

Finally, there are two other types of technique. "Rhythm" methods aim (not necessarily successfully) to avoid intercourse at those times of the month when sperm might find an ovum ready for fertilization. Sterilization methods are surgical operations to make one or both partners incapable of having children. Techniques can also be combined to give more effective contraception.

Before children

When a woman starts heterosexual activity, she will probably rely on the man to use a condom. But once regular relations are established, most young women prefer to use continuous methods like the Pill or one of the new IUDS.

Family planning

Many women take the Pill between having children. Others use an IUD, or (less effectively) diaphragm or condoms with spermicides. (An IUD can be removed by a doctor when conception is desired.) Some rely on the rhythm method, despite its failure rate.

After having children

Once a woman's family is complete, she may either return to a contraceptive that she has tried and liked, or she may at this point decide to be sterilized.

Efficiency of contraception
Given here are failure rates for different types of contraception. Figures, based on US surveys, refer to pregnancies per 100 users during their first year of use. Theoretical rates are given first, with actual-use rates given in brackets wherever appropriate.

☐ Actual-use failure rate

■ Theoretical failure rate

— Tubal ligation 0.04
Vasectomy 0.15
IUD 1.3 (5)
Combined pill 0.34 (4-10)
Minipill 1–1.5 (5-10)
Condom 3 (10)
Cap + spermicide 3 (17)
Rhythm (temp) 7 (20)
Rhythm (calendar) 13 (21)
Rhythm (mucus) 2 (25)
Spermicides 3 (20-25)
Withdrawal 9 (20-25)

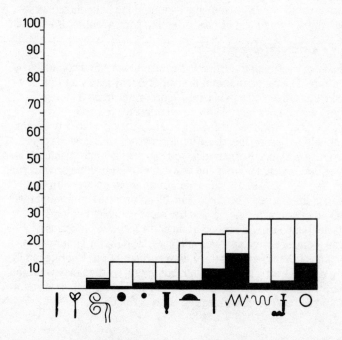

No other form of contraception has been as revolutionary as the Pill. It is easy to use, reversible, and nearly 100% effective provided a woman remembers to take it.

The Pill uses synthetic forms of the hormones estrogen and progesterone. These are produced naturally in the body for a few days in each menstrual cycle and continuously during pregnancy. In each case, they have the effect of inhibiting output of FSH and LH hormones. FSH and LH are needed if follicles are to ripen for ovulation, and this is why no ovulation occurs during pregnancy. The contraceptive pill has a similar effect; and as no ovulation occurs, no ovum is available for fertilization by a sperm. There are two main types of Pill: the **combined pill**, so called because each active pill in the package contains both hormones; and the **continuous or minipill**, in which all pills contain progesterone alone, and which works rather differently.

Contraceptive pill

TAKING THE PILL

The pill can be obtained on prescription from your doctor or from a family planning clinic; and since there are contraindications, you will need to seek guidance as to whether your medical history shows that it will be suitable for you.

Taking the pill is quite easy, the problem is to remember to do so. Most pills come in packets of 21 which are designed to aid memory. To start oral contraception, the first day of a period counts as day 1. Pill-taking begins on day 1 or day 5, whether bleeding has stopped or not. It continues for 21 days when the last pill is taken. A gap of 7 pill-free days follows before the next course, during which withdrawal bleeding occurs. For women who have difficulty in remembering this sequence, some pills are available in packs of 28. But the extra pills are dummies.

The first packet of pills may not give complete protection, and for the first 2 weeks an additional method of contraception should be used if you started on day 5 with the combined pill. (Beginning on day 1 usually gives complete protection.) When starting on the minipill, extra protection is always needed for the first 14 days.

If a combined pill is forgotten, it should be taken within 12 hours of the usual time even if it means taking 2 in 1 day. If more than 2 are missed and the gap between pills is more than 36 hours, then the pack should be finished but a second contraceptive also used. It is important not to forget to take the continuous pill, and it must be taken at the same time every day.

Doctors still disagree on how long a woman should stay on the Pill. On average, women tend to use it for 3 to 4 years. To regain fertility, a woman only needs to stop taking the Pill. But it may be some months before her ovaries are functioning normally and conception can occur.

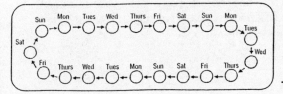

Typical contraceptive pill pack

©DIAGRAM

TYPES OF PILL

The **combined pill** is the most widely-used and effective type. The woman takes one standard pill each day for 21 days, starting on the 5th or 1st day after menstruation, and ending on the 25th or 21st. There is a gap of 7 days during which withdrawal bleeding occurs, then a new pack is started. As well as preventing ovulation, the combined pill affects the uterus lining, so implantation could not occur; and also causes the cervical mucus to thicken, forming a chemical barrier to sperm.

The **continuous** or **minipill** pack contains 28 pills, all active and all containing synthetic progesterone only. One is taken every day, even during menstruation. They work mainly by their effect on the uterus lining and cervical mucus, rather than preventing ovulation.

SIDE-EFFECTS

Most women experience some side-effects when on the Pill. There may be headaches, nausea, swollen or tender breasts, heavier periods although menstruation is generally lighter, and vaginal discharge. But not all women experience these, and most symptoms disappear within the first few months. If they do not, a change of brand may remove any unpleasant side-effects.

No women should take the Pill without consulting a doctor. Pills, and especially high-estrogen ones, carry a risk of blood clotting. The resulting thrombosis may be fatal. This is more likely in women over 35, and pregnancy, of course, itself carries higher risks. Other disorders a doctor must consider before prescribing the Pill include hepatitis, diabetes, migraine, and epilepsy. Opinions vary as to whether the Pill increases the risk of cancer of the breast and cervix, but it appears to protect against cancer of the ovary and endometrium (uterine lining). Estrogen can aggravate some types of existing cancer. Cervical smears are an important part of the medical examinations that accompany advice about taking the Pill.

INJECTABLES

Depo-Provera and **Noristerat** are based on similar hormonal principles to the oral pill, but are given by injection of progestogens every few weeks. They are given to women in about 70 countries, mostly developing ones. In their favor are their effectiveness, when other methods fail through lack of motivation or care. Against them are their possible side-effects and links with disease. Symptoms may include disruption of menstrual bleeding, which may be prolonged, heavy, unpredictable, or absent altogether; vomiting, dizziness, moodiness, headaches, and weight-gain; and rectal bleeding.

Links with disease include subsequent infertility in some women; blood-clotting disorders; and breast and cervical cancer.

Tests have shown that for every 100 women using injectable contraception, less than one will get pregnant in a year. It is most suitable for women who find it hard to remember to take the pill or who cannot use other methods.

Intrauterine devices

The IUD, also known as the "coil" or "loop", is a small plastic device inserted into the uterus by a doctor. It may be left there for several years, and while in place works as a contraceptive without requiring much attention. Intercourse can occur without restriction. Once the IUD is removed, fertility returns in 1 – 12 months.

Comparable practices date back to biblical times, when camel drivers inserted pebbles into the uteri of female camels to keep them from becoming pregnant. Yet how an IUD works is uncertain. Theories are that an IUD makes the ovum pass down the Fallopian tube too rapidly for either fertilization or implantation; that it interferes with the lining of the uterus, so that implantation cannot take place; or that it interferes directly with the implantation process.

The IUD is very effective while in place though some doctors advise use of a spermicide as well around the time of ovulation. But it may fall out, especially during the first few months or at menstruation. Early IUDs were too large for women who had not had children. Recently, smaller designs, usable by all women, have appeared. However, the failure rate may be a little higher.

Many women experience side-effects of heavy periods and/or pain with IUDs. IUDs may also aggravate infection, or (rarely) cause it. There is also a slight risk of perforation of the uterine wall, but significant damage is rare.

If pregnancy does occur, the IUD should be removed, as it increases the risk of miscarriage. Otherwise, though, most types have no effect on a fetus. Many doctors advise renewal of the IUD every 2-3 years.

IUDS
The plastic Lippes Loop (**a**) and Saf-T-Coil (**b**) are the most usual IUDS for women who have had children. The Copper T (**c**) and Copper 7 (**d**) are plastic wound with copper and are suitable for women who have not given birth. The Progestasert-T (**e**), not often used, releases progesterone into the uterus

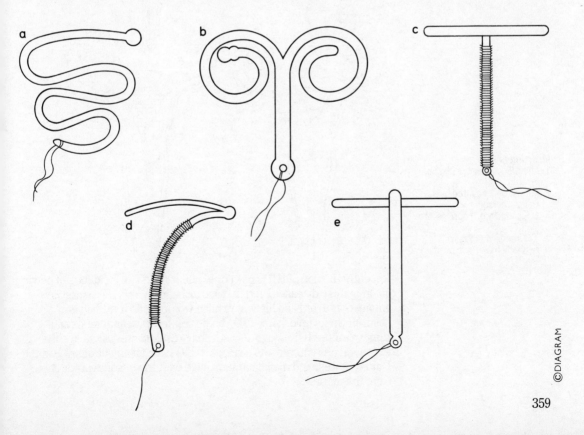

a b c d e

©DIAGRAM

An IUD must only be fitted by a trained person. Most are packed in a thin plastic inserter, which may be passed without difficulty through the cervical canal into the uterus. This is easiest during or just after menstruation. The IUD is pushed through the inserter and takes up its normal shape inside the uterus. This takes only a few minutes. Some women experience discomfort similar to a heavy period pain. This can last for 24 hours with some slight bleeding.

The IUD has nylon threads (or a stem projection) left hanging through the cervix into the vagina. As a result, a woman can – and should – make regular checks to ensure her IUD is still in place.

Tampons can still be used with the device in place, and it has no effect on lovemaking.

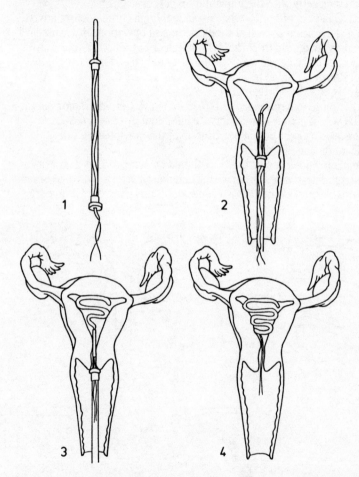

Inserting an IUD
1 The IUD comes in a plastic inserter
2 It must only be fitted by a trained person
3 Once inserted, it springs into shape
4 It is important to test regularly that it is in position

Recently the use of IUDs has come under fire. The incidence of pelvic inflammatory disease (PID) is twice as high among IUD-users as among non-users and highest of all in women who have had no children. In its mild form, PID can be treated with antibiotics and removal of the IUD. Severe cases may result in sterility; and surgery may even be required. As a result, IUDs have fallen out of favor in the United States, and manufacturers have withdrawn some products from the market.

Condoms

The condom (otherwise known as a "sheath," "rubber," or "French letter") is still probably the most widely used contraceptive. It has a long history, dating back some hundreds of years; and popularized mainly as a protection against venereal disease it is now widely recommended as a means of protection against AIDS. It should therefore be used whatever other form of contraception you have, particularly in any new relationship. When used carefully, preferably with a spermicide, it is an effective means of birth control. The condom consists of a thin rubber sheath, about 7in (18cm) long, open at one end and closed at the other. It fits tightly over the man's erect penis. When he ejaculates, his semen is trapped in the sealed end. This prevents sperms from entering the vagina.

Types of condom
There are various types of condoms: plain-ended or teat-ended, and they can be of different colors. Some people complain that condoms reduce sensitivity; but lubricated brands claim to be an improvement.

Using a condom
The condom is taken out of the packet rolled up, and is unrolled onto the erect penis just before intercourse. (This can be incorporated into lovemaking.)

At least 1in (2.5cm) at the tip should be left empty of air to help prevent bursting or leakage. After ejaculation, the man withdraws his penis before his erection subsides. While withdrawing, he should hold the condom so that it does not come off.

For easier insertion of the penis when a condom is used, it is better for a woman to use spermicidal cream or jelly, which gives the advantage of extra contraceptive effectiveness. Condoms have kept their popularity largely because they do not need medical supervision and can be obtained and carried around easily. They are sold in sealed packets and have a maximum shelf-life of 2 years, away from heat. Their chief disadvantage is that due to the annoyance of interrupting lovemaking, some couples may decide to "take the risk" of intercourse without contraception.

The female condom
This consists of a bag which is inserted into the vagina before intercourse to prevent semen from coming into contact with the cervix and vaginal walls. It is held in place by using rings. If used correctly, it should provide protection against pregnancy and sexually transmitted diseases comparable to that given by the male condom.

Types of condom
1 Plain ended
2 Teat ended
3 Teat ended

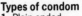

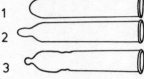

1
2
3

Putting on a condom
1 Carefully remove the rolled condom from its foil packet
2 Unroll about an inch of the condom and squeeze the tip between the thumb and forefinger, leaving an empty space beyond the penis to catch the sperm and prevent the condom bursting
3 Unroll the condom onto the erect penis; either partner can do this. Be careful not to damage the condom with your fingernails
4 After orgasm and before his erection subsides, the man must withdraw his penis from his partner's vagina, taking care to hold the rim of the condom close to his penis as he does so

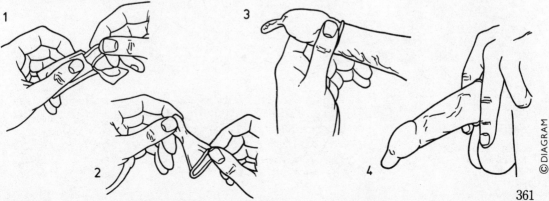

1

2

3

4

©DIAGRAM

The cap

The diaphragm is the best known example of caps that fit across a woman's cervix to act as a barrier to sperm. The diaphragm is a dome-like rubber device. Its rim contains a coiled spring. By itself, the cap is not particularly safe but, used carefully in conjunction with spermicides, it is quite effective. For most women, before the Pill was introduced, the diaphragm was the safest method of contraception available to them.

Putting a diaphragm in place is not very difficult, though at first it needs practice. The woman holds its edges together and pushes it by hand into the vagina so that the bottom edge rests against the vaginal wall behind the bladder. The spring causes the diaphragm to regain its circular shape so that it is held in place. Before insertion, 2-4in (5-10cm) of spermicidal cream or jelly should be squeezed onto the inside (closest to the cervix) or both sides of the cap. The cap should be put into the vagina not more than 2-3 hours before intercourse. After intercourse, it should be left in place for at least 6-8 hours while the sperm die. If intercourse occurs again in that time, more spermicide should first be introduced into the vagina without disturbing the cap which should remain in place for another 6–8 hours.

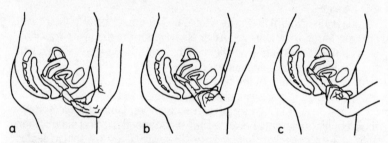

Inserting the cap
a Diaphragm being inserted into the vagina
b Placing the diaphragm over the cervix
c Checking the diaphragm

Diaphragms vary in size. An initial fitting by a doctor or nurse is essential, and the cap should be checked for fit every 6 months, after a pregnancy, or if more than 10 lb (4.5kg) is gained or lost in weight. At home, the cap must be washed after use, according to instructions, and checked carefully for holes.

The cervical cap is much smaller, and fits onto the cervix. It is no longer used except in special cases.

A vault cap is much more rigid than other caps. It fits across the top end of the vagina and is held in place by suction.

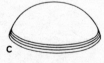
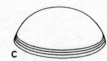

Types of cap
1a Diaphragm
 b Cervical cap
 c Vault cap

2a Diaphragm in place
 b Cervical cap in place
 c Vault cap in place

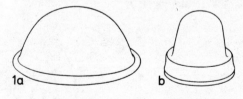
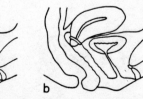
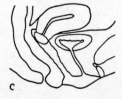

Spermicides

These are chemical products which are inserted into the woman's vagina before sexual intercourse. They act in two ways; by killing the sperm, and by creating a barrier of foam or fluid through which sperm cannot pass into the uterus.

Spermicides come in various forms: creams, jellies, aerosol foams, foaming tablets, suppositories, and C-film, a spermicide-impregnated plastic. But used by themselves, none of these is at all reliable as a contraceptive. If used, they should be combined with another method, such as a cap or condom.

Creams, jellies, and aerosols are sold with a special applicator. Using this, the woman squirts the chemical high up into her vagina. This should be done as near to intercourse as possible, and certainly no more than one hour before, as effectiveness is only temporary.

Suppositories and tablets come in solid form and must be inserted by hand deep into the vagina. Suppositories are cone-shaped and melt at body temperature: the tablets dissolve and foam in the vagina's moisture. Both should be inserted 15 minutes before intercourse.

C-film consists of a small square of soluble plastic which can either be inserted into the vagina or placed on the tip of the man's penis before it enters the vagina. It dissolves, releasing spermicide; but is no more reliable than other spermicides (and less so than some).

Some women find that spermicides irritate their genitals.

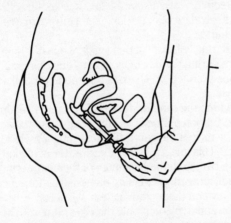

Using a spermicide applicator

THE SPONGE

This consists of a spermicide-impregnated sponge which is inserted into the vagina before intercourse and must be left there for 6 hours afterwards. The sponge can be bought from a pharmacy and is thrown away after a single use. Its effectiveness is likely to be about the same as that of other spermicides.

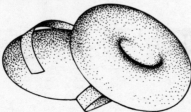

Contraceptive sponge

©DIAGRAM

Rhythm method

With this method, a couple do not have intercourse during the part of the woman's menstrual cycle when she can conceive – that is when a fertilizable egg is available.

The menstrual cycle lasts (in principle) 28 days. During this, the egg is available for fertilization for only about 1 day (the 24 hours that follow ovulation). However, there is no direct sign of ovulation, only of menstruation. Ovulation typically occurs halfway between the menstruation – on about the 15th day. So a woman can count forward 14 days from the start of her last menstruation, to guess when ovulation will occur. But the menstrual cycle is seldom perfectly regular. In most women, menstruation is erratic when periods return after the birth of a baby, and in a quarter of women it is always fairly erratic. (Other women may have a record of regular menstruation for years, followed by sudden unexpected irregularity.) Even where menstruation is regular, ovulation need not occur at the mid-point, the 15th day. It can occur anywhere from 16 to 12 days before the start of the next menstruation. (In fact, ovulation is sometimes induced by the stimulus of sexual intercourse). Finally, sperms can live in the woman's cervix for up to 72 hours and sometimes longer; so even if intercourse takes place four days before ovulation, it may on rare occasions cause conception.

The **calendar rhythm method**, just based on dates, is therefore not very effective, even if several days are kept free from intercourse around the likely date of ovulation. The **temperature rhythm method** is better.

A woman normally has a sudden small rise in her body's temperature during the day of ovulation, due to increased progesterone production. Use of a thermometer and a record chart show this rise.

But by the time the temperature rise is actually recorded, the possible fertilization period is usually over. (Also the action of the progesterone makes the cervical mucus unfavorable to sperm penetration.) This gives a "safe period" after ovulation, from the temperature rise up to the beginning of the next period. But it gives no safe period after the beginning of menstruation since there is no way of telling when the next ovulation will occur. Between menstruation and ovulation, only the **calendar method** gives any indication of safety.

Temperature method
a Menstruation
b Unsafe days ovulation likely
c Ovulation
d Safe days

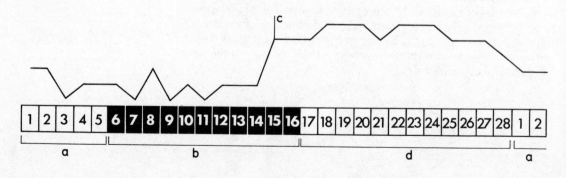

The mucus method

This natural method of birth control relies upon recognition of the changes in the nature and quantity of cervical mucus during the menstrual cycle. Like other natural methods, it is easier to practice if the woman has a regular menstrual cycle and a cooperative partner. A calendar is probably the best way of keeping track until the woman is familiar with the method and her own cycle. Intercourse on unsafe days must be avoided or some form of protection used.

Cervical mucus can be sampled by inserting a finger or speculum into the vagina, and *regular* examination of the kind of mucus being produced is important to the success or otherwise of the method. The signs described *below* relate to a *28-day cycle;* women with a shorter cycle should be aware of the fact that mucus may be harder to detect if it is mixed with menstrual flow.

For up to 3 days after menstruation has ceased, normally no mucus is produced and the woman may be aware of vaginal dryness; these days are fairly safe. When mucus starts to appear, it is at first cloudy and thick, and then becomes more profuse and thin for about 2 days (peak days). Days from first signs of mucus until 4 days after the peak days are "unsafe." Mucus production then tapers off toward the time of menstruation and becomes thick and cloudy once more; days from the 4th after peak until menstruation are "fairly safe."

In practice, most women using natural methods of birth control combine the rhythm and mucus methods in order to pinpoint as closely as possible the time of ovulation and "safe" days.

Mucus method
The diagram shows monthly changes in cervical secretions
a Menstruation
b Unsafe days
c Ovulation (unsafe)
d Fairly safe days
e Moderate amount, thick, cloudy
f Increasing amount, thick to thin, mixed cloudy and clear
g Maximum amount, very thin and slippery, clear
h Decreasing amount, thin, mixed cloudy and clear
i Tiny amount, thick, cloudy

▦ Thick mucus

⬚ Thin mucus

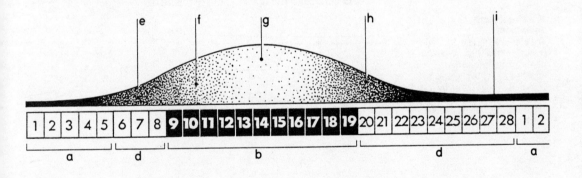

Withdrawal

Withdrawal (or "coitus interruptus") is the oldest and simplest method of birth control. The man takes his penis out of the woman's vagina just before his orgasm. His semen is ejaculated outside her body. Used with great care, withdrawal may be effective, but only if every drop of semen is not only kept out of the vagina but also right away from the vaginal lips. It is impossible to be sure of this, because some fluid containing live sperm may "weep" from the penis before orgasm; and in the pleasure of orgasm, the man may not withdraw properly.

Continued use of withdrawal can also be frustrating. The woman in particular may not be able to relax through fear that the man may not withdraw.

Post-coital methods

If a single act of unprotected intercourse takes place at around the time of ovulation, chances of conception are up to 20%; one act of unprotected intercourse at any time during an entire menstrual cycle carries about a 4% risk. If these risks are unacceptable, for example in cases of rape, there are three methods available.

The "morning after" pill

This method consists of taking large doses of synthetic estrogen. The pills must be started within 72 hours of intercourse and are 98% effective in preventing implantation of a fertilized ovum in the uterus, but the high doses of estrogen can cause unpleasant, even dangerous side-effects such as nausea and vomiting, headache, and tendency to form blood clots. Because of these side-effects, the morning after pill may only be prescribed once.

Insertion of an IUD

This can be effective up to 5 days after intercourse, by preventing implantation of the fertilized ovum in the lining of the uterus. It is not used if there is a possibility that the woman has a pre-existing infection or may have acquired one at the time of intercourse. Once inserted, the IUD may be left in place to provide long-term contraceptive cover.

Menstrual extraction may be used if conception and implantation have already occurred, and is in effect a very early abortion. It may not be widely available in some countries for this reason. Also known as menstrual regulation, it can be performed up to 2 weeks after a period was due. Suction is used to extract the uterus lining and also any embryo tissue that may be present. It takes about 10 minutes and a woman can leave the doctor's office unaided.

Menstrual extraction equipment
The uterus lining is extracted through a small hollow, flexible plastic cannula (**a**). This is attached either to a specially designed syringe (**b**) or, by means of a hose (**c**), to an electrically powered suction machine.

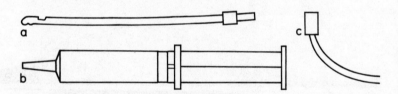

Extraction procedure
The doctor inserts a speculum (**a**) and washes the cervix with antiseptic. The cervix is held in place with a tenaculum (**b**), and a local anesthetic is then applied. A lubricated cannula (**c**) is next inserted into the uterus. Suction (**d**) is then applied, and the cannula moved around the uterine cavity until all the tissue is removed.

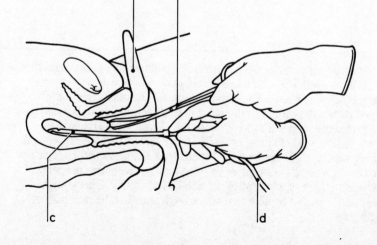

Sterilization

FEMALE STERILIZATION

Sterilization is the most effective form of birth control. But it is also the most final. As yet, no reversible method has been perfected, which means that a woman considering the operation must be absolutely certain of the decision before undergoing sterilization.

For women who are quite certain that they do not want any more children, sterilization is becoming more popular. The operation consists basically of cutting, tying, or removing all or part of the Fallopian tubes. As a result, eggs can no longer pass from the ovaries to the uterus and the sperm is unable to reach the egg. Provided that the operation is done correctly – there have been rare instances of the Fallopian tubes rejoining – sterilization is totally effective.

Sexual interest should remain unchanged and the menstrual cycle continues as normal. Some women, in fact, gain increased enjoyment from sex once the fear of pregnancy has been completely removed.

There are a number of different ways in which a woman can be sterilized. All require hospitalization but the time needed for recovery varies.

Tubal ligation

This is the most commonly used method of sterilization for women. It can be done in various ways. Traditionally, a general anesthetic is given and a 2-3in (5-7cm) incision made in the abdomen, just above the pubic hair. A piece is cut out of the Fallopian tubes, and the ends are then tied and folded back into the surrounding tissue. This operation is often performed after childbirth, although less reliable at this stage. After some days in hospital, a woman should then rest for some weeks (which for a working woman with children may be difficult). The same operation can be done by making a much smaller incision in the upper vagina. No scar is visible and the recovery period is much shorter. But it is a much more skilled and difficult operation.

Endoscopic technique

This is a more recent development in female sterilization. It involves the use of an instrument known as a laparoscope, which consists of a fine tube which conducts light and is connected to a telescope. This is inserted through a small cut in the abdomen. It can also be inserted through the vagina, and is used to light up and inspect the Fallopian tubes. Very fine forceps are inserted, either through the same cut or though a second smaller one, and an electro-current is passed along them to cauterize the Fallopian tubes. Only 2 tiny scars will remain and the recovery time is very short.

Hysterectomy

Until quite recently, a hysterectomy – which involves the complete removal of the uterus – was a fairly widespread means of sterilization. However, it is not now generally recommended for birth control purposes, though it is an operation that many women have to undergo for other reasons.

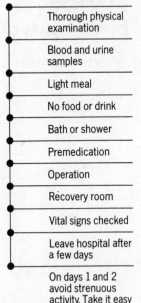

Timetable of events for laparoscopic sterilization

Thorough physical examination

Blood and urine samples

Light meal

No food or drink

Bath or shower

Premedication

Operation

Recovery room

Vital signs checked

Leave hospital after a few days

On days 1 and 2 avoid strenuous activity. Take it easy

MALE STERILIZATION

A **vasectomy** is a safe, simple, surgical operation in which each vas deferens – the duct leading from each testis to the penis – is cut and tied off. As a result, the semen a man ejects no longer contains sperm.

Apart from instances where the cut tubes have rejoined, the operation is always completely effective. It does not alter a man's ability to have an orgasm or to ejaculate. But the operation is rarely reversible, which again means that a man and his partner must be absolutely sure before undergoing a vasectomy.

The operation generally lasts under half an hour. For the majority of vasectomy operations, a local anesthetic only is needed. Either 1 or 2 very small cuts are made on or near the scrotum. A piece about 1½in (3.8 cm) long is removed from each duct, and the cut ends are then folded back and tied. Once the operation is over the man can generally return straight home and can be back at work within 2 or 3 days. The most common after-effects are likely to be some soreness and bruising.

A vasectomy is not immediately effective, however, as there are usually some sperms stored in the seminal vesicles, above the cut. For this reason, a second method of contraception must be used, until two successive follow-up tests of the semen show negative sperm counts (perhaps 2 or 3 months after the operation).

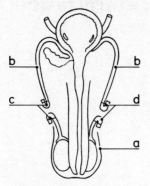

Vasectomy
Under a local anesthetic and through a small incision in the scrotum, each vas deferens is isolated and a small piece cut out. The cut ends are then folded back and tied. The scrotal incisions are then stitched.
a Scrotum
b Vas deferens
c Tied ends

Unsatisfactory methods of birth control

Breastfeeding mothers were once thought to be unable to conceive in the first 6 weeks after childbirth, if their periods had not returned. But, in fact, though the likelihood of conception is reduced, contraception is still necessary.

Douching – washing out the vagina after intercourse – is a completely ineffective method of birth control. Not only can sperm reach the cervix within 90 seconds, but the effect of squirting liquid into the vagina could be to help the sperm on their way.

It was once believed that if a woman did not have an **orgasm** she would not conceive. This is obviously untrue; many women do not have orgasms but still become pregnant.

Claimed to increase sensitivity, **American or Grecian tips** are short rubber condoms that fit over the tip of the penis only. Not only do they fail to increase sensitivity, they are also likely to come off in the vagina and so are an unreliable contraceptive.

The **gamic appliance** is also unsatisfactory. It consists of a small rubber bag attached to the end of a thin rubber tube. The tube is pushed down the urethra of a man's penis so that, when he ejaculates, the semen is held in the bag. Very rarely used, this method is likely to cause damage to the urethra or infection.

Recent developments

Research continues into alternative contraceptive methods which are better tolerated, less risky, more convenient and more reliable than existing ones.

Many experiments are aimed at contraceptives for women. Some of these are based on concepts already in use: sex hormones to inhibit ovulation or barrier methods. The **subcutaneous hormone implant** and the **contraceptive vaginal ring (CVR)** work by slowly releasing the hormone "levonorgestrel." The implant can be left in place under the skin for up to 7 years, but the CVR is removed after 3 weeks – before menstruation.

The **intracervical device** is a new approach to barrier contraception and can be used even by women with uterine and menstrual abnormalities. Positioned in the cervical canal, the mushroom-shaped cap blocks the entry of sperm into the uterus. But it also incorporates a one-way valve allowing the menstrual flow to be carried away, which means it does not have to be removed during periods.

The discovery and cloning of **inhibin** – a hormone secreted by the testes and ovaries – is particularly promising. It opens the door to a whole new generation of contraceptives. Indeed, this hormone, which plays an important role in regulating fertility in both sexes, could perhaps form the basis of a unisex pill. Inhibin features in the hormone cycle at a level where its use in this way would not suppress the libido. However, it remains questionable as to whether a woman would, indeed, trust that her partner had taken such a form of contraception.

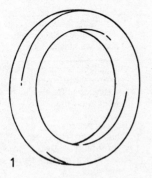

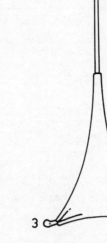

New developments
1 Slow-release progestogen-impregnated intravaginal ring
2 Small time-release hormone pellets for implantation into a woman's forearm or buttock
3 Intracervical device designed to release either progestogen or a spermicidal substance

Health hazards

The lists below contain symptoms which you may notice if you use the contraceptive methods concerned. Some, such as heavy menstrual bleeding with an IUD, are recognized to be common and to some extent inevitable; others marked in *italic* should cause you to seek a physician's advice.

	Hazards	Symptoms	Contraindications
Contraceptive pill	Higher risk than normal of: Thrombosis (up to 10 times greater than normal) Heart attack (up to 5 times greater than normal) and increasing with age High blood pressure Cervical erosion Subsequent temporary infertility Very small risk of liver tumor	Headache (*severe headache or migraine*) Nausea Fatigue Tenderness or swelling of the breasts Gain in weight Lessening of sexual response Increased vaginal discharge and susceptibility to moniliasis *Skin reactions* *Susceptibility to urogenital infections* *Chest pains* *Severe pain or swelling of the leg* *Breathlessness* *Visual disturbance*	Women who are more likely to suffer serious side-effects include: Over 35s Smokers Obese Diabetics Epileptics Those with varicose veins or family history of clotting disorder Those who have been taking the pill for more than 5 years
IUD	Ectopic pregnancy Infections Perforation of the uterus	Cramps Heavy menstruation *Signs of infection, such as heavy or malodorous discharge* *Abdominal pain*	Not suitable for women with: Pelvic inflammatory disease or other infections Heavy menstruation Endometriosis Bleeding disorders Abnormally shaped uterus (including fibroids)
Spermicides	Not very reliable unless used in combination with other methods	Vaginal irritation	
Diaphragm	None	Vaginal irritation from spermicides	Not suitable for women with prolapse of the uterus
Condom	Effectiveness relies heavily on proper use	Vaginal irritation	
Female sterilization	Risks associated with anesthetic and infection at operation Development of abdominal adhesions	Pain	Not suitable for women who might change their minds about wanting children
Vasectomy	Risk of infection at operation	Pain and bruising	Not suitable for men (or their partners) who might change their minds about wanting children
Injectables	Prolonged infertility (up to 2 years) Heavy or irregular bleeding (may be difficult to detect return of menstrual cycle or pregnancy) Increased risk of blood clotting disorders Possible adverse effects on fetus if given early in pregnancy Possible increase in risk of cervical and breast cancer	Gain in weight Bloating Vomiting Headache (*severe headache or migraine*) Depression Fatigue Lessening of sexual response Swelling or tenderness of the breasts *Heavy or continuous bleeding*	Not suitable for: Women who require only short-term contraception or who can use alternative methods Women who may already be pregnant Women who have just given birth or had a miscarriage or abortion Women who are breastfeeding

Termination of pregnancy

Weeks

(**4**) First missed period

(**6**) Clinical diagnosis of pregnancy possible

(**13**) Risks from abortion rise

(**17**) Fetal movements may be felt

(**28**) Fetus legally viable. Abortions are not generally carried out after this time unless continuation of pregnancy is the greater threat to the mother's life

40

Termination is a controversial and emotive issue, and the decision to end a pregnancy is rarely easy. For most women, however, whether the pregnancy has resulted from lack, misuse or failure of contraception, the problems of continuing with an unwanted pregnancy are generally greater than those of terminating it.

Confirming pregnancy
A missed period is usually the first sign of pregnancy. Others may be feelings of sickness, revulsion against some foods, and frequent urination. Fourteen days after the first missed period, a urine test can confirm pregnancy. Although there are home-testing kits, these are not always entirely reliable, and a sample of early-morning urine in a clean container can be taken to a doctor, clinic, or pregnancy-testing association. Results are often known within a few hours.

Choosing an abortion
Once a woman has decided to have an abortion, time becomes important. Although in some parts of the world abortions can be carried out until the 28th week (the fetus is then legally considered to have a separate existence), they are not often performed after the 12th week, and only very rarely after the 20th.

Abortion laws
Abortion is the most widely used method of birth control in the world. It has been estimated that nearly 1 in 4 pregnancies are terminated either legally or illegally. There has been a gradual liberalization of abortion laws and today well over 75% of the world's population live in countries where abortion is, to a greater or lesser extent, legal; but laws and facilities vary.

Abortion advice
If you do find you are pregnant but are not sure you want to be, your doctor, family planning clinic or a pregnancy advisory service are the people to see for guidance and information about abortion techniques and procedures.

Abortion techniques

ENDOMETRIAL ASPIRATION

Known also as "interception," "menstrual regulation," or "menstrual suction," this is a preemptive abortion technique – meaning that it can be performed for up to 2 weeks after a period was due – that is before a pregnancy can be positively confirmed. (See p.366 for its use as a post-coital method of contraception.)

Just occasionally, this process has been used not as an abortion technique, but as a means of avoiding menstrual discomfort by extracting the uterus lining in one quick operation. It is then given the different name of "menstrual extraction."

DILATATION AND EVACUATION (D&E)

Also called "vacuum curettage," "suction abortion," or "STOP" (suction termination of pregnancy), D&E is the most common method of abortion today. It is quick, easy to perform (it is increasingly carried out in outpatient clinics), and there is low risk of complication. Essentially, the fetus is removed from the uterus by suction through a narrow tube inserted through the cervix. D&E is normally carried out 7–12 weeks from the last menstrual period, after which time the fetus is too large for D&E to be performed safely.

Procedure

Very little preparation is needed. The woman's blood type is checked, and she should not eat for about 6 hours before the operation. Pubic hair need not be shaved. After an internal examination, the speculum is inserted and the patient given an anesthetic – local or general.

Recovery

The abortion takes about 10 minutes: the rest period afterwards, about 2–3 hours. When D&E is performed in hospital, patients often stay in overnight. Recovery is fast, though strenuous activity should be avoided for a couple of days. There is usually some bleeding, possibly with mild cramps, for up to 7 days. The normal period starts 4–6 weeks after the abortion. Most doctors advise that use of tampons and also sexual intercourse should be avoided for 2–4 weeks to prevent possible infection.

Dilatation and evacuation
1 Dilatation
a Speculum holding vaginal walls open
b Dilator to widen cervical canal
2 Evacuation
a Speculum
b Curette with plastic tube connected to suction apparatus and used to remove contents of the uterus

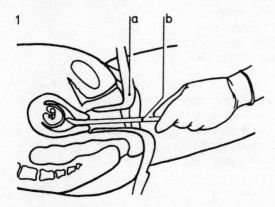

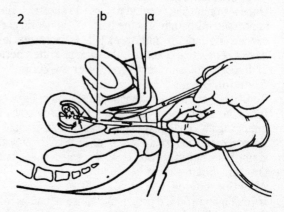

DILATATION AND CURETTAGE (D&C)

Before the development of suction abortion, D&C was the standard method used for pre-12th-week abortions. It is still a general gynecological procedure used for such problems as heavy periods. After dilating the cervix, the uterus contents are scraped away with a curette. D&C is more painful, requires general anesthetic, and carries more risks of perforation and infection than a suction abortion.

Dilatation

A series of polished metal dilators are used, the largest being about the width of a finger. A speculum holds the vaginal walls open. Once dilation is complete, the cervix is held steady with a tenaculum. A curette is then inserted into the uterus until it touches the fetus.

Curettage

When curettage only is used as an abortion technique, the cervix is first dilated as described above. A curette – a thin metal instrument with a spoon-like-tip – is then inserted into the uterus. The fetus and placenta are scraped loose and are removed with forceps.

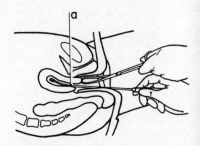

Curettage
Following dilation of the cervix, a curette is inserted and the uterus is scraped of unwanted material
a The curette

INDUCED MISCARRIAGE

Currently, the usual technique for late abortion is to induce miscarriage. Since it is so similar to normal childbirth, this can be a much more distressing experience than abortion methods for early pregnancy. There is also more potential risk, such as hemorrhage, shock, infection, and incomplete abortion. That is why late abortions are always carried out in hospital, and are rare.

Procedure

Under local anesthetic, an amniocentesis can be performed. Fluid is withdrawn and replaced by a miscarriage-inducing agent, normally a concentrated saline (salt) solution. The fetus dies, and in 6–48 hours the cervix dilates. Contractions occur and the fetus and placenta are expelled. Recently, use has also been made of prostaglandins (naturally occurring hormones). These stimulate contractions of the womb, causing miscarriage more rapidly than saline solution, and are safer. They are often given via the vagina in an easier, safer and more speedy method.

Induced miscarriage
a Amniotic fluid is withdrawn
b Saline solution is injected into the uterus

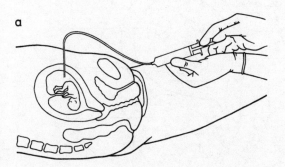
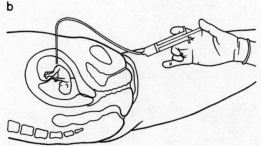

©DIAGRAM

HYSTEROTOMY

Hysterotomy (not to be confused with hysterectomy) is a method of late abortion that is rarely used today. It is similar to a mini-Cesarian section, and involves major surgery and hospitalization. It is the most complicated of all abortion techniques, and carries the highest risks.

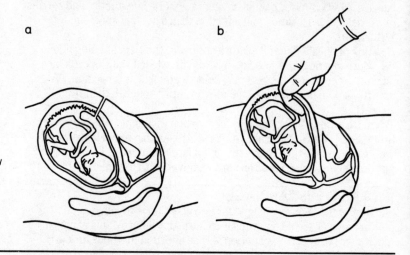

a   b

Hysterotomy
a Under general anesthetic, incisions are made in the abdominal wall, usually below the pubic hairline
b The contents of uterus – fetus and placenta – are removed through the incisions, which are then sewn up

Problems and health hazards

ILLEGAL TERMINATION

The diagram shows some of the physical damage that can result from illegal abortions. "Back-street" and self-induced abortions are still common: worldwide they cause 30–50% of all maternal deaths from pregnancy and childbirth. Various techniques are used, most of them either unsuccessful or highly dangerous. Inserting objects or pumping fluid and air into the uterus are among the most common methods and are often fatal. One argument for complete legalization is to prevent catastrophes that result from crude, unhygienic abortions.

Possible physical consequences of illegal abortion
a Punctured intestine, possibly leading to peritonitis, septicemia and intra-peritoneal hemorrhage
b Infection of Fallopian tubes
c Perforation into the peritoneal cavity
d Infection of the ovaries
e Intrauterine infection
f Perforation through placental site causing internal hemorrhage
g Blood clot (possibly infected) or air embolism (possibly lethal)
h Fetal malformation
i Laceration of cervix
j Laceration of vagina

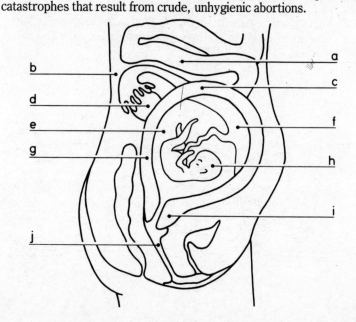

Emotional adjustments to termination

The decision whether to have an abortion is not lightly made. In many countries, the medico-legal restrictions governing the availability of abortion ensure that it is only performed for a definite set of "good reasons." Many women, therefore, have considerable difficulty in obtaining abortions through the state medical system and may even be determined enough to leave their home country. In view of these problems and the fact that a woman often has to struggle to do what she feels is the best thing for herself and others, emotions such as guilt and regret are less common sequels to abortion than might be imagined.

Problems are most likely to arise if the woman has been pressurized into making the decision to go ahead with abortion before she has come to terms with being pregnant, or because it is something that other people want for her and for themselves. If this is the case, it may be much harder for her to deal with the consequences of a decision which she feels was not her own. Anger at others may be directed inward and result in depression, and there may be long-lasting grief.

Women who make their own decision about abortion may also have mixed feelings. They may feel in some way guilty or inadequate for not having managed to prevent the pregnancy in the first place, and upset that they seem unable to maintain control over their fertility. Unless the abortion can be obtained on a day patient basis, the procedure causes some degree of disruption to routine, which can also be a source of stress. Rigid moral or religious codes also of course make the decision of women who would like children but are contemplating abortion on therapeutic grounds much harder.

However, once the decision has been reached and the abortion performed, the overwhelming sensation is likely to be that of relief that it is all over. But some women feel angry at the unnecessary distress they were subjected to in getting the abortion or the way in which it was carried out. It is not uncommon for there to be distaste for sex for some time afterward, particularly if the woman lacks confidence in the contraceptive method she is using. On the other hand, some women find that they gain awareness of a strength and resilience that they never recognized in themselves: having weighed the facts and made their decision, they have shouldered responsibility and done what they thought was right.

Sources of support

Pre-abortion counseling is extremely valuable in helping to sort out what to do about an unwanted pregnancy, but sadly it is not always available. Partners may be supportive, but are often too closely involved to understand fully the conflicting emotions a woman may be enduring both before and after abortion. Close friends or family who do not hold condemnatory views are likely to be the most easy people to talk to, especially if they have shared the experience of abortion themselves.

If depression develops and there is no-one else to talk to, helplines such as the Samaritans guarantee an unbiased, non-judgmental ear.

©DIAGRAM

THE MIDDLE YEARS

In the past, the approach of the menopause was usually viewed with alarm, particularly as women generally age so much more rapidly at this stage of life than do men. Today, by contrast, many women find that life improves greatly after the emotional and physical changes of their middle years. Some also say it is no longer the major hurdle it used to be, now that hormone replacement therapy is increasingly prescribed. But is HRT actually all it is cracked up to be? Are there any contraindications? And could it even be harmful in some instances? Be health-wise, and make these valuable years possibly the very best of your life.

Chapter seven

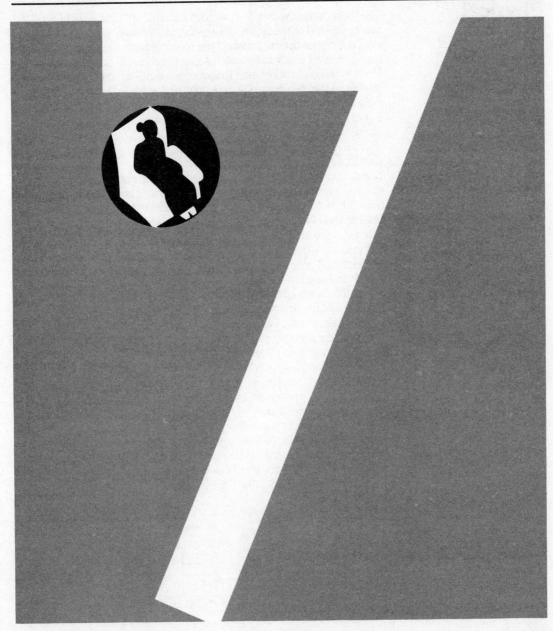

Physical changes

The menopause (also called the "climacteric" or "change of life") marks the end of the reproductive part of a woman's life. Its chief outward sign is the cessation of the monthly period. Some women also experience a variety of symptoms due to change in hormonal balance. Parts of the body may begin to age noticeably, but most women should be able to remain physically, mentally, and sexually as active after the menopause as before it. Some see the menopause as a time of regret. For others, it represents a welcome release from biological demands on the body.

ONSET OF THE MENOPAUSE

The menopause begins at different ages in different individuals. The usual age is around 50, though a few women start the menopause in their 30s, while onset in others is delayed into the 50s. But about half of all women lose their capacity to bear children by the age of 50, and only 5% remain capable beyond 55.

There are many reasons for variation in the time of onset. Race is one factor. White women of northern European stock tend to reach the climacteric late if they entered puberty early, and early if they entered puberty late. With Mediterranean and black women, both puberty and menopause come relatively early. Then, too, women of some families cease menstruating early, others late, for their racial group. Thus heredity plays a part; and a high living standard also tends to prolong a woman's reproductive life, while poor conditions shorten it. Childbirth is also relevant: if a woman has a child after she has passed 40, her menopause may be delayed; and the menopause may be hastened in women who have never given birth.

Abnormal variations

Some women experience exceptionally early menopause for no apparent reason. In the majority of cases, however, exceptionally early menopause occurs as a result of disease or medical treatment. Disease of the pituitary gland can trigger the event, as can medical irradiation of the ovaries, or their surgical removal; or, of course, a hysterectomy.

Onset of the menopause

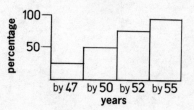

MENSTRUAL CHANGES

The first sign of the menopause is often periods becoming lighter, or later, than usual, and a woman may miss a period altogether. Sometimes periods are light one month and heavy the next; and this heaviness may be marked if the period is late although there may be other causes for heavy or irregular bleeding. This is why a woman should never put heavy or irregular bleeding down to the menopause but should see her doctor. Gradually, months or perhaps years later, the periods cease completely. (In some women, however, they may stop abruptly.)

Twelve months after the last period, a woman of 50 plus is estimated to be infertile. However, it is safest if she continues with contraception for 2 years after her last period to avoid any risk of pregnancy; and a woman under 50 should certainly do this.

Because women on the pill appear to continue menstruating, doctors often recommend periodic switching to another method of contraception after the age of 42 to see if the menopause has indeed begun; but it should be noted that the combined pill is not currently recommended for any woman over 45, or 35 if she smokes.

HOW THE CHANGE OCCURS

The diagram shown *bottom left* reminds us how the ovaries and uterus function in a normal 28-day menstrual cycle. FSH and LH hormones (produced by the pituitary gland at the base of the brain) stimulate one of the ovaries to release a ripened egg into the nearest Fallopian tube. That egg is then available for fertilization by a male sperm. Meanwhile, the follicle inside which the egg has developed is producing hormones too, first estrogen and then also progesterone. These cause the lining of the uterus to thicken in preparation for implantation if the egg is fertilized. If the egg is not fertilized, the thickened lining breaks down, and the woman experiences her menstrual period.

In middle age, aging ovaries cease to respond to FSH and LH, though secretions of these increase. As a result, fewer follicles are formed, and fewer release eggs; estrogen and progesterone output from the ovaries falls off; the uterus lining ceases to thicken, and menstrual bleeding changes pattern and eventually stops; and the uterus and ovaries start to shrink.

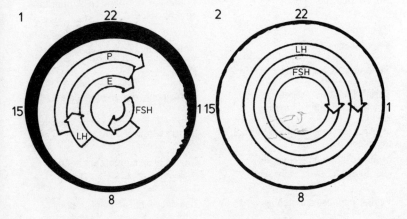

The menopause
1 Before the change
2 After the change
FSH Follicle stimulating hormone
LH Luteinizing hormone
E Estrogen
P Progesterone
◼ Uterine lining

©DIAGRAM

379

Menopausal symptoms

In many women, loss of periods is the only sign of the menopause. However, some women experience other symptoms for up to 10 years before the periods cease. Hot flashes, or flushes, are most common. These are a response of the hypothalamus gland to the falling estrogen level in the body. They often start as a warm feeling in the chest, moving to the neck and face, which color up. The rash may spread to the rest of the body, perhaps with a prickling sensation. Sweating sometimes follows. Hot flashes can last up to 15 minutes and may occur several times a day, or they may be transient and infrequent. Some coincide with the due dates of periods. Hot flashes may start before periods stop and recur over 2 or 3 years. The worst types cause discomfort and depression, and "night sweats" may even break up sleep.

Hormonal change may cause itching in any part of the body, but especially in the genitals. Vaginal dryness is also typical.

Many physical symptoms have been blamed on the menopause, and some doctors talk of a "menopausal syndrome." Apart from symptoms already described, this might include dizzy spells, headaches, and insomnia; fatigue and lack of energy; abdominal bloatedness; digestive troubles including pain, flatulence, constipation, and/or diarrhea; and breathlessness and palpitations.

But all these symptoms can be very variable from day to day, and many women do not experience them at all. In fact, no direct link with the menopause has been proved. (Some, though, can be signs of illness, so always check with a doctor.)

At the menopause, appetite often becomes variable and may increase, while the body's energy needs fall. Weight gain results unless food intake is controlled.

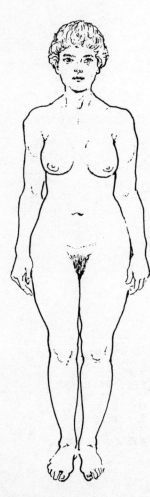

AT THE MENOPAUSE

Signs and symptoms	Treatment
Fatigue, headaches, dizzy spells, insomnia; moodiness, forgetfulness, irritability, anxiety, depression.	Normally no treatment; symptoms eventually disappear. Short-term prescription of tranquilizers or anti-depressants in severe cases; possibly control by hormone therapy in very severe ones
Hot flashes and sweating	Control by hormone treatment in severe cases
Palpitations	None if only due to menopause
Breathlessness	None if only due to menopause
Tendency to gain weight	Diet control
Variable appetite, digestive troubles, abdominal bloating	None if only due to menopause
Ovaries stop producing eggs and, therefore, estrogen	An irreversible change
Menstrual bleeding changes character and eventually stops	Normally no treatement needed. If bleeding occurs after the menopause, see a doctor
Vaginal dryness and itching	Use of creams and ointments.

Emotional changes

The menopause marks a changing point in a woman's life. From now on she is incapable of bearing children, and for those who had wanted to have children but were unable, it may be a sad time. The menopause is an unmistakable reminder that we are getting older; the physical symptoms may make some women feel exhausted, irritable and unattractive to their partner. Yet the middle years can be a very rewarding time of life: much depends upon non-physiological factors such as home life, work and the range of social activities available to each woman.

For many mothers, the menopause coincides with the teenage years of their children, when there may be worries about such matters as their emotional difficulties, examinations, antisocial behavior and leaving home. Long-term stress caused by these problems creates a background on which may be superimposed the physical stresses of the menopause, and it can sometimes be hard to be objective about where the real source of distress lies. Some women may be performing a balancing act with children and fruitful careers, and find that the menopause is one strain too much. Yet women who are busy, who have plenty of interests and little time to think, often seem relatively unaffected by "psychological" symptoms. There may be relief that worries about contraception are finally over, and some of the most distressing physical symptoms of the menopause can be banished by hormone replacement therapy, when appropriate.

A woman whose career has progressed well is likely to be at the height of her success in the middle years and a sense of self-confidence in one's abilities and optimism about the future can certainly help to alleviate stress caused by the menopause. But the woman whose life has revolved around her children and husband may be left feeling very lonely, redundant and depressed when the children leave home and her partner appears immersed in his career. On the other hand, if she has interests outside the home and welcomes the opportunity to stop being "Mom" and start being her own person again, her outlook will probably be entirely different.

It is not easy to generalize about the emotional changes that a woman will undergo at this time of her life; but if depression occurs, it is important to look closely at how social roots of illness (see pp.229–235) may be playing a part instead of blaming vague menopausal symptoms.

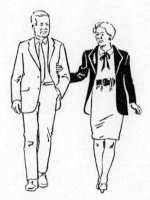

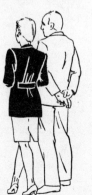

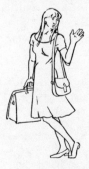

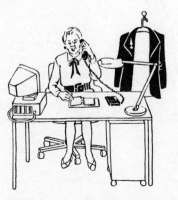

©DIAGRAM

Post-menopausal changes

Estrogen influences the growth and nourishment of the breasts, uterus, vagina, smooth muscle, and skin. It also tends to protect women against circulatory diseases, and possibly against loss of calcium from the bones. Thus the fall in estrogen accompanying the menopause heralds aging changes in the body.

Estrogen loss largely explains why muscles lose tone and the skin loses elasticity and becomes wrinkled. Deprived of estrogen, the breasts also gradually flatten and droop. The womb and ovaries shrink, and the vaginal wall becomes thinner. The vagina is also likely to become drier and lose some of its natural protective acidity, making it more prone to infections. In addition, sexual intercourse may become difficult and even painful. Tissues supporting the vagina and the muscles of the pelvic floor become less elastic and rather more flabby over the years. Prolapse of the uterus or vagina may follow.

Changes in secondary sexual characteristics include the loss of some pubic hair, and growth of hair on the upper lip and chin. More seriously, the risk of heart attack increases, while obesity, if it occurs, increases the risk of arthritis. Finally, well after the menopause, calcium loss from the bones can produce a curve in the spine. Many of these problems are treatable, however.

AFTER THE MENOPAUSE

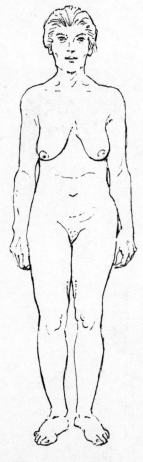

Signs	Treatment
Straggling hairs may begin to appear	Electrolysis or depilatory waxes
Skin loses elasticity	Skin care and massage help skin tone; hormone replacement therapy is possible treatment but mistrusted by some doctors
Bones lose calcium; spine eventually affected	Estrogen tablets may retard calcium loss from the bones; exercise and plenty of calcium in food is useful, too
Breasts eventually flatten and droop	Support sagging breasts with a well-fitting bra
Increased risk of circulatory disease	Circulatory disorders are best prevented by regular exercise and sensible diet
Ovaries and uterus shrink	No treatment needed.
Vaginal wall grows thin and is liable to irritation (less so if intercourse continues)	Application of estrogen cream helps, as does use of lubricants in intercourse
Vulval walls atrophy	Hormonal cream may help
Urinary infection and/or incontinence may occur	Drugs for infection; treatment of incontinence depends on cause
Pubic hair gets scantier	No treatment needed
Increased risk of arthritis	Arthritic pain is helped by anti-inflammatory drugs, such as aspirin. Surgery in severe cases

Hormone replacement therapy

The physical and emotional changes of the menopause can begin even before your periods finish and may include hot flushes, mood swings and a dry vagina, all of which are associated with the ensuing low levels of estrogen. The relationship with your partner may also be put under strain as your sex drive can be affected and intercourse may become painful due to lack of lubrication. However, the menopause does not need to be cause for depression: many of the symptoms are avoidable.

If you experience severe symptoms, your doctor may be able to prescribe Hormone Replacement Therapy (HRT), which many people claim has totally changed their lives. This is supplementary estrogen and/or progesterone in the form of pills, injections, implants, skin patches or creams: but it is usually taken in the form of a once-a-day estrogen pill which is combined with another progesterone pill on certain days of the month.

Many menopausal symptoms disappear with HRT, and there is the added benefit that it can aid depression, insomnia and irritability, as well as improving the quality of the skin and hair. It has also been linked to a reduction in arterial disease. However, perhaps one of the most important benefits of HRT is its effectiveness in the treatment of osteoporosis. Further deterioration of the bone mass can be prevented and it can even help to restore it.

But there may be risks. Although the long-term effects are still not known, certain studies have connected HRT with a higher incidence of cancer of the womb and breast, as well as circulatory problems such as heart disease. Minor side-effects can include bloating, nausea and, of course, monthly bleeding since periods continue during HRT, although they are usually light and pain free.

Everyone needs a thorough consultation before the prescription of HRT, and your doctor will be able to advise you of any possible side-effects or complications. HRT is unlikely to be prescribed if you have a history of breast, womb, vaginal or ovarian cancer, for instance, or if you have had breast cysts. It is also inadvisable if you have had any disease of the liver, kidneys or pancreas, or have circulatory problems or even high blood pressure. Diabetics, heavy smokers and those who are overweight are also likely to be advised against it.

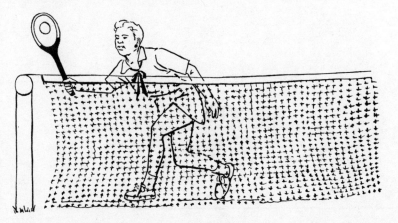

GROWING OLDER

In our part of the world, life expectancy for today's woman reaches well into the mid-seventies and beyond. But for many of us, increasing age often brings with it several new problems that must be faced: adjusting to retirement, the loss of a life partner, difficulties concerning suitable housing and a limited income, perhaps, as well as various physical conditions associated with being elderly. There are, however, many positive steps a woman can take in the attempt to make these years as healthy and as purposeful as possible. Many of the disorders of aging, so it seems, are not entirely inevitable.

Chapter eight

The changing body

Physical changes

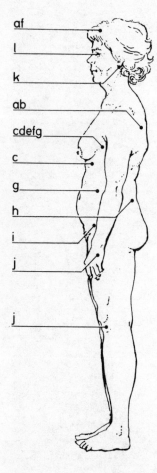

af

l

k

ab

cdefg

c

g

h

i

j

j

INSIDE THE BODY

As a person ages, there are general decreases in body efficiency. However, in the absence of disease, the natural changes that bring these about only occur very gradually and do not necessarily cause discomfort. Physical changes, shown in the diagram (*left*) are as follows.

a From about the age of 25, there is a continous loss of **nerve cells** ("neurons") from the brain and spinal cord. These cannot be replaced.

b With age, the **skeleton**, especially in women, becomes thinner and more brittle, as calcium is lost from the bones.

c This calcium tends to be deposited in other areas – especially the walls of the arteries and the cartilage of the ribs, causing **loss of elasticity**. Another effect can be a **restriction of lung capacity**.

d Hardening and narrowing of the arteries (**arteriosclerosis**) is also likely. This is responsible for a rise in blood pressure. The speed of blood flow also rises – though not excessively.

e When arteriosclerosis is combined with **atheroma** (fatty deposits on the arteries' inner lining), the condition is known as **atherosclerosis**.

f Disorders of the vascular system speed up **tissue decay**, through inadequate blood and oxygen supply. This especially affects the heart and brain.

g As aging proceeds, most internal organs – such as the liver, heart, and kidneys – become reduced in size and function. This is reflected in a reduction in the **basal metabolic rate** (that is, the energy production of the body at its lowest waking level). This means that the energy production of an elderly person is on average 2°F (1.1°C) lower than that of a 25 year-old.

h Deterioration of the vertebral disks causes a slight reduction in the length of the spine.

i Hormonal changes during the menopause mean that it is no longer possible for a woman to bear children, and in the subsequent years her uterus shrinks to approximately one-third of its former size.

j Muscles lose much of their strength, shape, and size. **Joints** become worn and lose some of their articulation. Combined with the degeneration of the nervous system, ease and often confidence of movement are lost.

k There may be deterioration in **hearing** and

l in **eyesight**.

CHANGING ABILITIES

It is possible to compare the physical abilities of a woman of 75 with the maximum abilities reached at her physical peak (usually some time between the ages of 20 and 30). Factors such as work rate and hand grip show up the decline. Some of these, in an average 75 year-old, are 50% less than at their peak. Underlying these changes are the declining efficiency of body processes (such as blood flow and oxygen uptake) and declining size of body organs. The degree of change ranges from a decline of only 10% (nerve conduction speed) to more than 60% (number of taste buds in the mouth).

CHANGES IN APPEARANCE

Many of the changes that take place inside the body as it ages have an effect on the individual's appearance (see *right*).

a The main alterations are brought about by the redistribution of **body fat.** In late life, and especially after the menopause, fat disappears from the breasts (giving them a more sagging appearance), and from the face (deepening wrinkles). But new fat appears around the chin, waist, hips, and bottom.

b At the same time, **skin** all over the body tends to become drier. It loses some of its elasticity and may chap readily in winter. It is this "drying out" process that quite early in middle age causes facial wrinkles to appear. Weakened blood capillaries beneath the skin may also cause it to bruise more easily.

c Hair is also affected by the aging process. Graying is caused by a decline in the production of natural coloring or pigment. For some, the process starts very early, while others retain their hair coloring well into old age. Balding is usually a male problem, but many women notice that their hair becomes thinner. Facial hair, though, may be more obvious in many women.

d The **features of the face** are changed not only by loss of fat, but also by atrophy of the facial bones, especially the jaw bone (making dentures less comfortable). The eyes may appear dulled, because of an opaque ring outside the iris (this does not interfere with vision) and recession of the gums may occur.

e Changes in the **vertebrae** and in **muscle strength** may cause the backbone to droop and the stomach to sag.

f Some **joints** – especially the wrists, knees, and hips – begin to enlarge. Small, temporarily painful knobs may also grow at the sides of the joints; but this is rare.

g Patches of red may appear on the backs of the hands and forearms due to harmless ruptures in **small blood vessels.**

h Tremor of the **hands** becomes common.

i Feet frequently develop corns, calluses, bunions, and hard, thickened, ingrowing or overgrown toenails.

While many of these changes are difficult, if not impossible, to reverse, several may be lessened by a sensible diet, a gentle keep-fit program, or – more controversially – hormone replacement (see p.383).

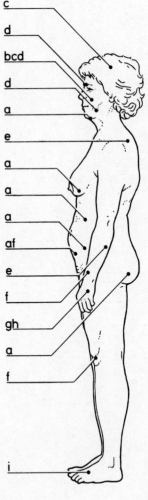

c
d
bcd
d
a
e
a
a
a
af
e
f
gh
a
f
i

©DIAGRAM

Emotional changes

SELF-IMAGE

Changes in temperament and behavior in old people may be accepted as inevitable. But how far they are really due to neurological and mental deterioration, it is often hard to judge since changes may also be due possibly to a woman's social, psychological, and physical situation. Declining physical ability and efficiency, perhaps involving being looked after by others; the end of working life; isolation, due to family remoteness; the disappearance of work contacts; and death of a spouse and friends – all can affect the elderly's self-esteem and lead to depression. Of course, many old people keep up a wide range of interests and have more spending power than ever before – but for others there can be difficulties, due to lack of money, loneliness, physical incapacity, and lack of mental stimulation. The rate of change in modern society adds to the elderly's disorientation; and the way of life in many old people's homes does little to help. All this can result in apathy, listlessness, resentment, alcoholism, and mental stagnation, which others then dismiss as inevitable senility.

On the positive side, early retirement, improved health care, multiple pension provisions, and the right form of housing choice can make old age a time of new opportunities and experiences. Obviously this desirable outcome is easier for couples who are both together, in good health and on a sound financial footing. Loneliness is the single old person's greatest enemy.

THE AGING BRAIN

With the onset of aging, memory, thought, and complex mental functions become slower and less reliable. Eventually, the individual may pass through a "second childhood," with finally only basic reflexes such as eating, walking, and coughing remaining. The frontal lobes of the brain – the first part to deteriorate – are less concerned with intelligence and intellectuality than with general personality, interest in life, deliberation, and consideration. Social inhibitions are often removed, and the person may become increasingly selfish, inconsiderate, obstinate, and emotional.

MENTAL DISTURBANCE

About 10% of people over 65 show some signs of organic brain disorder. Such mental illnesses due to old age were originally undifferentiated under the term "senility" – the loss of mental faculties with age. However, several main conditions are now recognized.

Interestingly, in dementia, for example, it is thought that a nutritional deficiency (in particular, of folic acid or Vitamin C) may at times be a cause. A sudden confused state can also be due to hypothermia (see p.391), unexpected change of environment or even a slight stroke, it should be remembered.

ACUTE CONFUSION
This is one of the most common mental disorders in old people. It is a disturbance of the brain due to physical illness elsewhere in the body, and is also known as "**acute brain syndrome.**" Strange surroundings and other psychological factors may also play a part. The symptoms are confusion, delirium, and disorientation in time and place. Perception is dulled, and the sufferer is frightened, often reacting violently to situations that have been completely misinterpreted. Speech becomes incoherent and rambling. The outcome depends on the preexisting mental state and the original cause of illness, but complete recovery is rare.

DEPRESSIVE ILLNESS
This is a mental illness, but organic nervous decline plays a part in its appearance. It is characterized by acute feelings of sadness, inadequacy, anxiety, apathy, guilt, and fear. It may be triggered off by internal factors (as in endogenous depression), or by external events such as bereavement and/or knowledge of an incurable disease (reactive depression).

SENILE DEMENTIA
This is the disorder that links most directly with the slow process of natural nerve cell loss. It usually begins to be noticeable between the ages of 70 and 80, and primarily affects the memory. It begins gradually with recent memory, and may proceed to the point at which the patient forgets her relations and even her own name. This forgetfulness leads to incompetence in personal care and management, and the person needs more and more attention as time goes on.
   Disorientation in time and place may also occur. Emotions are blunted, and there is increasing lack of consideration for others. There is usually no insight on the part of the patient into the fact that she is ill, which is partly why help may sometimes be rejected.

ALZHEIMER'S DISEASE
This is the most common form of dementia, in which heredity is thought to play some part but the cause is not yet known. However, recently an abnormal protein has been found in the brain of those suffering from Alzheimer's disease. The gene which controls it has been found on chromosome 21. It may also be related to a virus or to toxins in the environment.

ARTERIOSCLEROTIC DEMENTIA
This is also due to the death of brain cells, though in this case the cells die because blockage of the arteries impairs their blood supply. The onset may be gradual, or follow suddenly upon a major stroke. In either case, the effects in an old person are irreversible. Because the brain damage is restricted to areas affected by the blockage, the basic personality may remain more intact than in senile dementia. The person usually retains more awareness and insight into her condition, though this can result in depression and fear.

© DIAGRAM

Illness and aging

The atrophy of age reduces the body's efficiency, creating greater vulnerability and likelihood of malfunction. The body is still susceptible to all the usual disorders, while its maintenance, defense, and repair processes are all much weaker. Respiratory and heart disorders, for example, occur with much more frequency and intensity, skin wounds are more liable to infection, and bone fractures more difficult to heal. Cancer becomes more likely. But in addition, the deterioration of the body and its functions produces a number of ailments rarely found at a younger age.

NERVOUS DISORDERS

An old person's nervous system is likely to degenerate, since nerve cells cannot be replaced. The elderly are also more susceptible to strokes, and liable to falls that may damage the spinal cord or brain. All these may impair movement and the ability to think, see, hear, and express oneself.

Parkinsonism occurs fairly frequently in old age, though less often in women than in men. It is due to nerve cell degeneration in one part of the brain, usually as a result of arteriosclerosis. It manifests itself in trembling and muscular rigidity, and often begins in one hand and then spreads to other parts of the body. The body's rigidity interferes with all movement, from facial expression to locomotion, and brings increasing discomfort as the disease progresses. Treatment involves drugs, exercise, physiotherapy and possibly surgery.

INCONTINENCE

This inability to control the bladder and bowels is usually due to infection of the urinary tract or damage to controlling nerves. Atrophy or prolapse of the muscles is another cause. With old age, a woman may also lose awareness of her bladder, so that conscious control finally disappears and it empties of its own volition. Restricted mobility, emotional insecurity, and abdominal stress (caused by laughing, coughing or lifting) also contribute to precipitating incontinence.

Fecal incontinence is most often caused by impaction – the accumulation of a mass of feces in the rectum too bulky to be passed. This mass then acts as a ball valve, with fresh feces trickling round it and escaping in a continuous flow. Incontinence can also be due to diarrhea, as might occur in gastro-enteritis or rectal prolapse when the rectum wall collapses due to over-straining.

For the elderly who have difficulty in getting to a lavatory quickly, a commode or hand-held pot or urinal may be useful. Wearing a loose-fitting skirt or trousers that are easy to adjust can be helpful too. Special disposable pads are also available, and a doctor should be able to advise on other services that will make life easier both for the elderly person and for the carer.

HYPOTHERMIA

This very serious condition happens when body temperature falls below 95° F (35° C). It mainly afflicts old people who cannot afford adequate heating, food, or winter living conditions. The person becomes increasingly apathetic and lethargic, and below 90° F (32° C) coma usually occurs.

Direct heat must not be applied. The patient's surroundings should be warmed and a blanket wrapped around her to prevent further heat loss. Sadly, because of hypothermia, deaths among old people can rise by 30–50% in winter compared with summer. The harder the winter, the more dangerous the risk. The trend begins even in the 50–54 age group and becomes more marked over 60.

SPINAL DISORDERS

Slipped disk is the common name for prolapsed intervertebral disk. The spine is built up of a column of bones (vertebrae) separated by disks of cartilage that act as shock absorbers. (The disk interior is spongy but firm elastic tissue, held in place by the outer layer's strong fibrous tissue.) In a prolapse, one of these disks in the lower spine slips out of position, impairing mobility and exerting painful pressure on the spinal cord's nerves. **Cervical spondylosis** affects the upper spinal column by a degeneration that shortens the neck, forcing the vertebral artery to concertina, impairing the blood supply to the spinal cord and brain. Pressure is also exerted on the spinal cord's nerves, so their functioning and that of all connected nerves is affected.

JOINT DISORDERS

Joint degeneration results largely from the constant wear and tear of living, but injuries may accentuate and acclerate any disorders. **Osteoarthritis** affects most people over 60, though it occurs less in women than in men. It originates from loss of elasticity in the joint's cartilage. The cartilage breaks up with the joint's movement, and loose pieces may be deposited in the joint itself. These deposits may grow and become calcified, increasing discomfort. The bone around the joint hardens, and cysts may develop, with spurs of bone around the joint edges.

The knee, hip and hand are most commonly affected. The process cannot be reversed, but it can be delayed by gentle, regular exercise to loosen the joint and strengthen the muscles.

Surgery may be used to replace a severely deteriorated joint, such as the hip, with an artificial one.

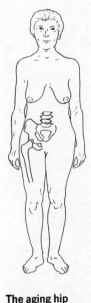

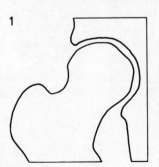

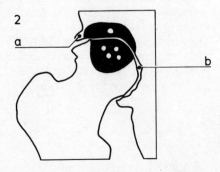

The aging hip

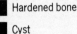 Hardened bone

 Cyst

1 Normal hip
2 Osteoarthritic hip
a Spur
b Reduced joint space

©DIAGRAM

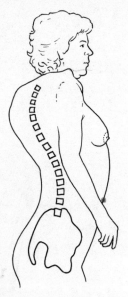

Rheumatoid arthritis usually begins in middle age, but its severity increases with time. It affects more women than men. The joint's tissues thicken so the cartilage becomes ulcerated and is eventually destroyed. There is overproduction of connective tissue, and ultimately the joint is swollen and may be fused solid.

The muscles waste with disuse. Special exercises, and rest in serious cases, are the main forms of treatment. The drug cortisone is now thought to cause many problems, though it does give temporary relief to some. Many other drugs can also be used but there is no cure.

Contractures are joint deformities due to a shortening (contraction) of the surrounding muscles and ligaments. Arthritic or neurological disorders, or simply prolonged inactivity, are the causes. If untreated, contractures become permanent and cause severe disablement. Treatment is with muscle-relaxing drugs and physical manipulation.

Osteoporosis is increased porousness of the bone, usually from unknown causes, but sometimes due to severe calcium salt deficiency. Hormonal changes after the menopause can also be the cause and hormone replacement therapy (see p.383) is thought to be helpful in preventing it, as is increased calcium in the diet. Exercise will also aid its absorption.

The skeleton becomes brittle and prone to fracture. The vertebrae are most often affected. They may collapse as they become weaker, and as they lose weight and size, the vertebral disks expand, producing increasing **curvature of the spine**. The condition may be triggered off by prolonged immobilization in bed. It is more common in women than in men.

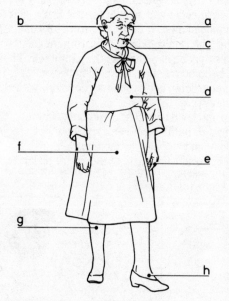

By the age of 60, most women in developed countries have retired or are thinking of retiring from work. If married, they may also be looking forward to the time when their spouse retires. Women who have interests outside work and home are more likely to anticipate their retirement with pleasure since it will bring increased time to spend on social activities, travel, hobbies, and visiting children and grandchildren. For single women whose career has been a mainstay of their social life, however, retirement may mean a less welcome change in life style: and whatever one's marital status, there may be financial concerns.

Preparation for retirement is of the utmost importance and should begin many years beforehand, particularly with regard to financial matters. Much stress in later life arises from health and money troubles; and even if only a little money is available, sound investment of capital to provide regular income together with health insurance will help give peace of mind in years to come. Couples may also wish to make adjustments to their wills, property matters and banking accounts to ensure that, if a spouse dies, the surviving partner will not be overburdened with legal or financial problems.

Friends, family and other social contacts take on a more important and potentially fulfilling role after retirement. For this reason, it is not always advisable to plan an immediate move to what seems an idyllic spot but is out of easy traveling range of familiar faces and places. How easy would it be to go shopping using public transport or with restricted mobility? Will the family be able to visit? These are among factors that should be given careful thought.

The weeks and months after retirement will almost certainly be stressful, no matter how well they have been planned. A single woman living alone may be lonely and feel very keenly the loss of status that went with her employment. Couples may have looked forward to spending more time together but find that they are irritated by each other's constant presence. But a woman who has earlier adjusted well to retirement is likely to be annoyed by a husband who appears to be depressed and aimless and always under her feet.

Not everyone stops working suddenly: it may be financially and socially more convenient to work part-time or freelance as a way of easing into retirement. In countries where the birth rate is decreasing, older people in key jobs are likely to be encouraged to stay on in an advisory or training capacity. Some companies also run active social programs for ex-workers so that people who have known each other for many years do not suddenly lose contact.

Adjusting to retirement

©DIAGRAM

LOSS OF STATUS

As a woman gets used to being officially a "senior citizen," other emotional adjustments have to be made. Women who have not had a job but concentrated on their homes and families may already have come to terms with the low status that society attaches to such activities. Other women, who have had successful careers, may feel that they have abruptly become invisible, a nobody. From being independent wealth creators, society now views them as dependants. Health problems which arise at this age are usually long-term conditions requiring elective surgery or the expensive services of health professionals such as dentists and chiropodists. The older woman often feels that her needs are given low priority relative to "productive" members of society, and she may find herself at the bottom of the surgical waiting list unless she has taken out insurance or is prepared to pay extra for treatment.

LOSS OF INDEPENDENCE

Many older women now live to an age where they suffer from chronic complaints such as arthritis, failing eyesight and heart disease, which gradually restrict mobility and will eventually result in some degree of dependence upon others. This inevitably entails some loss of self-respect and can be very distressing to those who have lived alone or themselves cared for an ailing partner for many years. Moving in with family can work out well, especially if the older woman can be semi-independent, but young families may be reluctant to care for an aging relative in the home, especially if nursing care is required or there are pre-existing tensions within the family. If there is no family to turn to, it is wise to assess as far ahead as possible what kind of accommodation will be most suitable in years to come. The most popular sheltered housing schemes often have a long waiting list.

In industrialized countries, society tends to disregard the value of older people as a source of knowledge and advice. They are instead lumped together and categorized as a "drain" on the state's economic resources. These attitudes are manifestly unjust and are beginning to be challenged by active senior citizens who campaign for better health provision and educational opportunities. Pre-retirement courses, now available to many employees, emphasize the importance of developing interests outside work and home long before retirement day arrives. The woman who already has extensive social contacts and commitments will be far less susceptible to the sense of loss of status commonly attached to leaving work. Women whose lives are hitherto revolved around home and family are also well advised to find new spheres of interest before a partner's retirement.

Surviving a partner

Most married women nowadays have the expectation that they will outlive their husbands, but may give little thought to how that will affect their lives until the event. If one partner has always relied upon the other to perform certain tasks like looking after financial matters or cooking meals, or only one partner is able to drive, bereavement will be complicated by additional worries which may seem minor beforehand but can cause considerable anxiety afterward.

As in any bereavement, grief proceeds in stages and initially is characterized by numbness and shock, followed by realization of what has happened and intense anguish with weeping. In western countries, the manifestations of grief are often suppressed – people are frightened of death and dislike to be reminded of its inevitability, so funerals tend to be hushed affairs and the bereaved person may even feel that others avoid her because they do not know what to say. But it is important that feelings of grief can be expressed openly to someone so that they can be properly worked through. If it is hard to talk to other family members who are dealing with their own grief, specialist support groups (including religious bodies) offer a sympathetic ear and can also give advice on how to handle the practical problems of funerals and wills.

Because the lives of the couple have been intertwined so closely, memories present themselves almost at every turn in the home. It is not uncommon to have the certain feeling that the lost partner is actually there in the room. Memories may be painful at first, particularly if the bereaved person is upset about the circumstances of the death – if it followed a family argument perhaps – but as time goes by happier memories can be recalled to bring some consolation. Guilt and anger are frequent accompaniments of grief and need to be talked about.

Grief tends to recur in waves, often provoked by apparently minor things, but may gradually give way to depression and feelings of listlessness. It is vital for the bereaved woman to take special care of herself, otherwise she runs the risk of becoming mentally and physically exhausted. If lack of sleep and depression become a serious problem, medication can help in the short term but it is better to seek different solutions such as counseling for anxieties and gentle exercise and fresh air for difficulty in sleeping. Friends and family need to be most supportive at this time; and time spent in talking and listening can greatly minimize distress.

It can be hard to resume social activities that one used to participate in as "half of a couple"; and keeping in contact with family and friends may be an easier way of maintaining a social life. Holidays and visits are excellent pick-me-ups, but a permanent move too soon after bereavement should be resisted.

©DIAGRAM

NEW WAYS OF WORKING

Retirement can also provide an ideal opportunity to start up a small business using skills previously acquired in the workplace or through recreational interests. However, any projected scheme that involves the risk of capital invested for security in old age should be considered very carefully with an independent financial adviser.

VOLUNTARY WORK

Nothing contributes more to a person's sense of self-esteem than the feeling that she is helping someone, and is needed. Older people always have some skill that they can offer, whether it is counseling, teaching, campaigning for better facilities or helping to look after people less able to help themselves. One activity that older people are particularly being asked to participate in is reminiscence work – students and historical researchers value the perspective that comes from a person who has lived through events instead of having to read bare facts in textbooks. Those who now live in a different homeland or culture than the one from which they originally stemmed can provide especially interesting information on family history and customs.

CREATIVE ACTIVITIES

Most people promise themselves that once they have stopped work, they will take up some form of creative activity – painting, novel-writing, or dress-making, perhaps. Although time for such pastimes may be short before retirement, it is a good idea to start classes, buy materials and put one's skills to the test as early as possible, so that the hobby is already in full swing by retirement day. As we get older, failing eyesight and lack of dexterity make things like knitting and sewing much harder, and it is useful to have a more passive alternative pastime, such as writing or reminiscence work, which help to keep the mind sharp.

EDUCATION

In Britain, 7% of students of the Open University are over the age of 60. Education represents both a challenge and an opportunity: it keeps the intellect honed and can open the door to new activities and a wider social circle. If formal schooling stopped at an early age because of the financial need to start work, retirement restores the chance to resume it. Many people study for college degrees, but the majority of older learners settle for short-term courses, perhaps at evening class or the local college. In large towns and cities, a wide range of activities may be available – academic subjects, craftwork, and more specialized courses for retired people, carers and voluntary workers. It can take a little while to get used to being a student again, but any lack of self-confidence should soon disappear and rusty skills can easily be brushed up. Enthusiasm and determination also compensate for a lot of minor deficiencies. With advancing age, it can, however, be more difficult to concentrate for long periods; so it is often a good idea to try alternating short bouts of study work with gentle exercise or the household chores.

Fitness

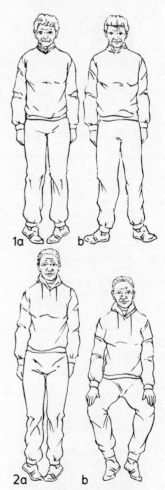

Exercise can be just as important for the elderly as for the young, if not more so. Even though bodily functions and processes are gradually slowing down, regular exercise of an appropriate kind helps to keep the joints supple and the muscles (including the heart) well toned. But inappropriate exercise includes anything that involves sudden unaccustomed strenuous activity. (Women of 60 who run marathons have mostly been runners for many years.) Similarly, anything that puts repeated strain on unused muscles is likely to result in damage that can take a long time to heal. The risk of falling should also be avoided.

Swimming and yoga, which encourage suppleness without stressing the joints, are particularly beneficial and should be continued for as long as possible: public swimming pools often have sessions limited to those over 60. Hobbies and pastimes like rambling and gardening help to maintain fitness, but bear in mind that a good walk each day is better than a 10-mile weekly hike, and heavy digging should either be left to someone else or done in small amounts.

Restricted mobility or failing eyesight limit participation in many activities, but exercise is still vital. A physiotherapist will be able to suggest special exercise regimes and maybe arrange for lessons in craftwork, such as basket-making, carving or weaving, which maintain dexterity and help keep the mind active.

General fitness, of course, also relies on a good diet. Vitamin supplements may be needed for those on a restricted diet, but are unlikely to be as important healthwise as fiber intake. It is a good principle to cut down on refined and processed foods and eat fresh or frozen fruit and vegetables wherever possible. A small vegetable plot, if available, provides both light exercise and a ready source of nutritious food.

The exercises shown here and on the next page are suitable for those in good health. If you have a chronic illness or condition such as a heart problem or hernia, consult your physician first. Try to get into a regular daily routine, choosing a time when you are unlikely to be interrupted and that is not too soon after a meal. Avoid wearing restrictive clothing and stop when you feel tired, or if you feel any twinges.

Exercises for feet and legs
These exercises will aid mobility and posture. Gradually increase the number each day.
  1 a Stand upright with your feet flat on the floor, then turn your toes and heels out, raising your heels
     b Turn your toes out and your heels in, raising your toes
  2 a Stand upright, then rise up on your toes
     b Bend your knees outward, lowering your body as if sitting; then rise slowly
  3 a Stand straight but relaxed
     b Raise your heels so that you stand on your toes
     c Continue rocking to and fro

©DIAGRAM

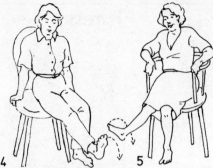
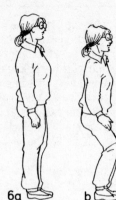
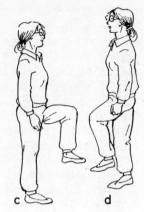

4 **5**

6a   b   c   d

More exercises for feet and legs

4 Sit on a chair with your right leg extended in front of you, your foot slightly off the ground. Wriggle the toes of your right foot. Repeat, changing legs

5 Sit with one foot raised. Turn your raised foot from the ankle to the right and to the left. Repeat with the other foot

6 a Stand upright with your arms by your sides
b Bend your knees, then straighten up
c Raise first one knee, then the other as high as possible, keeping your back straight

Exercises for hands and wrists

These exercises are useful for the bedridden, but they can be done by anyone, anywhere. Perhaps exercise with a friend or partner

7 a Sit up straight; close your fists up against your shoulders and keep your elbows well in
b Reach up with one arm, keeping the fist closed
c Repeat with the other arm

8 a Start with both arms resting on your thighs
b Reach up with both arms at the same time

9 a Sit with your arms stretched out as far as possible
b, c Raise one arm while lowering the other, then alternate

10 a Clench hands and bring them up to your chest, raising your elbows to the sides
b Push your left arm straight out in front
c Repeat with your right arm
d Raise, and then lower both arms

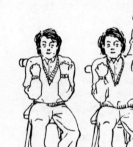
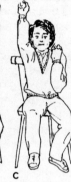
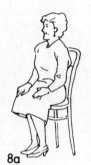
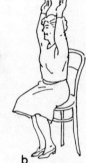

7a   b   c   8a   b

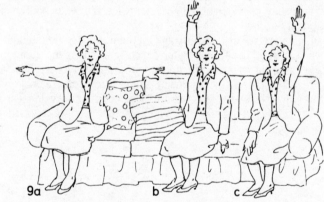

9a   b   c

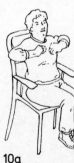
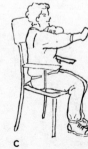
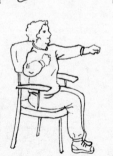
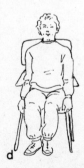

10a   b   c   d

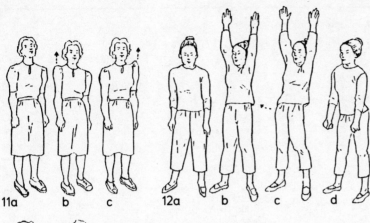

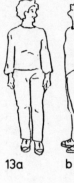

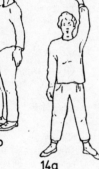

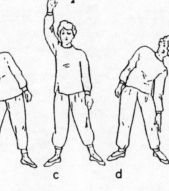

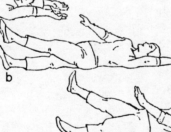

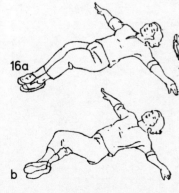

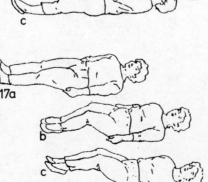

11a b c 12a b c d

13a b 14a b c d

15a b c

16a b 17a b c

Exercises for shoulders, neck and trunk

11 a Stand straight with your feet together, shoulders well back and fists clenched at your sides

b, c Raise and lower your right shoulder, then your left

12 a Stand with your feet apart, arms at your sides

b Raise your arms over your head

c Sway your hips backward and forward, keeping your knees straight as you sway

d When your arms get tired, put them by your sides and continue swaying your hips

13 a Stand relaxed

b Turn your head to the right, then to the left. Next let it fall forward and back Take care if you suffer from cervical spondylosis as dizziness may arise.

14 a Stand with your feet apart, arms at your sides. Raise your left arm above your head

b With straight legs bend from the waist, letting your right hand slide down the thigh

c Straighten up and repeat with the other arm

Exercises for trunk and back

With all floor exercises, if you don't have a carpet, put a blanket on the floor.

15 a Lie flat on the floor and stretch your arms out above your head

b Keeping your back flat on the floor, raise your left leg and then raise and reach forward with your right arm as though trying to touch your raised leg

c Repeat with your right leg and left arm

16 a Lie flat on the floor. Stretch your arms at right angles to your body; bend your knees, keeping your feet flat on the floor

b Swing your legs over to the right to touch the floor, then to the left

17 a Lie flat on your back with your arms at your sides

b Keeping your feet flat on the floor, raise your knees

c Twist your body very slightly and bump your left buttock 3 times on the floor, then the right buttock

©DIAGRAM

Calories

The following calorie counts are per ounce (28.5g)

Almonds		170
Apple	baked	10
	fresh	15
	stewed (no sugar)	10
Apricots	dried	50
Asparagus	fresh	5
Avocado pear		25
Bacon	fried lean	125
	grilled lean	90
Banana	peeled	20
Beans	baked	30
	green runner	5
Beef	burger	55
	steak, grilled	85
	stew	40
Biscuits	digestive	55
Bread	brown	63
	white	69
	wholemeal	78
Broccoli		10
Butter		225
Cabbage	boiled	5
Carrots	raw	5
Celery	raw	5
Cheese	Cheddar	120
	cream	230
Chicken	casserole	20
	roast	55
Chocolate	milk	160
Coffee	black	0
Coleslaw		40
Corn on the cob		35
Cornflakes		105
Cream	double	130
Duck	roast	90
Egg	boiled	45
	fried	70
	omelette	55
Figs	raw fresh	10
Grapes	green	20
Grapefruit	fresh	3
Haddock	fried	50
	steamed	30

Ham	boiled lean	60
Herring	fried	65
	grilled	30
Ice cream		60
Jam		80
Lamb chop	grilled	75
Lentils	boiled	25
Lettuce		5
Liver	calves', fried	75
Macaroni	boiled	30
Melon		5
Milk	fresh	20
	skimmed	10
Mushrooms	fried	60
Orange	fresh	10
Plaice	fried	65
	steamed	20
Pork chop	grilled	75
Potatoes	baked	30
	boiled	25
	chips, fried	65
	roast	35
Raisins	seedless	95
Rhubarb	stewed, fresh	0
Rice	boiled	35
Sardines	tinned	85
Sausages	beef, fried	80
	pork, fried	95
Semolina		25
Spaghetti bolognese		50
Spinach	boiled, fresh	5
Spirits		70
Strawberries	fresh	5
Swedes	boiled	5
Tea	white, no sugar	10
	lemon	0
Tomato	fresh	5
Tuna	tinned in oil, drained	70
Veal	fried	65
Watercress	raw	5
Wine		40
Yogurt	natural, low fat	60

This chart shows some of the diseases you may encounter worldwide, how they are generally contracted, and the necessary precautions.

Travel chart

	Risk areas	How caught	Vaccination	Additional precautions
AIDS	Worldwide	Sexual relations with an infected person or from injections with infected blood or use of infected needles	None available	Use a condom and, better still, avoid casual sex
Cholera	Africa, Asia, Middle East, especially where there is poor hygiene and sanitation	Contaminated food or water	Usually 2 vaccinations but not complete protection	Drink only mineral water, and watch what you eat, too
Viral Hepatitis A	Most of the world, especially where there is poor hygiene and sanitation	Contaminated food or water	Injection of immunoglobulin	Be very careful what you eat and drink
Viral Hepatitis B	Worldwide	Intimate contact with an infected person or from injections with infected blood or shared infected needles	Consult your doctor	Wear a condom and, better still, avoid casual sex
Malaria	Africa, Asia, Central and South America	Bite from infected mosquito	Anti-malarial tablets are available	Keep arms and legs covered after sunset; use insect repellants and mosquito nets when sleeping
Polio	Outside Australia, New Zealand, Europe and North America	Direct contact with an infected person and, rarely, via contaminated water or food	3 lots of drops taken 4–8 weeks apart. Additional dose may be necessary after 10 years	Be very careful about what you eat and drink
Rabies	Many parts of the world	Bite or scratch from an infected animal	Consult your doctor	Avoid contact with animals
Tetanus	Whenever medical facilities not adequate	Any wound	Vaccination will give fairly long-lasting protection	Wash any wound very carefully and consult a doctor right away
Tuberculosis	Asia, Africa, Central and South America	Airborne	Injection preferably 3 months before the proposed journey	You will probably not be at risk if your visit is short and if you are staying at a large international hotel
Typhoid	In areas of poor hygiene outside Australia, New Zealand, Europe and North America	Contaminated food or water	2 injections, 4–6 weeks apart. Revaccination by a single injection after 3 years	Be very careful what you eat and drink
Yellow Fever	Africa and South America	Bite from infected mosquito	Injection at a yellow fever vaccination center at least 10 days before your journey. Certificate valid for 10 years	As for malaria, above

©DIAGRAM

Expected date of delivery

You can use this chart to work out the expected date of delivery. Find the date of the first day of your last period. The date your baby is due is immediately underneath in bold.

January 1 2 3 4 5 6 7 8 9 10 11 12 13 14 15 16 17 18 19 20 21 22 23 24 25 26 27 28 29 30 31 — *January*
October 8 9 10 11 12 13 14 15 16 17 18 19 20 21 22 23 24 25 26 27 28 29 30 31 1 2 3 4 5 6 7 — *November*

February 1 2 3 4 5 6 7 8 9 10 11 12 13 14 15 16 17 18 19 20 21 22 23 24 25 26 27 28 — *February*
November 8 9 10 11 12 13 14 15 16 17 18 19 20 21 22 23 24 25 26 27 28 29 30 1 2 3 4 5 — *December*

March 1 2 3 4 5 6 7 8 9 10 11 12 13 14 15 16 17 18 19 20 21 22 23 24 25 26 27 28 29 30 31 — *March*
December 6 7 8 9 10 11 12 13 14 15 16 17 18 19 20 21 22 23 24 25 26 27 28 29 30 31 1 2 3 4 5 — *January*

April 1 2 3 4 5 6 7 8 9 10 11 12 13 14 15 16 17 18 19 20 21 22 23 24 25 26 27 28 29 30 — *April*
January 6 7 8 9 10 11 12 13 14 15 16 17 18 19 20 21 22 23 24 25 26 27 28 29 30 31 1 2 3 4 — *February*

May 1 2 3 4 5 6 7 8 9 10 11 12 13 14 15 16 17 18 19 20 21 22 23 24 25 26 27 28 29 30 31 — *May*
February 5 6 7 8 9 10 11 12 13 14 15 16 17 18 19 20 21 22 23 24 25 26 27 28 1 2 3 4 5 6 7 — *March*

June 1 2 3 4 5 6 7 8 9 10 11 12 13 14 15 16 17 18 19 20 21 22 23 24 25 26 27 28 29 30 — *June*
March 8 9 10 11 12 13 14 15 16 17 18 19 20 21 22 23 24 25 26 27 28 29 30 31 1 2 3 4 5 6 — *April*

July 1 2 3 4 5 6 7 8 9 10 11 12 13 14 15 16 17 18 19 20 21 22 23 24 25 26 27 28 29 30 31 — *July*
April 7 8 9 10 11 12 13 14 15 16 17 18 19 20 21 22 23 24 25 26 27 28 29 30 1 2 3 4 5 6 7 — *May*

August 1 2 3 4 5 6 7 8 9 10 11 12 13 14 15 16 17 18 19 20 21 22 23 24 25 26 27 28 29 30 31 — *August*
May 8 9 10 11 12 13 14 15 16 17 18 19 20 21 22 23 24 25 26 27 28 29 30 31 1 2 3 4 5 6 7 — *June*

September 1 2 3 4 5 6 7 8 9 10 11 12 13 14 15 16 17 18 19 20 21 22 23 24 25 26 27 28 29 30 — *September*
June 8 9 10 11 12 13 14 15 16 17 18 19 20 21 22 23 24 25 26 27 28 29 30 1 2 3 4 5 6 7 — *July*

October 1 2 3 4 5 6 7 8 9 10 11 12 13 14 15 16 17 18 19 20 21 22 23 24 25 26 27 28 29 30 31 — *September*
July 8 9 10 11 12 13 14 15 16 17 18 19 20 21 22 23 24 25 26 27 28 29 30 31 1 2 3 4 5 6 7 — *August*

November 1 2 3 4 5 6 7 8 9 10 11 12 13 14 15 16 17 18 19 20 21 22 23 24 25 26 27 28 29 30 — *November*
August 8 9 10 11 12 13 14 15 16 17 18 19 20 21 22 23 24 25 26 27 28 29 30 31 1 2 3 4 5 6 — *September*

December 1 2 3 4 5 6 7 8 9 10 11 12 13 14 15 16 17 18 19 20 21 22 23 24 25 26 27 28 29 30 31 — *December*
September 7 8 9 10 11 12 13 14 15 16 17 18 19 20 21 22 23 24 25 26 27 28 29 30 1 2 3 4 5 6 7 — *October*

©DIAGRAM

Glossary

Alopecia	Hair thinning or loss.
Amenorrhea	Absence of menstrual periods at an age when they should be regular.
Amniocentesis	Removal of fluid from the amniotic sac surrounding the fetus in order to check for abnormalities.
Amniotomy	Deliberate breaking of the amniotic sac or bag of waters in order to bring on or induce labor.
Anemia	A low red blood cell count, with symptoms of tiredness, headaches and sometimes dizziness. Usually due to iron deficiency.
Analgesic	A drug to relieve pain.
Anorexia nervosa	Form of self-starvation, with marked physical symptoms and psychological causation.
Areola	Ring of pink/brown skin around the nipple.
Arteriosclerosis	Hardening of the artery walls.
Atherosclerosis	Thickening of the artery walls by deposits of fatty substances.
Bartholin's glands	Pea-sized glands at the vaginal entrance that secrete muscus for lubrication during intercourse.
Benign	Not cancerous.
Biopsy	Removal of body tissue or fluid from a live person for purposes of diagnosis.
Break-through bleeding	Bleeding from the vagina between periods.
Bulimia	A psychological condition involving gorging followed by self-induced vomiting or use of laxatives.
Cancer	General term for many diseases characterized by abnormal cell division, and formation of a malignant tumor.
Candida albicans	A yeast infection of the vagina.
Carcinoma	A malignant or cancerous tumor.
Cervical smear	*See* **Pap smear.**
Cervix	Structure at the lower end of the uterus, protruding into the vagina.
Chancre	A sore that is the first sign of syphilis.
Chemotherapy	Treatment with drugs (usually for cancer).
Chronic	With a long duration and developing over an extended period.
Clitoris	A tiny, very sensitive organ at the front of the vagina above the urethral opening, stimulation of which can bring about orgasm.
Coitus interruptus	Withdrawal from intercourse by the man, sometimes still used as a method of contraception but with a very high rate of failure.
Colostomy	Artificial opening in the colon, created for disposal of feces when disease or injury have affected the colon or rectum, or both.
Colostrum	Yellow substance produced by the breasts prior to the milk coming through, and highly nutritious for the newborn.
Colposcopy	This painless technique is used to examine the cervix and vagina. The colposcope is a microscope that magnifies and thereby facilitates a view of possible abnormalities.
Cunnilingus	Sexual stimulation of a woman's genitals by a man, using his tongue.
Curettage	Scraping away of tissue from the uterus.

D&C	Abbreviation of dilatation (stretching) and curettage (scraping of the lining of the uterus). Chiefly to stop heavy bleeding, to remove unwanted tissue, to remove polyps or to diagnose an early cancer of the uterus.
D&E	Abbreviation of dilatation (stretching) and evacuation. Used only for termination of pregnancy.
Diabetes	Condition in which the pancreas fails to produce adequate supplies of insulin, characterized by excess glucose or sugar in the blood and urine.
Diuretic	A drug which helps to rid the body of excess fluid.
Douching	Cleaning the vagina with water or another solution, but rarely necessary.
Down's syndrome	Also known as mongolism, a condition caused by an extra chromosome and characterized by mental retardation and particular facial features. Incidence increases with maternal age (from 1 in 2,500 in those women under 20 to 1 in 40 in those over 44).
Dysmenorrhea	Painful periods.
Eclampsia	A serious condition following **pre-eclampsia** in pregnancy, with symptoms of convulsions and perhaps coma, sometimes fatal.
Ectopic pregnancy	Implantation of the fertilized egg outside the uterus, most frequently in a Fallopian tube.
Edema	Swelling due to fluid retention.
Embolism	Blood clot or air bubble blocking an artery.
Embryo	The fertilized egg, up to the 6-week stage, after which it is known as a **fetus**.
Endometriosis	Occurs when tissue from the lining of the uterus appears elsewhere: symptoms include painful periods.
Endometrium	Lining of the uterus.
Epidural anesthesia	Form of anesthesia sometimes used in childbirth and requiring injection of anesthetic into spaces in the spinal area.
Episiotomy	Cutting of the **perineum** to prevent tearing in childbirth.
Estrogen	The main female sex hormone produced by various glands but chiefly by the ovaries.
Fallopian tubes	Two tubes leading from the ovaries to the uterus.
Fellatio	Oral sex in which a man's partner uses his/her mouth to caress his genital area.
Fetus	The developing child in the womb, from six weeks after fertilization until birth.
Fibroid	A **benign** growth in the uterus.
Forceps	A surgical instrument, rather like tongs, sometimes used to assist the birth of a baby.
FSH	Follicle-stimulating hormone, playing a part in the ovulation process.
Gestation	Development period from conception to birth.
Gonorrhea	A common sexually transmitted disease.
Graafian follicle	The follicle releasing an ovum at ovulation each month.
Gynecologist	Doctor specializing in female health problems.
Hematuria	Blood in the urine, which can be a symptom of urinary infection or a tumor, among other conditions.

Hemophilia	Bleeding disorder in which the clotting factor is lacking or absent, found only in males but carried by women.
Hemorrhage	Bleeding.
Hemorrhoids	Also known as piles, these are a form of varicose vein occurring in the anus or rectum.
Herpes, genital	Form of venereal or sexually transmitted disease, caused by the herpes simplex virus.
Hormone	Chemical that acts as a messenger in the body, stimulating certain of its functions such as growth, metabolism and sexual response.
Hydatidiform mole	A form of abnormal embryo development.
Hymen	Also known as the maidenhead, a membrane partly covering the vaginal opening in a virgin, torn during first intercourse if not previously stretched by tampons or exercise.
Hyperglycemia	High blood sugar.
Hypertension	High blood pressure.
Hypoglycemia	Low blood sugar.
Hysterectomy	Removal of the uterus by surgery.
Hysterotomy	Termination of pregnancy by means of surgery via the wall of the uterus, but not commonly used unless other methods are contraindicated.
Ideopthatic	With no known cause.
Ileostomy	Opening in the abdomen made surgically, to facilitate passing of feces into a special bag.
Immunotherapy	Cancer treatment that involves stimulating the production of cells to fight the disease.
Incest	Sexual relations between parent/child or brother/sister.
Incompetent cervix	Cervix that dilates mid-way through pregnancy, resulting in loss of the fetus or premature birth.
Induction	The starting of labor by artificial means.
Intra-uterine vice (IUD)	Contraceptive loop or coil inserted into the uterus.
Kegal exercises	Exercises to strengthen the vaginal muscles with a view to improving sexual pleasure during intercourse.
Labor	The process immediately prior to birth.
Lactation	Milk production by the breasts.
Laparoscopy	Investigation of the pelvic area by means of the insertion of an optical instrument through the abdominal wall.
Leboyer method	Named after the French obstetrician, an approach to childbirth that emphasizes gentleness and gradual acclimatization for the baby.
Lesbian	Female who prefers a woman as a sexual partner.
Leucorrhea	Vaginal discharge.
Libido	Sex drive.
Liver spots	Freckling most often on the skin of the hands and arms, occurring at the menopause.
Lochia	Discharge from the vagina after childbirth.
Lymph	Body fluid containing white blood cells.
Malignant	Cancerous.
Mammography	X rays of the breasts, usually taken to identify presence of diseased tissue.
Manic-depressive	Someone suffering from a mental disorder involving extreme and cyclical mood swings.
Masectomy	Removal of the breast(s) by surgery, usually to prevent spread of cancer.
Mastitis	Inflammation of the breast(s).

Melanoma	Cancerous tumor, usually of the skin.
Menarche	The start of menstruation at puberty.
Menopause	The "change of life" when menstruation ceases.
Menstruation	The monthly period or shedding of the lining of the uterus.
Midwife	Specialist attendant at childbirth.
Miscarriage	Loss of the fetus.
Morning sickness	Nausea often experienced in early pregnancy.
Multigravida	Woman who has had more than one child.
Nausea	Feeling of sickness.
Obstetrician	Doctor specializing in pregnancy and childbirth.
Osteoarthritis	The most common form of arthritis, involving degeneration of the cartilage of the body's joints, particularly the fingers, knees, hips and spine.
Osteoporosis	Loss of bone mass, as they become more fragile.
Ovaries	The two sex glands that secrete both **estrogen** and **progesterone**, and also produce **ova**.
Ovulation	The release of an ovum from the ovaries each month from puberty to the menopause.
Ovum	Female egg cell produced by the ovaries.
Oxytocin	A hormone that stimulates the contractions of labor and also brings about milk production in the breasts.
Palpate	To feel the body's surface in order to detect lumps, or the position of the fetus in pregnancy, for instance.
Pap smear	Also known as a cervical smear, this test – in which a sample of the cells from the surface of the cervix is taken for investigation – should be performed regularly in order to identify the early stages of cancer.
Pelvic inflammatory disease (PID)	Infection of the Fallopian tubes and sometimes of the ovaries and womb.
Perineum	The area between the anus and the vagina. *See also* **Episiotomy**.
Pethidine	Narcotic used to relieve pain during labor.
Phlebitis	Inflamation of the veins, involving blood clots.
Piles	*See* **Hemorrhoids**.
Placenta previa	A placenta sited by the cervix instead of higher in the uterus.
Polyp	Soft growth that is **benign**.
Pre-eclampsia	Also known as **toxemia**, a condition that can occur in pregnancy and with symptoms of high blood pressure and fluid retention, which must be treated promptly.
Primigravida	A woman who is expecting her first child.
Progesterone	Hormone which has an important role in the menstrual cycle.
Prognosis	Forecast concerning the progress of an illness.
Prolapsed uterus	Dropping of part of the womb into the vagina due to deteriorated muscles.
Psychosomatic	A symptom with an emotional cause.
Puerperal fever	Infection, now rare, which can follow childbirth and which is caused by the streptococcus organism.
Puerperium	The period after childbirth (also known as postpartum period).
Quickening	Movements of the fetus in the uterus as felt by the mother.
Remission	Change in the course of a medical condition so that symptoms decrease in severity or even disappear.

Retroverted uterus	Uterus that is tilted backward instead of forward.
Rheumatoid arthritis	Disease in which the body's joints become painful and severely inflamed and which is far more common in women than men.
Rh factor	Substance which may or may not be present in the blood, so that every individual is either Rhesus positive or Rhesus negative. Of relevance in pregnancy, when Rh incompatibility may occur if an Rh negative mother has an Rh positive baby.
Rubella	German measles – an infectious disease which if contracted early in pregnancy may cause birth defects.
Salpingitis	Infection of the Fallopian tubes.
Schiller test	Test for the presence of vaginal or cervical cancer, using an iodine solution which stains normal cells brown.
Sickle cell anemia	Form of anemia affecting mainly blacks, and with symptoms of painful joints and ulcerated legs.
Sims-Hulver test	Test to examine cervical mucus to see whether it is hostile to sperm, as part of a fertility investigation.
Speculum	Medical instrument used during vaginal examinations.
Spermicides	Chemicals that will destroy sperm, used as contraceptives.
Suppository	A form of medication, shaped like a small bullet, inserted directly into the vagina or anus.
Syphilis	A sexually transmitted disease which can also affect a baby in the womb.
Testosterone	Male sex hormone, also produced in quantities by the ovaries and adrenal glands.
Thermography	Method for diagnosis of cancer, involving heat patterns that show up unhealthy tissue.
Thrombus	A clot forming in a blood vessel.
Toxemia	*See* **Pre-eclampsia.**
Toxic shock syndrome	Rare condition with symptoms of fever, vomiting and a rash, thought by some to be caused by tampons that encourage growth of certain bacteria.
Transition	The end of the first stage of labor in childbirth.
Trichomonas	A vaginal infection.
Tubal ligation	Cutting and tying or cauterization of the Fallopian tubes as a form of sterilization for the purpose of contraception.
Tumor	A growth of tissue which can be either **benign** and non-spreading, or **malignant** (cancerous).
Ultrasound	Sound waves forming pictures of the inside of the body, particularly useful during pregnancy and for diagnosis of pelvic complaints.
Urethritis	Infection of the urethra, the tube through which urine passes from the bladder.
Vacuum aspiration	Removal of tissue from the womb by suction, either for diagnosis or to improve menstrual problems; or to terminate a very early pregnancy.
Vaginismus	Condition in which the vaginal muscles contract so that sexual intercourse is rendered impossible.
Varicose vein	Bulging leg vein, quite common in women, which can be treated by the wearing of support hose or injections, or surgery, if necessary.
Venereal disease	Sexually transmitted disease (STD). Examples include syphilis, herpes, gonorrhea, and AIDS.

Useful addresses

Accidents and complaints

Action for the Victims of Medical
Accidents
24 Southwark Street
London SE1 1TY
(071 291 2793)

British Medical Association
BMA House
Tavistock Square
London WC1H 9JP
(071 387 4499)

Children's Legal Centre
20 Compton Terrace
London N1 2UN
(071 359 6251)

Commission for Racial Equality
Elliot House
10-12 Allington Street
London SW1E 5EH
(071 828 7022)

General Medical Council
44 Hallam Street
London W1N 6AE
(071 580 7642)

Adoption/Fostering

British Agencies for Adoption and
Fostering
11 Southwark Street
London SE1 1RQ
(071 407 8800)

Family Care
21 Castle Street
Edinburgh EH2 3DM
(031 2256441)

National Fostercare Association
Francis House
Francis Street
London SW1P 1DE
(071 828 6266)

NORCAP (National Association for
the Reunion of Children and
Parents)
3 New High Street
Headington
Oxford OX3 7AJ
(0865 750554)

Parents for Children
41 Southgate Road
London N1 3JP
(071 359 7530)

Aging

Age Concern
60 Pitcairn Road
Mitcham CR4 3LL
(081 640 5431)

Alzheimer's Disease Society
158/160 Balham High Road
London SW12 9BN
(081 675 6557)

Carers' National Association
29 Chilworth Mews
London W2 3RG
(071 724 7776)

Help the Aged
16-18 St James's Walk
London EC1R 0BE
(071 253 0253)

British Association for Service to
the Elderly
119 Hassell Street
Newcastle-under-Lyme
Staffordshire ST5 1AX
(0782 661033)

National Osteoporosis Society
Barton Meade House
PO Box 10
Radstock
Bath BA3 3YB

Allergies

Action Against Allergy
23/24 George Street
Richmond
Surrey GW9 1JY

National Society for Research into
Allergy
45 Hinckley
Leicester LE10 1JE
(0455 635212)

Hyperactive Children's Support
Group
71 Whyke Lane
Chichester
West Sussex PO19 2LD
(0903 725182)

Bereavement

Stillbirth and Neonatal Death
Society
28 Portland Place
London W1N 4DE
(071 436 5881)

Cruse
126 Sheen Road
Richmond
Surrey TW9 1UR
(081 940 4818)

Miscarriage Association
PO Box 24
Ossett
West Yorkshire WF5 9XG
(0924 830515)

The Compassionate Friends
6 Denmark Street
Bristol BS1 5DQ
(0272 292778)
For bereaved parents

Cancer

CancerLink
17 Britannia Street
London WC1X 9JN
(071 833 2451)

Bristol Cancer Help Centre
Grove House
Cornwallis Grove
Clifton
Bristol BS8 4PG
(0272 743216)

Women's National Cancer Control
Campaign
1 South Audley Street
London W1Y 5DQ
(071 499 7532)

Cancer Relief Macmillan Fund
15–19 Britten Street
London SW3 3TZ
(071 351 7811)

Marie Curie Foundation
28 Belgrave Square
London SW1X 8QG
(071 235 3325)

Cancer Aftercare
21 Zetland Road
Redland
Bristol BS6 7AH
(0272 427419)

BACUP
121/123 Charterhouse Street
London EC1M 6AA
(071 608 1785)

Childbirth

National Childbirth Trust
Alexandra House
Oldham Terrace
London W3 6NH
(071 992 8637)

Active Birth Movement
55 Dartmouth Park Road
London NW5 1SL
(071 267 3006)

Complementary Medicine

Anglo-European College of
  Chiropractic
13–15 Parkwood Road
Bournemouth BH5 2DF
(0202 431021)

British Naturopathic and
  Osteopathic Association
6 Netherhall Gardens
London NW3 5RR
(071 435 7320)

General Council and Register of
  Osteopaths
56 London Street
Reading RG1 4SQ
(0734 576585)

Incorporated Society of Registered
  Naturopaths
328 Harrogate Road
Leeds LS17 6PE

British Acupuncture Association
34 Alderney Street
London SW1V 4EU
(071 834 1012)

The Council for Acupuncture
Suite 1
19A Cavendish Square
London W1M 9AD
(071 837 8026)

Register of Traditional Chinese
  Medicine
19 Trinity Street
London N2 8JJ
(081 883 8431)

Yoga for Health Foundation
Ickwell Bury
Northill
Biggleswade
Bedfordshire SG18 9EF
(076 727 271)

British Herbal Medicine Association
PO Box 304
Bournemouth
Dorset BH7 6JX
(0202 433691)

Herb Society
PO Box 415
London SW1P 2HE

National Institute of Medical
  Herbalists
41 Hatherley Road
Winchester
Hampshire SO22 6RR

Faculty of Homeopathy
Royal London Homeopathic
  Hospital
60 Great Ormond Street
London WC1N 3HR
(071 837 3091)

Institute for Complementary
  Medicine
21 Portland Place
London W1N 3AF
(071 636 9543)

Association of Professional Music
  Therapists in Great Britain
The Meadow
68 Pierce Lane
Fulbourn
Cambridge CB1 5DL

British Association of Art Therapists
13C Northwood Road
Highgate
London N6 5TL

British School of Reflexology
92 Sheering Road
Old Harlow
Essex CM17 0JW
(0279 29060)

National Federation of Spiritual
  Healers
Old Manor Farm Studio
Church Street
Sunbury-on-Thames
Middx TW16 6RG
(093 2783164)

Shiatsu Society
19 Langside Park
Kilbarchan
Renfrewshire PA10 2EP
(05057 4657)

Society of Teachers of the Alexander
  Technique
10 London House
266 Fulham Road
London SW10 9EL
(071 351 0828)

British Hypnotherapy Association
1 Wythburn Place
London W1 5WL
(071 723 4443)

Contraception

Family Planning Information Service
27–35 Mortimer Street
London W1N 7RJ
(071 636 7866)

Women's Health and Reproductive
  Rights Information Centre
52–54 Featherstone Street
London EC1Y 8RT
(071 251 6580)

Margaret Pyke Centre
15 Bateman Buildings
Soho Square
London W1V 5TW
(071 734 9351)

Brook Advisory Centres
153A East Street
London SE17 2SD
(081 708 1234)
For under 25s

Dependencies

Alcoholics Anonymous
PO Box 1
Stonebow House
Stonebow
York YO1 2NJ
(0904 644026 or 071 351 3001)

ASH (Action on Smoking and
  Health)
5–11 Mortimer Street
London W1N 7RH
(071 637 9843)

Women's Alcohol Centre
66A Drayton Park
London N5 1ND
(071 226 4581)

ACCEPT (Drugs Helpline)
(071 286 3339)

Narcotics Anonymous
PO Box 417
London SW10 0RN
(071 351 6794)

DAWN (Drugs, Alcohol and Women
  Nationally)
39–41 North Road
London N7 9DP
(071 700 4653)

Families Anonymous
(071 731 8060)

Disabled

RADAR (Royal Association for
    Disability and Rehabilitation)
25 Mortimer Street
London W1N 8AB
(071 637 5400)

British Sports Association for the
    Disabled
The Mary Glen Haig Suite
34 Osnaburgh Street
London NW1 3ND
(071 383 7277)

Union of Physically Impaired Against
    Segregation
Flat 2
98 Woodhill
London SE18 5JL
(081 854 8431)

Eating Problems

Overeaters Anonymous
PO Box 19
Streatford
Manchester H32 9EB
(061 981 9363)

Compulsive Eating Groups
Women's Therapy Centre
6 Manor Gardens
London N7 6RA
(071 263 6200)

Anorexia Anonymous
24 Westmoreland Road
Barnes
London SW13 9RY
(081 748 3994)

Eating Disorders Association
The Priory Centre
11 Priory Road
High Wycombe
Bucks
(0494 21431)

Fat Women's Group
London Women's Centre
Wesley House
4 Wild Court
London WC2B 5AU

Female Health

Wellwoman Information
24 St Thomas Street
Bristol BS1 6JL
(0272 221925)

Endometriosis Society
65 Holmdene Avenue
London SE24 9LD

PID Support Group
c/o WHRRIC
52–54 Featherstone Street
London EC1Y 8RT
(071 251 6580)

Breast Care and Masectomy
    Association
26A Harrison Street
London WC1H 8JG
(071 837 0908)

General Health

British Diabetic Association
10 Queen Anne Street
London W1M 0BD
(071 323 1531)

British Heart Foundation
102 Gloucester Place
London W1H 4DH
(071 935 0185)

Arthritis and Rheumatism Council
41 Eagle Street
London WC1R 4AR
(071 405 8572)

Health Education Authority
Hamilton House
Mabledon Place
London WC1H 9TX
(071 631 0930)

Coronary Prevention Group
60 Great Ormond Street
London WC1N 3HR

Infertility

National Association for the
    Childless
318 Sumner Lane
Birmingham BI9 3RL

Single and Infertile
293 Meadgate Avenue
Chelmsford
Essex

British Pregnancy Advisory Service
Austy Manor
Wootton Wawen
Solihull
West Midlands B95 6BX
(05642 3225)

Marriage and Family

The Parent Network
44–46 Caversham Road
London NW5 2DS
(071 485 8535)

Marriage Guidance Council (Relate)
76A New Cavendish Street
London W1M 7LB
(071 580 1087)

Divorce Conciliation and Advisory
    Service
38 Ebury Street
London SW1 0LU
(071 730 2422)

Mental Health

British Association for Couselling
37a Sheep Street
Rugby CV21 3BX
(0788 78328)

Mental After Care Association
Bainbridge House
Bainbridge Street
London WC1A 1HP
(071 436 6194)

Samaritans
17 Uxbridge Road
Slough SL1 1SN
See telephone directory for local
    branch number

MIND
22 Harley Street
London W1N 2ED
(071 637 0741)

Schizophrenia Association of Great
    Britain
Bryn Hyfryd
The Crescent
Bangor
Gwynedd LL57 2AG
(0248 354048)

Richmond Fellowship
8 Addison Road
London W14 8DL
(071 603 6373)

Fellowship of Depressives
    Anonymous
36 Chestnut Avenue
Beverley
N Humberside HU17 9QU
(0482 860619)

Action on Phobias
89 The Avenue
Eastbourne
Sussex BN21 3YA

Sexual Abuse/Rape

Rape Crisis Centres
PO Box 69
London N6 5BU
(071 837 1600)

Childline
(0800 1111)

Incest Crisis Line
(081 890 4732)

National Society for the Prevention
  of Cruelty to Children
67 Saffron Hill
London EC1N 8RS
(071 242 1626)

Criminal Injuries Compensation
  Board
Whittington House
19–30 Alfred Place
Chenies Street
London WC1E 7LG
(071 636 2812)

Suzy Lamplugh Trust
14 East Sheen Avenue
London SW14 8AS
(081 392 1839)

Kidscape
82 Brook Street
London W1Y 1YG
(071 488 0488)

Sexual Problems

Herpes Association
41 North Road
London N7 9DF
(071 609 9061)

Terence Higgins Trust
52–54 Grays Inn Road
London WC1X 8JU
(071 831 0330)

Sexual and Personal Relationships
  of the Disabled
286 Camden Road
London N7 0BJ
(071 607 8851)

Association of Sexual and Marital
  Therapists
PO Box 62
Sheffield S10 3TS

SIGMA
BM Sigma
London WC1N 3XX
(071 837 7324)
Advice for non-gay partners of
  bisexuals

Lesbian Line
BM Box 1514
London WC1N 3XX
(071 251 6911)

GEMMA
BM Box 5700
London WC1N 3XX
Lesbian support group

Positively Women
(071 837 9705)
For women who have HIV

Single Parents

Gingerbread
35 Wellington Street
London WC2E 7BN
(071 240 0953)

Termination

Brook Advisory Centres
223 Tottenham Court Road
London W1P 9AE
(071 580 2991)
Branches in Bristol, Burnley,
  Birmingham, Liverpool, Coventry,
  Edinburgh

British Pregnancy Advisory Service
Austy Manor
Wooton Wawen
Solihull
West Midlands B95 6BX
(05642 3225)

Margaret Pyke Centre
15 Bateman Buildings
Soho Square
London W1V 5TW
(071 734 9351)

Pregnancy Advisory Service
11–13 Charlotte Street
London W1P 1HD
(071 637 8962)

Vegetarianism

Vegetarian Society
Parkdale
Dunham Road
Altrincham WA14 4QG
(061 928 0793)

Vegan Society
33–35 George Street
Oxford OX1 2AY
(0865 722166)

Women at Work

The Trades Union Congress
Congress House
Great Russell Street
London WC1B 3LS
(071 636 4030)

Equal Opportunities Commission
Overseas House
Quat Street
Manchester M3 3HN
(061 833 9244)

Working Mothers Association
77 Holloway Road
London N7 8JZ
(071 700 5771)

Workplace Nurseries Campaign
77 Holloway Road
London N7 8JZ
(071 200 0281)

Index